Introduction to Communication Disorders

A Multicultural Approach

Introduction to Communication Disorders

A Multicultural Approach

Charlena M. Seymour, Ph.D.
Dean of the Graduate School, University of Massachusetts, Amherst

E. Harris Nober, Ph.D.
Professor of Communication Disorders, University of Massachusetts, Amherst

Butterworth–Heinemann
Boston   Oxford   Johannesburg   Melbourne   New Delhi   Singapore

Recognizing the importance of preserving what has been written, Butterworth–Heinemann prints its books on acid-free paper whenever possible.

 Butterworth–Heinemann supports the efforts of American Forests and the Global ReLeaf program in its campaign for the betterment of trees, forests, and our environment.

Library of Congress Cataloging-in-Publication Data

Introduction to communication disorders : a multicultural approach /
   [edited by] Charlena M. Seymour, E. Harris Nober.
      p.   cm.
   Includes bibliographical references and index.
   ISBN 0-7506-9559-5
   1. Communicative disorders--Cross-cultural studies.
   2. Communicative disorders--Social aspects. I. Seymour, Charlena
M.   II. Nober, E. Harris
   RC429.I58 1997
   616.85'5--dc21   97-26063
                                                                    CIP

British Library Cataloguing-in-Publication Data
A catalogue record for this book is available from the British Library.

The publisher offers special discounts on bulk orders of this book.
For information, please contact:

Manager of Special Sales
Butterworth–Heinemann
313 Washington Street
Newton, MA 02158-1626
Tel: 617-928-2500
Fax: 617-928-2620

For information on all Butterworth–Heinemann publications available,
contact our World Wide Web home page at: http://www.bh.com

10 9 8 7 6 5 4 3 2 1

Printed in the United States of America

Contents

Contributing Authors

Mary V. Andrianopoulos, Ph.D.
Assistant Professor of Communication Disorders, University of Massachusetts, Amherst

Jane A. Baran, Ph.D.
Professor of Communication Disorders, University of Massachusetts, Amherst

Ruth Huntley Bahr, Ph.D.
Assistant Professor of Communication Disorders, University of South Florida, Tampa

Carolyn Conrad, Ph.D.
Private Practitioner in speech-language pathology, Chicago

Myrna P. Cronen, Ph.D.
Adjunct Assistant Professor of Communication Disorders, University of Massachusetts, Amherst; Consultant in Speech Pathology, Veterans Affairs Medical Center, Northampton, Massachusetts

Karen S. Helfer, Ph.D.
Associate Professor of Communication Disorders, University of Massachusetts, Amherst

Patricia A. Mercaitis, Ph.D.
Associate Professor of Communication Disorders and Director, Center for Language, Speech, and Hearing, University of Massachusetts, Amherst

E. Harris Nober, Ph.D.
Professor of Communication Disorders, University of Massachusetts, Amherst

Linda W. Nober, Ed.D.
Professor of Education, Westfield State College, Westfield, Massachusetts

Charlena M. Seymour, Ph.D.
Dean of the Graduate School, University of Massachusetts, Amherst

Harry N. Seymour, Ph.D.
Professor and Chair of Communication Disorders, University of Massachusetts, Amherst

Luciano Valles, M.A.
Lecturer, Department of Communication Disorders, University of Massachusetts, Amherst

Judy Perkins Walker, Ph.D.
Assistant Professor of Communication Disorders, University of Maine, Orono

Toya A. Wyatt, Ph.D.
Associate Professor of Speech Communication, California State University, Fullerton

Preface

This book is primarily intended as an introductory text for the beginning student in speech-language pathology and audiology. It will also serve as an excellent reference resource for any professional directly or indirectly involved with the habilitation, rehabilitation, remediation, and education of people with disabilities. The text is structured to provide basic information and advanced details for the reader with additional specific needs. Hence, the overall divisions of the book include: (I) Background and Foundation, (II) Normal Processes, (III) Speech-Language Pathology in Children and Adults, and (IV) Audiology in Children and Adults. At the end of the chapters, study questions are presented for the student as well as scholarly references for in-depth study.

Perhaps the most distinguished feature of this book is that each author weaves the current, comparative information on the multicultural and multiethnic attributes of communication disorders into the fabric core of the context. Consequently, the information is not a self-contained, stagnant orientation but a dynamic treatment of communication variances from the past into the future.

The text employs a perspective of totality in which the field of communication disorders is viewed from the outset in an historical context reflecting the social, political, educational, and economic forces driving the culture of the time and the treatment of the disabled. The relationship between the normal processes of communication and the differences and subsequent disorders of communication are traced in detail decade by decade; this historical chronicle includes an outline of major U.S. legislation relative to the educational management programs for the young and the adult disabled. Acoustic, physical, and physiologic substrates of the speech, language, and hearing mechanisms are addressed in context when pertinent to the topic and not as separate sections or chapters. This is a departure from other texts; our intent is to provide a more meaningful and cohesive style.

We thank the contributors and all family and colleagues who assisted us throughout the development of the text.

C.M.S.
E.H.N.

Introduction to Communication Disorders

A Multicultural Approach

I   Background and Foundation

1   Social Forces and United States Legislation for the Disabled: Effects on Communication Disorders

E. Harris Nober

Throughout the centuries in the United States and elsewhere, disabled people have been subject to the political, social, economic, and religious forces of the community. As a consequence, the terminology, assessment, and treatment of the disabled reflect these forces. This chapter focuses on the last 90–100 years of education and service to the disabled in the United States, with emphasis on the last 5 decades.

Development of Treatment, Terminology, and Advocacy for the Disabled

Origins of Treatment of the Disabled

People with a communication disorder, whether a receptive type (e.g., deafness) or an expressive type (e.g., stuttering), were historically among the earliest of the disabled to receive treatment. Some treatments date back to 1550 BC, when scribes in Egypt and Mesopotamia assisted the disabled with communication disorders for social, political, and religious reasons. For example, scribes treated the deaf and the blind to establish their legal and religious rights (Moores et al. 1990). Aristotle addressed property ownership rights of the deaf and dumb (speechless). The Romans developed a separate code for the deaf regarding property ownership rights.

During this same period, stutterers in various nations were treated for rhythm control. With no formal professional training available to serve the speech and language disabled, the treatment was conducted by clergy or monks who used creative personal techniques that were developed through experimentation and experience. The origin of a formal program to educate deaf children is attributed to a meeting of the French Academy of Sciences in 1749.

Origins of Treatment in the United States

In the United States, a deaf social community was established at Martha's Vineyard, MA, around 1715. Other early organizations for the disabled in the United States comprised the disabled, their parents, and a few professional advocates. The professional advocates organized into early political action groups that prompted entitlement acts for the disabled in the United States. In time, the legislation for entitlements and services was based on the fourteenth amendment of the U.S. Constitution, which mandates equal opportunities to all citizens. The resolve and perseverance of political action groups prompted other nations to pass protective acts and entitlements for their citizens with disabilities.

Origins of the Study of Communication Disorders in the Twentieth Century

Early in the twentieth century, people with speech or hearing disorders were served by speech correction teachers, teachers of the deaf, teachers of children with special physical disabilities, psychologists, and, occasionally, physicians. The Chicago public school system employed as many as 10 speech correction teachers in 1910 (Matthews and Frattali 1994). In 1914, a Cornell University instructor of speech, Dr. Smiley Blanton, completed a medical degree at Cornell University and was hired by Dr. Robert West of the University of Wisconsin to establish the first speech clinic in the United States. In 1921, Sara Stinchfield and Robert West received the first and second doctorates, respectively, in the field that evolved over the years. As the field expanded, the name of the field varied from speech correction to speech-language pathology; then to speech-language-hearing pathology; and finally to audiology, speech-language pathology, and communication disorders. Soon after the first doctorates were awarded, academic programs in speech and learning science, speech-language pathology, and audiology were established at Columbia University, the University of Iowa, and the University of Pennsylvania (Paden 1970). Programs and clinics were then established across the country.

The first national organization dedicated exclusively to the broad spectrum of speech-language and (later) hearing disorders was the

American Academy of Speech Correction.* It was founded by 11 people on December 29, 1925, at the conference of the National Association of Teachers of Speech. It came about as a result of grievances related to the limited opportunities for speech correction scientists to disseminate their research at speech conferences or to publish in the *Quarterly Journal of Speech Education*. Robert West was elected as its first president.

In contrast with the medical focus established by Robert West at the University of Wisconsin, a group of psychologists and linguists at the University of Iowa explored the linguistic (at that time termed *general semantics*) characteristics of communication disorders during the 1920s. The research led to early psycholinguistic directions in speech and language correction and voice therapy. In 1923, the University of Iowa established its first speech correction clinic and enlisted Lee Travis and Wendell Johnson to run it. Afterward, communication disorders programs opened in other universities throughout the East and Midwest. Many programs added experimental phonetics research, which is now called *speech and hearing science*.

Changes in Terminology

Over the years, the disabled population has been identified and categorized by an array of diagnostic terminology that reflects the social milieu of each period. The term *disability* is the current politically correct term in the United States. It has superseded *crippled, insane, mentally retarded, deaf-dumb mute, deaf-mute*, and *handicapped*. Accordingly, terminology related to educational treatment changed from *drill* and *training*; to *therapy, conditioning*, and *behavior modification*; to the current term *special education*. Even the terms related to measurement (e.g., *testing, ongoing diagnosis, prescriptive teaching, evaluation*, and *assessment*) have vacillated. Such changes in terminology reflect both the social and political dynamics and the prevalence of medical priorities or educational descriptive priorities.

These changes in disability terminology also clearly reflect the interactions of economic, social, political, educational, and technological forces of the period for all fields of disability (Sage and Burrillo 1994). In that light, it is interesting to consider the following

---

*The American Academy of Speech Correction has undergone a number of name changes. In 1935, it was renamed as the American Speech Correction Association. In 1947, it was renamed as the American Speech and Hearing Association. In 1978, it was again renamed as the American Speech-Language-Hearing Association (ASHA). In 1997, the ASHA membership exceeded 87,000 workers who served millions of people of all ages. ASHA is the official certifying and accrediting agency for speech-language pathologists and audiologists. The current roles of the speech-language pathologist and the audiologist have increased and are detailed in both the *Dictionary of Occupational Titles* (U.S. Department of Labor 1991) and as an ASHA statement (Flower 1994).

examples. The terms *exercise* and *practice* were replaced by *therapy*, which was replaced by *teaching*, which is currently called *service*. The term *crippled* was changed to *impaired*, then to *handicapped*, and then to *disabled*. Even the term *disability* is being renamed by some as *dysfunctional* or (more recently) *challenged*. In this way, for example, cerebral palsied persons are described as physically challenged; sensory impaired, hard of hearing, or deaf persons are described as hearing-impaired; and the blind are described as visually impaired. The earlier terms *amentia* for a cognitive disability and *dementia* for an emotional disability are virtually defunct. The spectrum of cognitive levels once described by *idiot, imbecile*, and *moron* have been replaced by *mental retardation*, then by *developmentally delayed* and *mentally challenged*; and most recently by *environmentally challenged*.

Dissenting Disabled Advocates

It is, however, important to note that some disabled persons and their advocate groups have been intolerant of labels that allude to motor, sensory, or cognitive limitations; dysfunction; or abnormality. They contend that such labels foster the disability. One such example is the perception of Deaf Power. Deaf Power advocates insist the "Deaf" (they always use a capital D) are an ethnic group who are biologically equipped to do everything but hear. Dolnick (1993) stated that deaf culture is construed as a shared affirmation, not a denial of the conditions of the deaf. Dolnick also stated that the Deaf Power advocates contend that deafness is not tantamount to deprivation and is not a disability like blindness. Deaf culture advocates nurture a sense of pride so intense that some wish for a deaf baby to maintain family identity, congruity, and harmony (Dolnick 1993). Some deaf culture advocates maintain that the educational management responsibility of a deaf child born to hearing parents belongs to the deaf community and not the hearing parents. Their rationale is that the deaf child is a linguistic minority in the hearing family—a contentious attitude considering that more than 90% of deaf children have hearing parents and siblings. Finally, Deaf Power advocates vehemently reject "being altered" by a hearing aid or, even worse, a cochlear implant (i.e., a device that invades and rewires the inner ear). The cochlear implant is perceived as the ultimate retrofit to nature's choice (Dolnick 1993).

Overview of Major United States Acts for the Disabled

The first federal laws in the United States that assisted disabled people pertained to the blind and the deaf. In 1827, Public Law (PL) 19-8 enabled Florida and Kentucky to purchase land to build asylums for the deaf and dumb; however, the bill did not provide funding. Federal construction funds were not provided to Florida and Kentucky until 1847 with the passage of PL 29-1. In 1857, Congress established the Columbia Institution for the Deaf and Dumb with PLs 34–36. Within 20–30 years, schools for the deaf, blind, and mentally retarded opened in New York; Philadelphia; Boston; Providence, RI; and Hartford, CT. In 1879, PL 45-186 was passed to promote education of the blind. By the end of the 1800s, there were 14 federal acts and entitlements for the disabled; however, a significant federal priority shift toward children occurred since rehabilitation for adults was not construed to be a federal responsibility. Not until the Soldier's Vocational Rehabilitation Act of 1918 (PL 65-178) was vocational rehabilitation funding appropriated for disabled veterans on a national scale. A year later, the Vocational Rehabilitation Act (PL 66-236) of 1920 extended vocational rehabilitation to nonveteran citizens.

In 1935, the landmark Social Security Act authorized all newspaper stands in federal buildings to be operated exclusively by blind people. In 1943, the Citizen's Act (PL 78-113) entitled the mentally retarded and emotionally disturbed to financial assistance. There were subsequent amendments in 1954 (PL 83-565) and 1961 (PL 87-276) that pertained to research, model programs, and training. In 1967, PL 89-105, establishing the National Commission on Architectural Barriers and the National Center for Deaf-Blind Youth, was passed. The Medicaid and Medicare programs for the disabled were subsequently established.

From 1920 to 1959, 51 acts were passed that provided a range of entitlements. However, a cohesive, national plan to study and serve mental retardation and other disabilities occurred only when President Kennedy facilitated a series of acts for new programs and institutes. During the Kennedy presidency, the Title I program (PL 89-313) was established and was followed by a plethora of federal acts in the 1960s. These acts established the following:

- The National Technical Institute for the Deaf
- Mental retardation, mental health, and community health centers
- Federal assistance for state-operated and state-supported schools for the disabled
- The Vocational Rehabilitation Act (PL 89-333) to train disabled persons for the workplace
- Model Secondary School for the Deaf Act (PL 89-694), with amendments to the Elementary and Secondary Education Act to develop innovative educational programs for deaf children
- The National Eye Institute to treat the blind
- Disabled Children Early Education Assistance Act (PL 90-538) to provide funds for preschool programs
- The National Center in Educational Media for the Disabled (PL 91-61) to enhance educational training materials

In 1965, a milestone entitlement act, the Elementary and Secondary Education Act (PL 89-10), was passed that supplemented costs for local education agency (LEA) programs designed for educationally deprived children. The act defined new federal responsibilities in education and addressed individual needs, planning, consumer participation, personnel development, public and nonpublic participation, and supplemental services. During the 1960s, 54 laws for the disabled were enacted, as compared with the 51 acts passed between 1920 and 1959.

Overview of Communication Disorders by Decades*

1900–1929

Before the 1900s, the residential school model was popular for disabled children. From 1900 to 1920, however, community-based special classes began in local schools. Also during the 1920s, many professional organizations were formed, including organizations for the disabled.

The 1920s was also a pivotal period for research that subsequently was applied to the study of disabilities. Foundations of behavioral, experimental, and clinical research in psychology are rooted in this period. Pavlov's experiments on conditioning were presented in 1926. Classic studies appeared on cognitive development, sensory mechanisms, neural excitation in the brain, and psychophysical measurement. A few of the classic research scholars of the period are Scripture (1902) in psychology; Head (1926) in aphasia; Dewey (1923) on the classic frequency count of English sounds; Negus (1929) on the anthology on the larynx; and Fletcher (1929), who performed baseline research on speech acoustics.

1930–1939

During the 1930s, including the time of the Great Depression, employment for professionals working with the disabled was relatively stable, because President Roosevelt provided special funds for these workers. The 1935 Social Security Act was revised to include disability insurance for disabled workers and with an allocation of up to 1.5% of its trust fund to assist the disabled.

Also during the 1930s, ground-breaking texts appeared in speech pathology, psychology, medicine, linguistics, engineering, special education, and research methodology. Normative data were collected to

---

*The decade-by-decade boundaries are not absolute in all instances, as range overlaps occur. Even federal acts overlap these periods from enactment to implementation.

calibrate diagnostic instrumentation, i.e., the audiometer for hearing threshold levels relative to a normal standard. Research in speech pathology continued to focus both on nonorganic speech disorders (e.g., stuttering and articulation) and organic disorders (e.g., voice dysfunction [dysphonia], cerebral palsy, and aphasia). Preschool language development was expanded from the original 1926 Piaget language and thought treatise for the young child. In 1937, a physician named Orton related cerebral dominance to language disorders.

Leaders in medicine, psychology, and neurophysiology provided basic research on brain mechanisms, behavior function, homeostasis and endocrine function, instinctive behavior, and learning and individual differences. Although the depressed economy diminished research funds, construction and equipment expansion in universities, and research centers, the momentum was evident.

1940–1949

In the 1940s, basic research expanded further in (1) the neurophysiology of perception, (2) stimulation of motor areas of the brain, and (3) neural facilitation and reciprocal innervation of muscle activity. During this period, development also occurred in the study of maturation, learning, operant conditioning, Mowrer's learning drives, group decision models, galvanic skin conductivity, cochlea physiology, the cochlear microphonic, Bekesy's traveling wave theory, aural rehabilitation, and hearing aid fitting. Research pertaining to educational models for deaf children favored the oral-aural model.

In 1943, Grace Fernald founded a clinic for disabled children in California. In 1947, physician Alfred Strauss and psychologist Laura Lehtinen challenged the prevailing diagnostic assessment and management of disabled children. They identified children who were previously labeled as behaviorally maladjusted, hyperkinetic, or perceptually impaired as minimally brain damaged (MBD) (Strauss and Lehtinen 1947). The diagnosis of MBD was accepted by service providers with enthusiasm in the 1940s; however, it was then called into question in the 1950s and openly disputed in the 1960s. Strauss and Lehtinen also developed psychomotor tests to identify behavioral, language, and conceptual symptoms as "soft signs" of central nervous system dysfunction. These soft signs included perseveration, perceptual aberrations, psychomotor dysfunction, figure-ground confusion, speech defects, antisocial behavior, hyperkinesis, sleeping problems, learning problems, impulsiveness, pugnacious behavior, poor organization, and distractibility. Collectively, these behavioral symptoms comprised the Strauss syndrome. The movement was so pervasive that a child with these soft sign symptoms was labeled a *Strauss child*.

The diagnosis and rehabilitation of hearing disorders were the underpinnings for the field of audiology, the study of hearing and hearing disorders. Training programs for brain insult and aural rehabilitation were fine-tuned to serve World War II veterans with language and hearing disorders, but stuttering and articulation remained the dominant fields of exploration. Collaboration of linguists, psychologists, neurologists, speech-language pathologists, and speech and hearing scientists produced the classic rehabilitation models that are in use today. During this time, the term *lip reading* was renamed *speechreading* to include facial and body language.

The prevailing expectation was that World War II would produce excessive traumatic and psychogenic (pseudohypacusis) hearing loss problems among the troops. In preparation for the postwar returning veterans, several aural rehabilitation and diagnostic centers were set up in the United States in Veteran's Administration hospitals and centers. Additionally, federally funded research centers, such as the Harvard Psycho-Acoustic Laboratory, provided a foundation for auditory perceptual research. At the Psycho-Acoustic Laboratory, a "master hearing aid" explored different circuitry combinations on returning veterans who sustained an array of conductive and sensorineural hearing impairments. This laboratory also developed the bisyllabic Spondee word lists to ascertain the speech recognition (formally speech reception) threshold and the monosyllabic, phonetically balanced word lists to measure auditory discrimination ability. Audiology also benefited significantly from surgical advances in otology and from engineering technology.

1950–1959

During the 1950s, the U.S. Congress passed the Cooperative Research Act that fostered gainful research between the federal government and universities. Two-thirds of the funds appropriated were earmarked for the study of mental retardation. In 1951, Arnold Gesell and Catherine Amatruda, both physicians, published their classic maturational and developmental research of infant and toddler development (Gesell and Amatruda 1951). Following the Sputnik launch by the Soviets in 1958, federal funds expanded for research and development centers and government-supported programs. Education funds increased services and research for the disabled, jobs for professionally trained people, and student internships. Inventions and technical innovations that emanated from space and health care research were often modified to serve the disabled. An example of this was the development of the transistor and, later, painted circuits. Both were adopted for hearing aids and other assistive devices. During this period, training programs and clinics to serve the disabled flourished throughout the country.

Experimental, physiologic, and clinical psychology advances provided benefits to various speech and language disorders. A multitude of books on speech, language, and hearing disorders were published. Physiologists and psycholinguists extended their research on auditory neuronal pathways, mental retardation, cerebral palsy, and aphasia. Aural rehabilitation benefited from surgical ear restoration for people with conductive middle ear pathology. The hallmark linguistic theory of Noam Chomsky, which eclipsed prevailing linguistic theories, became the foundation for the Lenneberg biolinguistic theory of language acquisition. The research of Chomsky and Lenneberg continued to challenge most language theories for decades.

From a sociopolitical perspective, the role of the doctor, professor, teacher, therapist, or any authoritarian figure fell out of favor in the late 1950s due to a rise in the individualistic perspective. Hence, the acceptance of one's self became a dominant deterrent to the authority protocol, which in turn impacted therapy protocol. Decision making often emanated from small encounter groups of people sharing similar problems. In educational settings, the reward-contract model prescribed a predetermined set of behavioral objectives used to reach goals. In this way, performance was not defined by a group norm. Individualism permanently altered treatment strategies for the disabled. Success was considered relative and modular, and criterion-referenced assessments were used.

The attitude of self-determination fostered a perspective of objectivity and, subsequently, accountability. Objectivity, however, had multiple connotations. In audiology, the quest for objectivity gave rise to objective hearing tests, in which the person remained passive or asleep as head electrodes scanned the brain for a response to an induced sound. In a different type of objective test, skin electrodes measured galvanic skin response changes that were innervated via the autonomic nervous system.

This sociopolitical movement was also the climate for the civil case of *Brown v. Board of Education of Topeka*, in 1954, which subsequently impacted federal entitlements for the disabled. The suit challenged racial discrimination toward black children in public schools. The ruling contended that education was the means to achieve other constitutional rights ensured by a democratic society; hence, no person could be denied an education using exclusion or any devious means that violate the equal protection guaranteed by the fourteenth amendment of the Constitution. This case gave the federal government the legal authority needed to intervene when education was denied to any person or group.

1960–1969

Socially and professionally, the 1960s were a turbulent period in the United States. As respect for authority eroded further, individuals and advocacy groups demanded more responsibility and accountability at all societal levels. This attitude generated consumer protection and consumer rights entitlements and the further demise of authoritarianism. Parents of disabled children insisted that educators justify their program strategies by showing demonstrable evidence of improvement and progress. Behavioral objectives, which quantified the incremental gains toward the overall goal, formed the core of therapy plans. The achievements of the early civil rights movement also impacted on the federal entitlement acts for the disabled.

Sensitivity and humanistic directions prevailed at all levels of society, including among the disabled. Universities and government agencies established human subjects committees to protect people and, later, animals against research exploitation. The authoritative and revered physicians and other clinicians were inundated with malpractice suits that held them accountable for their services. There was a social thrust for privacy, confidentiality, and nondiscriminatory testing and an aversion to some teachers' negative images and low expectations of disabled students, which were seen as self-fulfilling prophesies.

Although the categorical labels of children were replaced in some states, many states and the federal government retained medical and diagnostic categories such as cerebral palsy, aphasia, deaf, blind, MBD, and so on. Other classifications (i.e., mild, moderate, and severe) emerged that reflected the magnitude or severity of the disability. Another classification was based on the prevalence of the disability, such as high incidence or low incidence. Some states preferred a noncategorical classification, such as special needs children. The category *learning disability* (LD) had the greatest impact on educational management for the remainder of the century.

In 1963, the term *LD* was introduced in Chicago by Sam Kirk at a joint meeting of parents of disabled children and leading special educators (e.g., William Cruickshank, Newell Kephart, Helmer Myklebust, Ray Barsch, and Marion Frostig). The goal of this Chicago meeting was to consider and replace the medical and diagnostic labels attached to disabled children. The group aspired to a descriptive term that related to behavioral performance. Agreeing that the universal weakness of these children involved some form of learning, the category LD was conceived. At this meeting, the Association for Children with Learning Disabilities was established. This organization was renamed in later years as the Learning Disabilities Association.

The category LD includes dyslexia (reading problems), language problems, perceptual motor problems, hyperkinesis, and MBD.* From its inception, it was clear that the boundaries between LD and other heterogeneous learning deficits would be blurred. Indeed, the most prevalent specific learning disability, dyslexia, is a reading deficit that is rarely outgrown in its entirety but compensated for throughout life.

---

*In the decades to come, the terms *attention deficit disorder* (ADD) and *attention deficit hyperactivity disorder* (ADHD) were considered LD subgroups. In general, LD became so prevalent that in the mid-1990s it accounted for more than one-half of all disabled U.S. school children. In 1996, the prevalence of ADD and ADHD had escalated such that 25% of the school-age children in the United States received methylphenidate hydrochloride (Ritalin) for their ADD and ADHD symptoms.

During the 1970s, advocate groups for disabled children proliferated. Parents brought class-action lawsuits against state educational agencies (SEAs) and LEAs. In 1972, two important lawsuits were tried: (1) *Pennsylvania Association for Retarded Children v. The Commonwealth of Pennsylvania* (PARC) and (2) *Mills v. The Board of Education of the District of Columbia*. Subsequent lawsuits followed throughout the nation. Collectively, the PARC and *Mills* decisions produced important civil rights benefits for the education of disabled and minority children. In the PARC case, it was decided that every child could benefit from an education. Retarded children were, therefore, entitled to a free and appropriate education that could not be delayed since, according to the decision, education is a continuous and individualized process. The *Mills* case included all disabled children and required tests, hearing procedures, and time limits for service, as well as prohibiting exclusion.

Following *Mills*, PARC, and other related court decisions was the enactment of the Education of All Handicapped Children's Act of 1975 (PL 94-142). The act was nicknamed the *Educational Bill of Rights for Handicapped Children* or the *Quiet Revolution*. PL 94-142, which was a revision of part B of the Education of the Handicapped Act (PL 91-230), heavily impacted all educational management phases for disabled children. No institution, group, or agency was spared from mandated compliance. Compliance required accountability and direct family intervention for all school-age (i.e., 5- to 18-year-old) disabled children. The following are some primary provisions of PL 94-142:

- A constitutional right to a free and appropriate education
- A redistribution of resources and revenue sharing
- A right to due process
- A requirement for nondiscriminatory testing and assessment
- A right to individual educational planning
- A requirement for least-restrictive environment educational placement
- A requirement that individual educational planning teams include parents or advocate substitutes
- A requirement that service providers be well trained and competent

During the 1970s, Congress also amended the Elementary and Secondary Education Act (PL 93-380), increasing funds sixfold, guaranteeing due process, and requiring state goal commitments and timetables to serve all disabled children. In addition, the Vocational Rehabilitation Act of 1973 (PL 93-112) prioritized services for the disabled, added joint client-counselor decision-making policies, and prohibited any form of discrimination. Overall, 84 acts were legislated for the disabled in the 1970s: These acts affected education, health, housing, income maintenance, budget laws, nutrition, civil rights, social services, transportation, and vocational rehabilitation. The focus of these acts was on education, health and vocational rehabilitation, and civil rights. Civil rights alone accounted for 11 acts.

In the field of audiology, technologic advances improved diagnostic audiometry and hearing-aid fidelity. For deaf education, the oral-aural (oralism) model, an approach adapted in 1880 at the Milan Congress on Deafness, was supplanted by the total communication model.* The total communication model used all relevant sensory modalities simultaneously with the manual language format.

Also during the 1970s, research progressed on the psychological implications of deafness; on language development; on public access for the disabled; on state licensing, certification, and accreditation; on in-service training and continuing education for service providers; and on new diagnostic and assessment instruments.

1980–1989

During the 1980s, entitlements for the disabled increased in education, health, housing, income maintenance, budget laws, nutrition, civil rights, social services, transportation, and vocational rehabilitation. Seventy-six additional acts passed during this decade focused on education, health, vocational rehabilitation, and civil rights.

In 1986, Congress enacted the Education of the Handicapped Amendments Act (PL 99-457), which became effective September 1, 1991. It added comprehensive service and educational management for disabled infants, toddlers, preschool children, and their families. It contained two new provisions that precipitated changes for educational and health care institutions: (1) the Handicapped Infants and Toddlers Program for children age birth to 2 years and (2) the Preschool Grant Program for children age 3–5 years. PL 99-457 required each state governor to appoint an interagency coordinating council and to identify a lead agency. Other primary provisions of the act required the state to

- Define *developmentally delayed*
- Provide due process protection and a service timetable
- Provide multidisciplinary assessment of child and family needs
- Provide a data bank of early intervention programs
- Prepare an individual family service plan with a case manager
- Promulgate a public awareness program

---

*By the 1990s, the total communication model was superseded by the American Sign Language (ASL) model. It was found to be perceptually and cognitively difficult to employ the auditory language modality and visual information input concurrently as required by the total communication model. Because they are two different language systems, processing hand motion and lip movements concurrently was confusing; therefore, only one system prevailed.

- Develop a central directory of resources, services, experts, and programs and a "Child Find" operational referral system
- Develop a comprehensive service personnel development plan
- Establish personnel standards and requirements for service providers

The Handicapped Infants and Toddlers Program required an early intervention case manager for better interdisciplinary family and professional coordination. This required the development of a comprehensive, multidisciplinary, individual family service plan for infants identified as at risk. The definition of at risk depended on the infants' case histories, developmental delays, physical and mental maturity, cognition, and diminished speech and language communication. PL 99-457 provided funds that enabled early identification of disabled children, family training, and interagency collaboration. Hearing-impaired infants were, therefore, identified during the first few weeks or months rather than at 2.0–2.5 years of age, which was the former national average (Nozza 1996).

The 1990s

Through 1995, 17 acts, mostly in education and vocational rehabilitation for the disabled, had been passed. During the 1990s, the parameters of LD were expanded for funding and legal purposes by PL 101-476, the Individuals with Disabilities Education Act (IDEA) in 1991. IDEA provides detailed definitions of the criteria required to identify the LD child.* In 1992, the U.S. Department of Education reported that 96% of disabled school-age children, who represent 12% of all school-age children, are classified according to four of the ten types of disabilities (U.S. Department of Education 1992). The 1992 report listed learning disability incidence at 49.1%, speech impairment at 22.7%, mental retardation at 12.7%, and serious emotional disturbance at 9.0%. The remaining 6.5% was comprised of six low-incidence groups (i.e., deaf-blind, multiple handicapped, orthopedic impaired, hard of hearing, visually impaired, and other health problems).

IDEA reauthorized the PL 99-457 and substituted the word *individuals* for the word *children* and the word *disabled* for the word *handicapped.* IDEA added autism and traumatic brain injury to the list of

---

*IDEA defined specific learning disabilities as "a disorder in one or more psychological processes involved in understanding or using language spoken or written, such disorder may manifest itself in imperfect ability to listen, think, speak, read, write, spell, or do mathematical calculations. Such disorders include such conditions as perceptual handicaps, brain injury, minimal brain dysfunction, dyslexia, and developmental aphasia. Such term does not include children who have learning problems which are primarily the result of visual, hearing, or motor handicaps, of mental retardation, of emotional disturbance, or of environmental, cultural, or economic disadvantage."

disabilities. It also added provisions for adolescents' transitions into the workplace. Furthermore, IDEA stipulated that an attention deficit disorder was a symptom of a learning disability, not a separate disability. IDEA therefore enabled children with attention deficit disorder to receive aid. IDEA also defined traumatic brain injury as an acquired brain injury from an external physical force that causes perceptual, cognitive, sensory, motor, language, or social disabilities that adversely affect educational performance.

The hallmark act of the 1990s has been the Americans with Disabilities Act (ADA) of 1990 (PL 101-366). ADA is a sweeping bill that ensures that 40 million Americans have equal opportunities in education, employment, transportation, public accommodations, and telecommunications. ADA defined *disability* as (1) a physical or mental impairment that substantially limits one or more of the major life activities, (2) a record of such an impairment, and (3) being regarded as having such an impairment. In addition to defining disability, two terms were specified in ADA: *reasonable accommodation* and *undue hardship.* Reasonable accommodation includes modifying existing facilities, policies, examinations, and work schedules; ensuring consideration of the disabled when assignments to vacant positions are made; applying new technology to improving the quality of life for the disabled; and using qualified readers and interpreters for the hearing or sight impaired. Undue hardship denotes a significant expense associated with a modification, the type of modification, and the number of disabled persons affected.

The ADA evolved from decades of acts designed to protect the disabled. Also based on the fourteenth amendment to the Constitution, ADA preserved the collective benefits of preceding acts that provided disabled children and adults with medical treatment, protection from abuse, accessibility to public facilities, and protection against employment discrimination. The ADA contains the following five titles:

- Title I prohibits employers from discriminating against disabled persons by denying reasonable accommodations for the limitations of any given disability in employment tests, hiring practices, advancement, discharge, compensation, and job training.
- Title II prohibits discrimination in delivery of public services, in transportation vehicles, in older and newly constructed buildings, and in state and local activities.
- Title III prohibits discrimination in delivery of private or public services open to the public (e.g., hotels, restaurants and bars, movies and theaters, concert halls, stadiums, shopping centers, health facilities, museums, libraries, parks, schools, nurseries, day-care centers, and exercise and recreation centers).
- Title IV requires telephone companies to install telecommunication equipment for the hearing impaired and some speech and hearing disorders.

- Title V specifies that no other laws, state or local, can invalidate, negate, or reduce the ADA and that the federal government has congressional authority to enforce these titles. Title V authorizes the Architectural and Transportation Barriers Compliance Board to issue minimum accessibility guidelines. It also authorizes the attorney general and the National Council on Disability to spell out and enforce these guidelines.

The incidence and prevalence of communication disorders, in addition to issues concerning multiculturalism, have also changed in the 1990s. *Incidence* is defined as the number of new cases of a disorder in a time period. *Prevalence* is defined as the current number of cases for a designated time period. Statistics vary widely among experts because data depend on the manner of data collection, sampling procedures, disorder categories and specifications, test conditions, datelines, counting methods, and age classifications (Shewan 1994).

Prevalence of communication disorders has increased during the 1990s (Shewan 1994). Expanded awareness of exposure to fetal alcohol syndrome, acquired immunodeficiency syndrome, human immunodeficiency virus, cytomegalovirus, and toxic substances have affected the data (National Institute on Deafness and Other Communication Disorders Advisory Board 1992). Adams and Benson (1992) contend that age is a primary factor in the prevalence of hearing impairment. This is supported by data showing that the prevalence of hearing impairment is 1.6% in children younger than 18 years of age and 40.3% in adults older than 75 years of age, with the latter population increasing in size. Adams and Benson also stress that the incidence and prevalence of communication disorders vary by ethnic and cultural composition (e.g., the African-American population who are older than 45 years of age in the United States have a higher prevalence of cerebrovascular accident) (Adams and Benson 1992).

The Inclusion Model

During the 1990s, the inclusion (or inclusive) model has expanded nationwide as a component of the educational school reform movement. The inclusive model places the disabled child in the regular classroom with the regular classroom teacher as the primary instructor. With full inclusion, there is no tracking, e.g., moving students into sections based on test or performance scores. The classroom teacher is solely responsible for the disabled student and his or her classmates (see Chapter 2).

The inclusive model has sociopolitical implications. Indeed, the National Joint Committee on Learning Disabilities opposes the "idea that all students with learning disabilities must be served only in regular education classrooms" (American Speech-Language-Hearing Association 1993a). The committee claims that because of the unique needs of the

LD child, an individualized program is required for maximum performance. This group further asserts that "responsibility for developing plans must be shared by regular and special educators, parents, and student consumers of the services" (American Speech-Language-Hearing Association 1993b). Indeed, many special educators, speech-language pathologists, and teachers of the deaf oppose full inclusion.

A 1993 statement from the Council for Exceptional Children supports a rich variety of educational and vocational program options and experiences in community-based, nonschool environments and special schools for disabled children. The statement further stresses the importance of placement in mainstream classes for part of the day and views inclusive schools as the "first and foremost call for a change in attitudes and values ... a new ethos that celebrates diversity, promotes accountability, culturalism, and professional collaboration, values the strengthening of social relationships among children, and explores strategies for pursuing excellence without sacrificing equity" (Council for Exceptional Children 1993).

Projection for Future Decades

The professions centered around communication disorders reflect the social, political, and economic forces of the times. They also interact with and are affected by changes in health care and educational and technologic advances in product research. Because of these multiple forces, the future of these professions is sure to be fraught with change.

For example, by 2010 more than one-third of the U.S. population will be of non-European background, and by 2050 about one-half of the population will be persons of color (Taylor 1994). There must, therefore, be an increase in cultural diversity research and recruitment relative to intracultural variation in communication disorders.

Research in this area has begun. Taylor (1994) studied language boundaries (limits of normalcy or difference) for cultural context, cognition, and communicative development. In this study, Taylor found that language and culture are reflected in dialect, Creole language, indigenous ethnography, communication competence, behavior, and purpose. It has also been found that ethnic groups differ in attitudes about the nature and significance of communication disorders (Taylor 1994; Bebout and Arthur 1992; Buchanan 1993).

Conclusion

Treatment of the disabled has been reported for centuries. Professional fields in the United States will continue to reflect the social, political, economic, and educational forces of the future. The rights of individuals will continue as a strong underlying force to encourage educational and vocational benefits for the disabled.

It is likely that the inclusion model will expand, increasing the classroom teacher's responsibility for both disabled and nondisabled students. Concurrently, it is likely that tracking will be eliminated. Inclusion will pose even greater restrictions on the child who is hearing impaired due to the need for special equipment, seating, and other services (Nober 1993; 1996).

Changes in health care, education and social services, and entitlements continue to be debated in the United States Congress and in many state legislatures. Because of imposed budgetary restrictions, reductions of direct federal and state support for programs to assist the disabled are likely to occur. The following are some predictions for persons with communication disorders and other disabilities:

- Special education will be altered to place greater emphasis on persons with low-incidence disabilities and the severely disabled.
- Educational training and research funds will be modified and reduced, thereby generating more need for paraprofessional aides.
- The Internet and the World Wide Web will become central avenues to assist the disabled as multimedia computer technology expands.
- Acts for the disabled will stress state and local autonomy.
- Research and training will emphasize multicultural and multiracial issues in speech-language pathology and allied fields.
- Audiology will separate from ASHA into an independent field.

Technology and telecommunication advances will significantly alter professions like those that study communication disorders, special education, educational management, and vocational rehabilitation. The computer is being used for research, diagnosis, rehabilitation, teaching, surgical intervention, and as assistive devices. Interactive multimedia and telecommunication advances have already precipitated distance learning through the Internet and the World Wide Web.

All fields that deal with communication disorders are undergoing dynamic development changes. These changes are affecting (1) education and special education, (2) medicine, (3) psychology, (4) physiology, (5) genetic engineering, (6) electrical and mechanical engineering, (7) computer science, (8) linguistics, (9) vocational rehabilitation, and (10) physical and occupational therapy. By using the past as an index of the future, it can be predicted that new advances in the study of communication disorders will significantly enhance the lives of disabled people (Minifie and Flower 1994).

References

Adams PF, Benson V. Current Estimates from the National Health Interview Survey. Vital and Health Statistics, Series 10 (176). National Center for

Health Statistics. Public Health Service. Washington, DC: U.S. Government Printing Office, 1992.

American Speech-Language-Hearing Association. National Joint Committee on Learning Disabilities. Reaction to "Full Inclusion": A Reaffirmation of the Rights of Students with Learning Disabilities to a Continuum of Services. Rockville, MD: American Speech-Language-Hearing Association, 1993a;63.

American Speech-Language-Hearing Association. Preferred Practice Patterns for the Professions of Speech-Language Pathology and Audiology. Rockville, MD: American Speech-Language-Hearing Association, 1993b;35.

Bebout L, Arthur B. Cross-cultural attitudes toward speech disorders. J Speech Hear Res 1992;35:45–52.

Buchanan H, Moore E, Counter A. Hearing Disorders and Auditory Assessment. In D Battle (ed), Communication Disorders in Multicultural Populations. Boston: Andover Medical Publishers, 1993;256–286.

Council for Exceptional Children. The Council for Exceptional Children's Draft Statement on Inclusive Schools [reprinted]. Reston, VA: Masstream, 1993.

Dolnick E. Deafness and culture. Atlantic Monthly 1993;272:37–53.

Flower RM. Introduction to the Professions. In F Minifie (ed), Introduction to the Communication Sciences and Disorders. San Diego: Singular Publishing Group, 1994;1–41.

Gesell A, Amatruda C. Developmental Diagnosis: Normal and Abnormal Child Development. New York: Paul B. Hoeber, 1951.

Matthews J, Frattali C. The Profession of Speech-Language Pathology and Audiology. In G Shames, E Wiig, W Secord (eds), Human Communication Disorders. New York: Merrill Publishing, 1994.

Minifie FD, Flower RM. A Vision for the Future. In F Minifie (ed), Introduction to the Communication Sciences and Disorders. San Diego: Singular Publishing Group, 1994;673–690.

Moores D, Cerney B, Garcia M. School Placement and Least-Restrictive Environment. In D Moores, K Meadow-Orland (eds), Educational and Developmental Aspects of Deafness. Washington, DC: Gallaudet University Press, 1990;115–136.

National Institute on Deafness and Other Communication Disorders Advisory Board. In the 1991 Annual Report (NIH Publication No. 92-3317). U.S. Department of Health and Human Services, Public Health Service. Rockville, MD: National Institutes of Health, 1992.

Nober EH. PL 99-457 and Its Effects on Educational Management of Hearing-Impaired Children. In Service, Training, Research and Assistive Warning Device Programs for the Hearing-Impaired in Australia and New Zealand. Washington, DC: World Rehabilitation Fund International Exchange of Experts and Information in Rehabilitation, 1993.

Nober EH. Audiology and Education. In SE Gerber (ed), The Handbook of Pediatric Audiology. Washington, DC: Gallaudet University Press, 1996;314–342.

Nozza RJ. Pediatric Hearing Screening. In FN Martin, JG Clarke (eds), Hearing Care for Children. Boston: Allyn & Bacon, 1996;95–114.

Paden EP. A History of the American Speech and Hearing Association, 1925–1958. Washington, DC: American Speech and Hearing Association, 1970.

Sage D, Burrillo LC. Leadership in Educational Reform: An Administrative Guide to Changes in Special Education. Baltimore: Paul Brookes, 1994.

Shewan CM. Incidence and Prevalence of Communication Disorders. In R Lubinski, C Frattali (eds), Professional Issues in Speech-Language Pathology and Audiology. 1994;89–104.

Strauss A, Lehtinen L. Psychopathology and Education of the Brain-Injured Child. New York: Grune & Stratton, 1947.

Taylor OL. Communication and Communication Disorders in a Multicultural Society. In F Minifie (ed), Introduction to the Communication Sciences and Disorders. San Diego: Singular Publishing Group, 1994;43–76.

United States Department of Education. To Assure a Free Appropriate Education of All Handicapped Children: Fourteenth Annual Report to Congress on the Implementation of P.L. 94-142, The Education of All Handicapped Children's Act. Washington, DC: U.S. Government Printing Office, 1992.

United States Department of Labor. Dictionary of Occupational Titles [revised] (4th ed). Washington, DC: U.S. Government Printing Office, 1991.

Chapter 1   Study Questions

1. Trace the origins of how people with communicative disorders were treated and the sociological reasons for that treatment.
2. Review how diagnostic terminology labels and clinical intervention changed relative to the social, political, and economic forces in the United States.
3. Discuss some key U.S. acts that have impacted treatment of the disabled.
4. List the basic provisions of the Americans with Disabilities Act and discuss their implications for extending integration of the disabled into the mainstream.
5. Discuss the role of the fourteenth amendment of the U.S. Constitution in legislation passed during the past 40 years regarding the disabled.

2 Professional Collaboration and Management

Linda W. Nober

"The goal of the professions of speech-language pathology and audiology is the provision of the highest quality treatment and services consistent with the fundamental right of those served to participate in decisions that affect their lives" (American Speech-Language-Hearing Association 1996a). According to the American Speech-Language-Hearing Association (ASHA) Scope of Practice policy statements, speech-language pathology professionals serve patients and their families and work to prevent speech, voice, language, communication, swallowing, and related disabilities (American Speech-Language-Hearing Association 1996a). Additionally, audiology professionals identify, assess, and manage disorders of the auditory, balance, and other neural systems. Detailed descriptions of these roles and functions provide the theoretical framework for services to persons of all ages with, or at risk for developing, communication problems (American Speech-Language-Hearing Association 1996b).

Speech-language pathologists and audiologists are professionals who have training in the allied fields of medicine, psychology, education, linguistics, and other disciplines that contribute to the treatment of communication disorders. Within medicine, specialties such as pediatrics, neurology, otology, psychiatry, and gerontology contribute to the content knowledge of communication disorders. Within psychology, specialties such as neuropsychology, counseling, educational psychology, cognitive psychology, and developmental psychology are important and related subdisciplines. Within education, reading, regular and special education, deaf education, and learning disabilities are areas of study that contribute information. Linguistics, psycholinguistics, physical therapy, occupational therapy, and numerous other disciplines also provide speech-language pathologists with important information that facilitates an integrated understanding of the role of communication in the lives of children and adults. Such transdisciplinary knowledge provides the core for professional collaboration and professional development activities for speech-language pathologists and audiologists.

Speech-language pathology and audiology job descriptions frequently include the requirement of good oral and written communication skills. These abilities are basic prerequisites of communication disorders professionals. Oral and written communication skills relate to the practice of speech-language pathology and audiology in several interactive situations:

- With parents, caregivers, patients, or any combination of these
- With other professionals working within a team (e.g., individualized educational plan [IEP] or medical), both in the school and the clinic
- In report writing for dissemination to other professionals, insurers, or referral sources
- In consulting
- In developing programs
- In identifying, assessing, and evaluating service delivery systems

Additional human relationship skills are required for a successful practice in communication disorders. These skills include (1) interpersonal problem solving, (2) interviewing, (3) giving and receiving feedback, (4) managing resistance, (5) observing, (6) collecting data, (7) following through on interactions, (8) paraphrasing, (9) listening empathetically, (10) communicating nonverbally, (11) resolving conflicts, (12) making decisions, (13) managing time, (14) in-service training, (15) contracting, and (16) negotiating.

Basic Principles of Professional Collaboration and Consultation

Lerner (1993) and Idol and colleagues (1986) define the differences between consultation and collaboration in the following manner: Consultation occurs when a person with expertise interacts with someone with less competence, and collaboration occurs when a problem is addressed by persons of equivalent levels of expertise.

Lerner integrates the pioneering work of human relations theorists and special educators who used a collaboration model. In doing so, she identifies as important to successful collaboration the need to (1) set common goals, (2) schedule time and facilities so that planning and evaluation can occur, (3) provide for face-to-face communication, (4) address problems that require resolution collaboratively rather than through top-down management, and (5) evaluate the effectiveness of the collaboration efforts.

Professional Development

During the 1990s, the emphasis on in-service education and continuing education programs has grown. Professional development programs have evolved such that teachers, therapists, medical personnel, and most persons in the helping professions participate at required or voluntary levels. Local education agencies, unions, school districts, state departments of education, colleges and universities, and professional societies provide opportunities for in-service education and professional development activities. Professionals earn continuing education units to corroborate their participation in these educational activities. This emphasis has broadened to include professional development activities that are designed and implemented by local or regional practitioners rather than by visiting scholars.

Each agency or state determines professional development requirements independently; however, there is a trend toward mandating professional development as part of recertification requirements (Massachusetts Department of Education 1994). Professional development activities overlap professional collaboration activities in many areas.

Individual Education Plans

Currently, disabled students are educated through systems of collaboration that involve IEPs. There is a clear rationale for good professional collaboration and consultation among communication disorders personnel—to facilitate improved learning and attainment of educational achievement for students and families. IEP teams are comprised of personnel from different disciplines who are able to contribute their areas of expertise and work cooperatively together to plan instructional techniques for students with communication disorders. This team model, or case management group, has been commonly used in the medical and health care professions; however, until the 1975 enactment of Public Law (PL) 94-142, educational IEP teams were not uniformly used to plan programs for individual students. The passage of this landmark legislation (and its subsequent amendments) altered the involvement of speech-language pathologists and audiologists in education programs. It also created new issues for preparation of communication disorders professionals (Nober 1984).

Employment Settings of Speech-Language-Hearing Professionals

According to the omnibus survey statistics gathered by ASHA in 1994, almost 53% of the 86,000 members of ASHA were employed in public or independent schools in grades ranging from prekindergarten to twelfth grade (American Speech-Language-Hearing Association 1994). Hospital and medical practices employed an additional 27% of the membership. Additionally, because teacher certification is a state function, many states certify speech-language pathologists who are not members of ASHA (but who meet similar requirements) for employment in the schools. Almost 25 states have licensure requirements for clinical practitioners (non-teachers) that parallel the ASHA requirements. These data indicate that the majority of speech-language pathologists and audiologists are employed in settings that require professional collaboration and consultation rather than single-practice settings.

The employment settings of speech-language pathologists or audiologists are related to the age of the population to be served. Age factors affect professional collaboration because settings that serve young children require different interactive skills than settings that serve young adults or elderly persons.

According to data given by the U.S. Department of Education in its Sixteenth Annual Report to Congress in 1994 (U.S. Department of Education 1994), almost 1 million students from 6 to 21 years of age received speech and language special education services in schools. Almost 885,000 students 6–11 years of age and 100,000 students 12–17 years of age received speech-language services for their difficulties. Within the 18- to 21-year-old age group, almost 4,000 students received speech and language services. Data were not collected, however, by category of service for students younger than 6 years of age. Clearly, the elementary-age students engaged the largest number of practitioners serving the largest number of students, with almost 200,000 students 6–8 years old being served. There is considerable reduction in the number of students served older than 10 years.

In 1994, the U.S. Department of Education also estimated that approximately 8% of the school-age population received special education services under the Individuals with Disabilities Education Act (PL 101-476) (U.S. Department of Education 1994). Of this total, 1.83% were identified as having speech, language, or hearing disabilities, second only to the specific learning disabilities category. Additionally, 50,500 speech-language pathologists and audiologists were employed nationally to serve students with speech and hearing difficulties (U.S. Department of Education 1994). The report also projected that 4,700 additional speech-language and hearing professionals were needed to serve these students' needs more completely. The large proportion of speech-language pathologists or audiologists needed to serve school-age students with disabilities has created a need that affects professionals, e.g., paraprofessionals.

This chapter describes professional collaboration relative to early childhood programs (infancy and preschool); to elementary, middle, and secondary school programs; to clinical programs for young adults; and to programs for persons older than 65 years of age. The age and the work environment of the speech-language pathologist or audiologist has been described, because the problems of each work situation present unique opportunities for professional collaboration.

Early Childhood Issues

Infants and Toddlers

Factors That Contribute to Disabilities

The birth of a baby is, for most families, a significant life experience filled with elated family support and jubilance. Occasionally, this fact is belied by circumstances unique to the new mother, father, or the baby. Families of newborns with birth defects often describe difficult family interactions and acceptance patterns (Widerstrom et al. 1991; Batshaw and Perret 1992). The most common birth defects that significantly impact the family involve genetically transmitted disorders (e.g., Down syndrome, Hurler's syndrome, Klinefelter's syndrome, fragile X syndrome) (Widerstrom et al. 1991). Typically, birth disorders that result in developmental disability occur early in life, are not likely to be outgrown, and affect two or more basic developmental domains (e.g., communication, cognition, motor skills, social-emotional development) (Billeaud 1993). Parents of newborns with developmental disabilities face long-term responsibilities for the care and education of their children. While information regarding the transmission of genetic disorders is available, many families are not prepared to provide for a child with a significant birth disorder.

Prematurity contributes significantly to developmental disabilities (Frey 1995). Other factors that contribute to developmental disabilities are designated as risk factors. The most significant risk factor is the socioeconomic status of the mother (Thurman and Widerstrom 1990). Children born to young, economically disadvantaged, poorly educated mothers are at significant risk for disabilities. Birth weight and gestation period compound the risk factors, particularly when limited prenatal care is provided (Frey 1995). Unplanned or unwanted pregnancies are common among young women, and young mothers-to-be may be unable or may elect not to seek medical support and prenatal care. Poor nutrition, alcohol abuse, or substance abuse during pregnancy are also added risk factors for newborns. Maternal toxicity, illness, drug reactions, excessive weight gain or loss, and many other factors can also contribute to the birth of a child with disabilities (Widerstrom et al. 1991; Batshaw and Perret 1992). Research on low-birth-weight, very low-birth-weight, and extremely low-birth-weight babies, as well as on gestation period, has found that these conditions are significant factors in the birth of a baby with disabilities (Thurman and Widerstrom 1990). Several researchers have also reported that cultural differences tend to (1) enhance the developmental acquisition of the infant with a disability or (2) exacerbate the difficulties of the child (Ivey et al. 1993; Thurman and Widerstrom 1990).

Early Intervention Programs

Early intervention programs vary from state to state under the regulations of PL 99-457, but almost all state programs provide services to children born with disabilities through their respective departments of public health, education, mental retardation, or developmental disabilities. These programs are based on years of federally funded support under the Handicapped Children's Early Intervention Program (Thurman and Widerstrom 1990).

A typical early intervention team includes an early childhood specialist skilled in developmental programs, a speech-language pathologist, an occupational therapist, a physical therapist, a social worker (who is often the case manager), and a nurse liaison, linking medical and psychoeducational interventions for the family (Billeaud 1993). PL 99-457 also required the individualized family service plan, which is a written program to provide needed services to the child and family. The speech-language pathologist, audiologist, or both is almost always part of the early intervention team providing services to newborns and their families. A primary goal of the speech-language pathologist on the team is to help parents stimulate communication skills in their newborn. This is done by training mothers, fathers, and siblings to facilitate receptive and expressive language (e.g., sounds, cries, babbling, and echolalia) as near to the developmentally appropriate age as possible (Luterman 1987). According to data collected by the U.S. Department of Education, which monitors the implementation of PL 99-457, the speech-language pathologist is almost always a primary service provider for disabled and developmentally delayed infants (Thurman and Widerstrom 1990).

The literature in child development is replete with articles on parental concerns about the development and acquisition of good language skills (Thurman and Widerstrom 1990). In this literature, parents with backgrounds that are culturally, linguistically, and socioeconomically diverse recount their concerns about their child's language acquisition patterns. Within African-American, Hispanic, Asian, and Native American (AHANA) groups, the developmental milestones of motor skills and communication skills are preeminent among the concerns expressed by parents of children with disabilities. Speech-language and hearing professionals communicate to the family the potential impact of the birth disorder on the child's language development (Billeaud 1993; Bricker 1986).

Hearing loss and cleft palate present more complex problems for speech-language pathologists or audiologists who are members of an early intervention team (Johnson-Martin et al. 1990). The diagnosis and education plan for an infant or toddler with an identified hearing loss presents many special concerns for the speech-language pathologist and the audiologist (Maxon and Brackett 1992). Typically, decisions regarding the method of communication (manual or oral) to be used by the family are determined at the time of the diagnosis, which is between the ages of 18 and 24 months in the United States (Nober and Nober 1992). Explaining the different approaches to language acquisition for hearing-impaired youngsters to parents or caregivers is one of the major responsibilities of speech-language and hearing professionals. Deciding which approach to take carries with it lifelong consequences (Paul 1993). The audiologist or speech-language pathologist often helps the parents explore options and select a method of communication for their child. Speech-language pathologists or audiologists also have major responsibilities in cases involving children with cleft palate (Shames et al. 1994). Parents need advice from medical personnel to understand the development of oral skills of children with cleft palate. While other diagnostic categories present difficulties for early intervention teams, hearing loss and cleft palate present special concerns for the professional role of the speech-language pathologist or audiologist in case management of very young infants and toddlers.

Preschoolers

The provision of preschool education, typically center-based, for all disabled children 3–5 years old is a cornerstone of PL 99-457. (Nondisabled preschoolers are not included in federal mandates for public education.) Public, free, and appropriate preschool education is intended to help compensate for the developmental difficulty of a young disabled child and to make an effort to resolve problems early in life, when the potential for effective intervention is greatest. Twenty years of research consistently affirms the benefits of early intervention (Thurman and Widerstrom 1990).

Studies have found that the most frequent reason for referral for special education services by a parent of a 3- to 5-year-old child is speech and language delay (Johnson-Martin et al. 1990; Beaty 1994). Typical referrals include questions to the family doctor or, if there is no personal family physician, questions to the social service provider. Mothers and fathers refer their children for screening or evaluation due to concern about their children's speech and language development. Untrained and linguistically and culturally diverse families are anxious when a child does not meet the broad expectations of the linguistic community (e.g., saying "Momma," "Dadda," and "bottle" by age 3).

Parents often compare their child with others in the park, playground, baby-sitting center, or family celebrations. Parents become concerned, because in most cultures early language acquisition is identified as being directly related to intelligence (Thurman and Widerstrom 1990). Programs for mothers and preschool children (e.g., Mommy and Me, Head Start, church play groups, and day-care centers) emphasize developmental milestones and their importance. Programs for mothers seeking job skills or transition to work from welfare stress parenting skills, which also include knowledge of developmental milestones. Language acquisition is easily assessed by most new mothers as an indicator of their child's normal developmental progress. It is far more difficult for many new parents to identify motor skills development or socioemotional milestones relative to the expectations of what is considered normal (Thurman and Widerstrom 1990).

Training for health care and medical professionals has changed to offer greater exposure to developmental differences. These personnel are less likely to project that a child will outgrow a delay in speech, as was the custom into the 1970s (Billeaud 1993).

The differences between countries with a universal maternal and child health care system and the splintered system within the United States have been compared at international meetings (Gerber 1988). In the United States, preschool programs for disabled children are provided by the local education agency (LEA) where the child resides. A team of school-based personnel and the parent(s) of the preschool child determine the type and extent of services needed by the child. If the team determines that the child has a disability or is at risk for a disability, an IEP is prepared. Typically, an educational preschool program is provided that is similar to a private nursery school program (Johnson-Martin et al. 1990). Speech and language service is most commonly provided either within the preschool classroom (through the language-based or inclusion model) or as a pull-out service (Nober 1994). The speech-language pathologist is required to assess the child's speech and language needs, communicate those needs to the team members (including the parents), and design a program of intervention. Professional collaboration requires the speech-language pathologist to use standardized assessment tools that are age appropriate for preschoolers. Collaboration also requires that the oral and written reports of the assessment are understood by team members, particularly the parents (Prelock et al. 1995).

Articulation and language assessment tests use terms unique to speech-language pathologists and audiologists. Explanation of the term *alveolars* or *morphemes* is important to team members and requires that the speech-language pathologist describe their meaning and significance. The explanation of hearing loss presents problems for nonaudiologists, because decibel loss is often confused with percentage of hearing loss (Nober and Nober 1992). Trends in early childhood education are focusing on developmentally appropriate interventions that meet goals developed for each child (Johnson-Martin et al. 1990). There is, therefore, a strong need for the speech-language pathologist to convey to team members and parents the relevance of developmental differences in the receptive and expressive language of the preschool child (Prelock et al. 1995). In time, an IEP team, which works together on screening and assessment, becomes familiar with the tests and techniques of each specialty. In-service education programs provided by speech-language pathologists and audiologists help each IEP team member learn about the unique assessment tools of the communication disorders discipline and help broaden the planning and intervention skills of the entire preschool IEP team and its programs.

Elementary, Middle, and Secondary School Programs

The landmark federal legislation, the Education of All Handicapped Children's Act (PL 94-142) enacted in 1975, is now termed the *Individuals with Disabilities Education Act* (IDEA, PL 101-476). It mandated special education services to all disabled children 5–18 years old. Speech-language and audiology programs have been included as a major part of those special education services. A review of the statistics summarized in the Sixteenth Report to Congress on the Implementation of PL 94-142 demonstrates the extent to which speech-language and hearing services have been expanded within the schools to meet the mandates of free, appropriate special education, regular education services, or both to all disabled students (U.S. Department of Education 1994).

The need for speech-language and hearing personnel to work effectively on interdisciplinary teams of special educators has been consistently affirmed in the literature, at state speech and hearing association meetings, at ASHA annual conventions, at the Council for Exceptional Children annual conferences, and at meetings of the U.S. Department of Education Office of Special Education and Rehabilitation Services (National Association of State Boards of Education 1992). As the trends and themes of education for disabled persons have developed over the 20 years since the enactment of PL 94-142, the professional educators who work with disabled persons have changed their therapies to better address the needs of the population they serve (Clark 1994).

Professional collaboration and communication problems are different for professionals working in middle and secondary schools, because each student receiving speech-language and hearing services may have as many as five different teachers for various subject areas. Teacher-to-teacher communication by the speech-language and hearing professional is complicated. It is not unusual for middle and secondary building–level speech-language professionals to work with students who display the most severe disabilities. In these settings, students are educated in a segregated school class or setting in which the curriculum is geared to life skills and vocational needs. In such situations, the speech-language pathologist emphasizes vocabulary skills and interpersonal communication (Clark 1994).

Inclusion Models

In the mid-1990s, the direction of special education services changed once again based on several landmark court cases, research reported in the literature, and themes presented by parents and teacher advocates (Sage 1993). Although speech-language and hearing programs in schools have expanded over the past 20 years, they have largely been traditional pull-out programs that serve speech-handicapped students in individual or small group therapy sessions outside of the regular classroom programs. In 1996, the remediation emphasis was to provide elementary school speech and language services to students within the regular classrooms, a model termed *inclusion*. Inclusion programs vary from providing services in the classroom within a separated physical area to team teaching by the teacher and speech-language pathologist. They have been assessed as being more appropriate for students with some types of communication disorders, particularly language-processing difficulties (Nober 1993).

The following reasons have been presented for moving away from pull-out programs toward inclusion programs:

1. Pull-out programs cause students to miss regular education instruction by the regular teacher whose instructional language, assessment techniques, and classroom management techniques are different from those of individual or small-group instruction. It is estimated that a 30-minute, pull-out session for speech-language therapy results in only 14 minutes of service after preliminary, organizational activities are completed (Nober 1994).

2. The presence of the speech-language pathologist in the regular classroom, providing instruction to students with speech and language difficulties, provides the important curricular framework for the language-delayed student. While special services can be an asset to the student who needs reduced visual or auditory stimulation, the student can miss the contextual clues given by the teacher in the curriculum areas of reading and language arts, including written language assignments (Falk-Ross 1995).

3. It is estimated that for every student with a speech-language problem IEP, two other primary grade students in a classroom of 28 can benefit from instruction provided by a speech-language pathologist. Students with language problems involving generalizations, cate-

gorization, similarities and differences, and parallel construction are not referred for speech and language services; however, these students could benefit from placement within a group of students who are working on these specific, language-based tasks (Nober 1994; Eger 1992; Huffman 1992).

Elementary school-age students are the largest age group receiving speech and language services. Inclusion programs serve as an alternative to traditional speech-language pull-out programs in many school districts. Some LEAs mandate all services within the inclusion model for elementary-age students. Some LEAs mandate a written rationale before providing speech and language services to students who do not clearly demonstrate that the speech or language deficit impairs academic learning. Many LEAs refuse to provide speech and language intervention for students with fluency disorders, unless there is a demonstrated psychoeducational impact from the disorder. There is still controversy surrounding inclusion programs. This controversy is highlighted by the concerns expressed by parents and teachers who think that the reduced stimulation of a small therapy room is the best environment for providing speech and hearing therapeutic interventions (Lozo 1993).

Traditional Pull-Out Programs Versus Inclusion Programs

A comparison of the traditional pull-out programs and the inclusion programs highlights the factors that present challenges for speech-language pathologists working in primary or elementary school grades. Collaboration among the speech-language pathologist, teachers, and other team members varies depending on which of these two ecological service delivery models is used.

Collaboration in the Traditional Pull-Out Model

Traditional pull-out programs require that the speech-language pathologist assess the student, design instruction, evaluate the student's progress, and communicate these assessments at an annual team meeting involving teachers, parents, an administrator, and, occasionally, the student. There is minimal case management by supervisors. A typical case load for an elementary school–based speech-language pathologist varies from 30–100 students (Peters-Johnson 1992). The speech-language pathologist is responsible for the paperwork for each student he or she serves, even in LEAs where a specialist writes all of the IEPs.

Communication between and among team members, the student, and the regular or special education teacher varies from weekly oral progress reports to annual written reports presented at team meetings. There are different communication models for different LEA programs; however, most speech-language pathologists work with the classroom teacher to incorporate curricular topics in the vocabulary and language aspects of therapy. A caseload of 50 students representing 20 different regular class teachers, however, prohibits extensive communication between the speech-language pathologist and teachers. Even reduced caseloads of 30 students make it difficult for the speech-language pathologist to communicate effectively with every teacher. It is not unusual to restrict communication about individual students to team meetings, lunchroom pick-up conferences, or brief written notes (Huffman 1992).

Speech-language pathologists have developed effective communication skills with resource personnel or related services personnel in schools (e.g., physical therapists, occupational therapists, school guidance counselors, or counseling psychologists) (Minifie 1994). This communication model is enhanced by providing direct service to the same students, typically those with more severe special needs. Over the years, the same team of specialists provides direct services, communicates with parents, works interactively with regular classroom teachers, and is known to the special education administration. The more diverse the needs of the student, the greater the likelihood of good, ongoing communication among the resource staff members.

Collaboration in the Inclusion Model

Inclusion programs require ongoing communication between and among teachers and resource staff (Lozo 1993). Team teaching requires planning time, support staff, and conference time. When the speech-language pathologist serves six second graders in one classroom beside a regular second grade teacher willing to share a classroom with another professional, there is increased communication and sharing of ideas and information (Nober 1994). In ideal situations, teachers and speech-language pathologists have enough autonomy to select with whom they will work and share a classroom, but various styles and administrative mandates prevail throughout the country. There is growing evidence that communication and collaboration are more time-consuming and more rewarding for disabled students, professionals, and parents, when an inclusion model is selected (U.S. Department of Education 1992). Specific ideas for improving communication and collaboration and for fostering good team teaching models are available.

On-site, within-classroom models have been found effective for a segregated classroom of small groups of students with similar speech and language difficulties (e.g., developmentally disabled primary grade students or students whose primary diagnosis is severe mental retardation or pervasive developmental disability). Additionally, all students in the classroom benefit from the materials prepared by the speech-language pathologist (Nober 1994). Ten to twelve students compose an on-site, segregated class. Daily therapeutic sessions for language can be built into the schedule to serve this large number of students. A similar model is effective for classes of hearing-impaired students or segregated classes of students with severe motor difficulties. There is a growing body of information from speech-language pathologists about the benefits of work in these classrooms, including the design of instruction, the interaction between and among students, and the use of paraprofessionals with students with severe disabilities (Lozo 1993). Positioning, feeding, oral-motor skill development, and the use of sign or other augmentative communication systems are all models of instruction that are enhanced by on-site classroom instruction by the speech-language pathologist working within a segregated classroom for students with severe disabilities.

Middle and secondary school–aged students present different problems for communication and collaboration among professionals, including the speech-language pathologist (Sapier and Gower 1987; Lerner 1993). Lerner identified several specific problems encountered by adolescents with language and learning difficulties. These problems include passivity about learning, poor self-esteem or self-concept, difficulty in social situations, and lack of motivation (Lerner 1993). These problems are exacerbated by the complexities of family pressures, cultural differences, and expectations (particularly regarding curriculum demands, minimum competency tests, and graduation requirements) (National Association of State Boards of Education 1992). The National Association of State Boards of Education summarized these difficulties with the following data: only 57% of students in special education graduate with a diploma and 49% of disabled youth are employed 2 years after leaving school. A typical large, urban school district may document that 50–60% of students entering ninth grade successfully complete twelfth grade and graduate (National Association of State Boards of Education 1992).

Traumatic Brain Injury

Communication and education professionals are significantly challenged when providing services to secondary school students who have had a traumatic brain injury (TBI) (Minifie 1994). Almost 400,000 new patients with TBI are admitted to hospitals in the United States each year. Most of these patients are between the ages of 15 and 24 years. Falls and accidents involving automobiles, motorcycles, off-road vehicles, and firearms are the most frequent causes of the more than 50,000 TBI incidents that have caused permanent changes in the lifestyle and neurologic function of adolescents and young adults each year. More than 70% of TBI patients are boys, probably due to risk taking and associated aggressive behavior (Minifie 1994; Batshaw and Perret 1992).

Adolescents and young adults with TBI are treated in an acute-care facility for less than 3 months or until the patient is medically stable. The long-term need for rehabilitation and training for TBI patients continues to be a critical problem for families. Regional rehabilitation centers have developed programs to serve adolescents and young adults, rather than commingling these patients with neurologically impaired elderly patients in nursing homes. Speech-language and hearing services have become a focal treatment service, because TBI patients can have near-normal cognitive skills with impaired psychomotor function (Ylvisaker 1985). Assistive communication devices are needed as a therapeutic tool for TBI patients until they are able to regain independent, communicative function.

A part of PL 101-476 emphasized the importance of TBI as a category of disability requiring a transition plan designed and developed by an educational and rehabilitative team. Professional collaboration in the design and development of the transition plan emphasizes family and individual needs, because the young TBI patient must move from an acute-care medical facility to a long-term care rehabilitative medical facility to a family-life situation (which may include secondary or post-secondary schooling). Supportive counseling for the family and rehabilitation counseling for the TBI patient are bipolar foundations of the transition plan (Shames et al. 1994). The goal of the transition plan is to return the adolescent or young adult to a school program to reasonably accommodate the student's social, educational, and vocational needs. Within the school, the adolescent or young adult assumes an important role in planning for his or her educational and vocational future. This type of team planning is significantly different from the IEP team planning for an elementary-age student and presents numerous challenges for all team members. Several research studies have indicated that the presence of an adolescent or young adult at his or her IEP meeting alters the professionals' interactions (Lerner 1993).

Elderly Adults

While many neurologic problems affect elderly persons, by far the greatest contributor to neuropathology is a cerebrovascular accident (CVA), or a stroke (Minifie 1994). According to the National Stroke Association, strokes affect 500,000 Americans every year (Minifie 1994). Seventy-two percent of these strokes occur in persons older than 65 years of age. Nursing home care is required for about 180,000 victims of stroke each year. Holland (1980) and Swindell and colleagues (1994) have written effectively about the different types of aphasia that result from CVAs and how these language impairments are categorized and treated.

Each family's personal situation is unique regarding financial circumstances, primary language, expectations for longevity, and the support network. A long-term study of persons who have had a CVA details the effects of the changes in communication abilities on families (Holland 1980). The literature is replete with explanations of the difficulty in understanding the stroke patient's language patterns. For the stroke victim, Medicare or Medicaid will typically support speech-language and rehabilitation services in acute-care hospitals, in rehabilitation centers, and at home with follow-up care after a CVA.

The speech-language pathologist's visits at home are awaited by a CVA patient's family, because the service is seen as a lifeline to communication between and among family members and the community. Medicare, Medicaid, or both provides speech-language rehabilitation services to persons who have had a CVA for only a finite period of time, unless the patient continues to make significant progress at reevaluation periods. It is, therefore, of paramount importance to provide the stroke patient with alternative communication modes, so that families can continue to care for their loved one, hopefully in a home-based setting (Swindell et al. 1994).

Within medical-rehabilitative communities, many multidisciplinary rehabilitation centers that coordinate services to the elderly are emerging. These group practices provide occupational and physical therapy, as well as speech-language, nursing, and social service interventions. This team model is used to ensure improved coordination of services for families and CVA patients.

For some elderly persons, particularly those with neurologic deficits too great for home-based care, nursing homes provide skilled nursing care, as well as occupational, physical, and speech-language therapy, for clients who require 24-hour monitoring. In addition to stroke, many patients in nursing homes exhibit dementia, Alzheimer's disease, post-traumatic amnesia, and additional neuromotor speech disorders (e.g., dysarthria and dysphagia). These disorders challenge the speech-language pathologist to provide ongoing assistance to the family members responsible for the changed, disabled family member (Minifie 1994).

Conclusion

The diversity of employment settings and the broad patient age ranges with which speech-language pathologists and audiologists work complicates professional interpersonal communication and collaborative efforts. Team participation in planning and evaluation are necessary to the successful communication disorders professional in any setting.

References

American Speech-Language-Hearing Association. Scope of practice in speech-language pathology. ASHA 1996a;38:1–4.
American Speech-Language-Hearing Association. Scope of practice in audiology. ASHA 1996b;38:1–4.

American Speech-Language-Hearing Association. Omnibus Survey Facts. Rockville, MD: American Speech-Language-Hearing Association, 1994.

Batshaw M, Perret Y. Children with Disabilities. Baltimore: Paul Brookes, 1992.

Beaty J. Observing Development of the Young Child. New York: Merrill-Macmillan, 1994.

Billeaud F. Communication Disorders in Infants and Toddlers. Boston: Butterworth–Heinemann, 1993.

Bricker D. Early Education of At-Risk Handicapped Infants, Toddlers, and Preschool Children. Glenview, IL: Scott, Foresman, 1986;47–49.

Clark G. Is a functional curriculum approach compatible with an inclusive education model? Teaching Exceptional Children 1994;26:36–39.

Eger D. Why now? Changing school speech-language service delivery. ASHA 1992;34:40–41.

Falk-Ross F. Addressing Language Difficulties in the Classroom: A Communication Competence Perspective. Presented at the American Speech-Language-Hearing Association, Orlando, FL, December 1995.

Frey D. Does anyone here think this baby can live? New York Times Magazine July 9, 1995;22–47.

Gerber S. The State of the Art in Pediatric Audiology. In S Gerber, G Mencher (eds), International Perspectives on Communication Disorders. Washington, DC: Gallaudet University Press, 1988.

Holland A. Communication Abilities in Daily Living: A Test of Functional Communication for Aphasic Adults. Baltimore: University Park Press, 1980.

Huffman N. Challenges of education reform. ASHA 1992;34:41–44.

Idol L, Paolucci-Whitcomb P, Nevin A. Collaborative Consultation. Rockville, MD: Aspen Publishers, 1986.

Ivey A, Ivey M, Simek-Morgan L. Counseling and Psychotherapy: A Multicultural Perspective. Boston: Allyn & Bacon, 1993.

Johnson-Martin N, Attermeier S, Hacker B. The Carolina Curriculum for Preschoolers with Special Needs. Baltimore: Paul Brookes, 1990.

Lerner J. Learning Disabilities: Theories, Diagnosis, and Teaching Strategies. Boston: Houghton Mifflin, 1993.

Lozo D. Inclusion: implications for speech-language programs in the schools. Lang Speech Hear Serv Schools 1993;24:4.

Luterman D. Deafness in the Family. Boston: Little, Brown, 1987.

Massachusetts Department of Education. Massachusetts Regulations for Certification of Educational Personnel. Quincy, MA: Massachusetts Department of Education, 1994.

Maxon A, Brackett D. The Hearing Impaired Child. Boston: Butterworth–Heinemann, 1992.

Minifie F. Introduction to Communication Sciences and Disorders. San Diego: Singular Publishing Group, 1994.

National Association of State Boards of Education. Winners All: A Call for Inclusive Schools. The Report of the NASBE Study Group on Special Education. Alexandria, VA: National Association of State Boards of Education, 1992.

Nober L. Models of Speech Services and Statewide Delivery Systems. Presented at the Council for Exceptional Children Conference, Washington, DC, April 1984.

Nober L, Nober EH. Programs for Hearing-Impaired Children Under PL 99-457. A G Bell Presentation, San Diego, CA, May 1992.

Nober L. Inclusion Programs in Schools. Presented at the American Speech-Language-Hearing Association, New Orleans, LA, November 1994.

Paul P, Jackson D. Toward a Psychology of Deafness. Boston: Allyn & Bacon, 1993.

Peters-Johnson C. Caseloads in schools. ASHA 1992;34:12.

Prelock P, Miller B, Reed N. Collaborative partnerships in a language in the classroom program. Lang Speech Hear Serv Schools 1995;26:286–292.

Sage D (ed). The parent perspective. Inclusion Times 1993;1:1.

Sapier J, Gower R. The Skillful Teacher. Carlisle, MA: Research for Better Teaching, 1987.

Shames G, Wiig E, Secord W. Human Communication Disorders. New York: Merrill, 1994.

Swindell C, Holland A, Reinmuth O. Aphasia and Related Adult Disorders. In G Shames, E Wiig, W Secord (eds), Human Communication Disorders. New York: Merrill, 1994;520.

Thurman S, Widerstrom A. Infants and Young Children with Special Needs. Baltimore: Paul Brookes, 1990.

United States Department of Education. To Assure the Free Appropriate Public Education of All Children with Disabilities: Sixteenth Annual Report to Congress on the Implementation of the Individuals with Disabilities Education Act. Washington, DC: U.S. Department of Education, 1994.

United States Department of Education. OSERS: News in Print, Inclusion. Washington, DC: U.S. Department of Education, 1992.

Widerstrom A, Mowder B, Sandall S. At-Risk and Handicapped Newborns and Infants. Englewood Cliffs, NJ: Prentice-Hall, 1991.

Ylvisaker M. Head Injury Rehabilitation. Children and Adults. San Diego: College Hill Press, 1985.

Chapter 2 Study Questions

1. Describe the effects of birth weight and gestation period on children with disabilities.
2. Why have inclusion programs become popular in elementary school speech-language programs?
3. Identify the elements of collaboration that are required to work in inclusion programs.
4. Describe the needs of families of an adult with a cerebrovascular accident.
5. Young adults with traumatic brain injury require special treatment by the speech-language pathologist. Explain some issues facing the school-based, speech-language pathologist regarding this population.

II   Normal Processes

3 Language Structure and Function

Toya A. Wyatt

To effectively identify and remediate language disorders in children, speech-language pathologists must be knowledgeable about the course of normal language development. They must not only understand the process by which children develop language but also the order and sequence in which various aspects of language are acquired. In addition, it is important for speech-language professionals to understand the basic structure and rules of language. These rules specify (1) how words are arranged within sentences (syntax), (2) how smaller units of words (e.g., suffixes and prefixes) are used (morphology), (3) how sounds are combined within words (phonology), (4) how the linguistic symbols of a language are used to mark certain ideas and concepts (semantics), and (5) how language is used to accomplish certain communicative goals (pragmatics). This is the type of knowledge a child must possess if he or she is going to become a mature, competent speaker of his or her native language.

Language Defined

Language is "a complex and dynamic system of conventional symbols that is used in various modes for thought and communication" (American Speech-Language-Hearing Association 1983). The American Speech-Language-Hearing Association's definition of language further states that

> *language evolves within specific historical, social, and cultural contexts; language, as rule-governed behavior, is described by at least five parameters—phonologic, morphologic, syntactic, semantic, and pragmatic; language learning and use are determined by the interaction of biological, cognitive, psychosocial,*

and environmental factors; effective use of language for communication requires a broad understanding of human interaction including such associated factors as nonverbal cues, motivation, and sociocultural roles.

Bloom and Lahey also define language as "a code whereby ideas about the world are expressed through a conventional system of arbitrary signals for communication" (Bloom and Lahey 1978).

Taken together, these two definitions of language emphasize the following key aspects that must be considered when discussing the language development of children from diverse cultural and language backgrounds:

1. Language is an important means for expressing or communicating ideas or thoughts.

2. Languages use organized sets of symbols (i.e., linguistic code) for conveying these ideas and thoughts.

3. The symbols and rules of a language are arbitrarily determined and agreed on by a given community of speakers (i.e., the speech community). Each language has its own unique symbols, as well as rules for using and combining these symbols. The specific symbols and code used vary among speech communities. They depend on key cultural, historical, and social factors, such as the geographic location and historical origins of the speech community and the amount of social contact that speech community has had with other speech communities. This arbitrariness explains why the same concept (e.g., dog) is expressed with so many different words (e.g., *dog, chien, perro*) throughout the world.

4. For a language to be considered a language, it must have a set of symbols and rules that are agreed on by two or more persons. This idea concurs with Bloom and Lahey's (1978) statement that languages represent conventional linguistic systems. The speakers of any language must use the agreed-on symbols if they wish to be understood by other speakers of that language. Because a language per se only requires two native users, the term *twin language* can often be applied to the communication used between twins (even when it is comprehensible only to the twins who use it).

5. All languages are rule-governed. Every language in the world, whether it is English, Spanish, French, German, Wolof, Swahili, Tamil, Japanese, or Guayanese, has a set of rules agreed on by its community of speakers. These rules govern how the sounds, words, and sentences of that language are constructed to form meaningful messages. They also dictate how language users within a given speech community are to use that language in various social situations.

6. Dialects constitute slightly different varieties of a given language and are also rule-governed. All English-speaking children, regardless of whether they speak African-American English, Hawaiian Pidgin English, Appalachian English, or some other variety of English, use a linguistic code that is valid and rule-governed. This is also the case with varied Spanish dialects (e.g., Mexican-American, Puerto Rican, and Castilian). In addition, contrary to popular thought, there are only slight grammatical, phonologic, and lexical differences between dialects within the same language.

7. Language can be conveyed through a number of communication channels, or modalities, including oral (speech), written (reading and writing), and manual (sign language) channels. It is for this reason that American sign language and other manual communication systems such as SEE1 (Seeing Essential English) and SEE2 (Signing Exact English) are considered as legitimate and rule-governed languages.

Different Components of Language

Languages can be described in terms of five parameters: phonology, morphology, syntax, semantics, and pragmatics. The terms *content*, *form*, and *use* have also been used to delineate these parameters (Bloom and Lahey 1978). Form is also used to refer to the phonology, morphology, and syntax parameters collectively. Content represents the semantic parameter, and use refers to the pragmatic parameter. Each of these components constitutes an important aspect of communicative competence and must be understood by those both acquiring and studying language. Communicative competence involves understanding the rules for using each of these components in an integrated manner to communicate effectively with others.

Phonology

The phonologic component of language refers to its sound system. Each language has a finite set of sounds that can be used for producing meaningful words and sentences, as well as rules for combining sounds within words. These rules specify which sound combinations are acceptable and the word positions in which sounds can occur. Each language has a set number of sounds, or phonemes. The number and types of sounds that make up a language's phonologic system vary from language to language. For example, while English has 24 consonants, Spanish has 18. In addition, English has 14 vowels, but Spanish has five (Langdon 1992). Another key difference is that English contains some sounds that are not found in Spanish and vice versa. Examples of sounds occurring in English but not in Spanish include /z/ as in *z*ebra, /v/ as in *v*iolin, /ð/ as in *th*at, /dʒ/ as in *j*ump, /θ/ as in th*i*nk, /ʃ/ as in *sh*ip, /ʒ/ as in mea*s*ure, and /n/ as in *n*o. English vowels that are not found in Spanish include /ɪ/, /e/, /æ/, /ʊ/, and /o/. This explains why some native Spanish speakers produce the English word "peas" as "pea*ce*" and the word "s*i*t" as "s*ea*t." Likewise, the trilled /r/ that is found in Spanish words, such as "pe*rr*o," is not found in English and is likely to be difficult for most native English speakers.

Languages also vary in terms of their sound distribution and sequencing rules. Distribution rules dictate the positions in which sounds can occur within words. For example, according to the sound distribution rules of English, the *ng* sound (/ŋ/) can never be used in the beginnings of words (initial word position). It can only occur in the middle of words (medial word position) as in fi*ng*er or at the ends of words (final word position) as in ki*ng*. Other sounds (e.g., /b/) can occur in all three word positions. By comparing sound distribution rules of Spanish and English, we can once again see some very important differences. English and Spanish share the sounds /b/, /p/, /g/, /m/, /t/, /k/, /tʃ/, and /f/. All of these sounds can occur in all three word positions in English; however, none of these sounds can occur in the final positions of words in Spanish.

Sound sequencing rules delineate sound combinations that are allowable in a given language. For example, according to the sound sequencing rules of English, /str/ is an acceptable sound combination in words, but /tlf/ is not.

Morphology

Languages also have rules for how individual words are to be structured in terms of word endings and beginnings. In English, there are several different affixes (i.e., suffixes and prefixes) that can be added to root words to convey additional meaning. Each of the word parts (i.e., root words, suffixes, and prefixes) represent meaningful units known as *morphemes*. Morphemes cannot be broken into smaller portions without destroying meaning.

There are two different types of morphemes in English: free morphemes and bound morphemes. The primary distinction between these two types is the fact that free morphemes can stand alone, while bound morphemes cannot. The morphemes *ball* and *toy* are examples of free morphemes that do not need to be combined with any other morphemes to convey meaning. The plural marker -*s*, which is used in English to convey the concept of more than one when attached to a free morpheme, is an example of a bound morpheme. Bound morphemes are also commonly referred to as *inflectional markers*.

Languages differ in the use of inflectional markers. For example, in Chinese, which is considered to be a noninflectional language, one would not find equivalent forms of the English plural -*s* and past tense -*ed* markers within words. This is because both of these concepts (i.e., plurality and time) are inferred, instead, from the preceding discourse context (Cheng 1993).

Syntax

The term *syntax* refers to the sentence construction or grammatical rules of a language. Syntax specifies the order in which words must appear to form a meaningful utterance. For example, according to the grammatical rules of English, it would be unacceptable for an English-speaking child to produce the sentence *In flower is cup yellow.* In producing such a sentence, the child would be violating several rules of English word ordering. In this case, he or she would have violated the rule that requires an article to precede the noun (i.e., *flower* and *cup*) and the rule that requires the preposition (i.e., *in*) to follow the verb (i.e., *is*). Knowledge of the syntactic rules of a language helps a child determine what is grammatical and what is ungrammatical in his or her language.

What is considered to be grammatical in one language or dialect, however, may not be considered grammatical in another. For example, in Spanish adjectives generally follow the noun they modify. In addition, they must agree in gender and number with the noun they follow. Therefore, in Spanish if one wants to talk about a black cat, one would have to say "el gato negro." However, the literal translation of this phrase in English is *the cat black.* In English, this is considered ungrammatical, because it violates a very basic syntactic rule of English (i.e., that adjectives must precede the nouns that they modify). Similarly, in Spanish if one wanted to say "the black cats," it would be necessary to mark the gender (masculine) and number (plural) of the noun (i.e., *cat*) on every word in the noun phrase including the article, adjective, and noun. Therefore, it would be necessary to say "los gatos negros," which literally translates to *these cats blacks* in English. Once again, this would be incompatible with the syntactic rules of English that do not require that English speakers mark articles and adjectives for gender and number. Likewise, if one said "el gatos negro" in Spanish, it would be considered ungrammatical according to the syntactic rules of Spanish.

Semantics

The term *semantics* refers to the conceptually based aspects of a language. The conceptual basis of a language is expressed through individual and combined word meanings. To become competent communicators of a language, speakers must not only be familiar with a language's phonology or grammar but must also possess a good understanding of word meanings (i.e., receptive vocabulary). They must also have the ability to accurately express meaning through appropriate word choices (i.e., expressive vocabulary). The vocabulary of language has also been referred to as a language's *lexicon.* Most of us have had the experience of going to a different part of the country or world where a different language is spoken and having a difficult time both in understanding what is being said and trying to get our points across. The majority of misunderstandings in such situations are probably related to the vocabulary differences between languages.

Even within a language, there can be vocabulary differences between dialects of that language. This explains why the English word *bad*, which is typically used for referring to something negative in mainstream or Standard American English, can have a different connotation in the African-American speech community (particularly among some teenagers who use the word *bad* to refer to a positive extreme [i.e., very good]). It also explains why there are at least 19 different ways of saying *ballpoint pen* in the various Spanish speaking communities of the world (Langdon 1992).

Pragmatics

It is not sufficient for persons to learn the linguistic code of a community and the meanings expressed by that code if they do not know how to use the code to meet their everyday needs. For a person to be an effective communicator in his or her speech community, he or she must also know how to use the native language system effectively to express wants, desires, and intentions. The term *pragmatics* refers to this aspect of linguistic competence.

One of the most important aspects of pragmatics is understanding the ways language is used to control the behavior of others and accomplish other important speech tasks (e.g., commenting on something that has just been said, refuting something that has just been said, or describing an object or event to someone else). Each of these tasks are commonly referred to as *speech acts* or *language functions*.

While researchers have proposed a number of different taxonomies for describing the different uses of language, there is a general consensus that these various uses of languages are basic and universal to all speech communities (Bloom and Lahey 1978). Some language researchers, however, have also shown differences in how various communities use language (Heath 1986; Kochman 1972). Heath (1986), for example, describes six uses of language (i.e., language genres) that are important to success in mainstream American classrooms and are commonly found in mainstream American homes (Table 3.1).

While Heath acknowledges that each of these genres appears, to some extent, in all communities, she also provides evidence of cross-cultural variation not only in frequency of use but also in the nature of use. As one example, she states that in some Mexican-American homes, primarily those of recent immigrants, adults primarily use label quests (asking for the names of objects, people, etc.) with children to identify body parts, family members' names, and immediate activities (Heath 1986). According to Heath, it is much rarer for children to be asked to label distant or secondary items, such as pictured objects in books. In addition, label quests occur most frequently during large

TABLE 3.1   Language Genres

Label quests
> Language activities in which adults either name items or ask for the name of an item.
> *Examples:*
>> An adult pointing to a dog asks the child, "What is that?"
>> Adult holds up a ball and says to a child, "See ball?—Ball."

Meaning quests
> Language activity in which an adult attempts to either (1) infer the meaning of a child's utterance, (2) interpret his or her behavior for the child or interpret the child's behavior, or (3) ask the child to explain what the child's utterance means.
> *Examples:*
>> A baby points to a cookie, and the adult says, "You want cookie?"
>> Adult says to the crying baby, "Oh, don't cry. Mommy didn't mean to yell."

Recounts
> When a speaker retells an experience or information already known to both the teller and listener (often for the sake of performance).
> *Example:*
>> Retelling a story that was just read to a child.

Accounts
> Means for providing information that is new to the listener or new interpretations of information that the listener already knows.
> *Example:*
>> Child who comes home to tell his parents what he did in school that day.

Eventcasts
> When a person provides a running narrative of events that are currently within the attention of both the teller and listener.
> *Example*
>> Mother who says as she dresses her child, "OK, now we put on our shoes, now we put on our coat. ..."

Stories
> Fictional accounts that involve some animate being moving through a series of events with goal-directed behaviors.

Source: Adapted from SB Heath. Sociocultural Contexts of Language Development. In Bilingual Education Office (ed), Beyond Language: Social and Cultural Factors in Schooling Language Minority Students. Los Angeles: Evaluation, Dissemination, and Assessment Center of California State University, 1986;168–170.

family gatherings and are rarely a part of daily mother-child interactions. In contrast, label quests occur more frequently in many mainstream American homes, usually within the context of daily feeding routines and book-reading activities. They also occur as a normal part of daily classroom routines, particularly in the primary grades, when teachers frequently ask children to answer *what* and *what-kind* questions during book reading and picture-labeling tasks. According to Heath, differing language-use patterns such as this often result in a home-school mismatch for children who have been exposed to language socialization experiences different from those of peers from mainstream cultural backgrounds.

The pragmatics of language also govern how conversations are organized and maintained. In every speech community, there are rules for how one initiates a conversation, keeps a conversation or topic going (i.e., topic maintenance), initiates a new topic within a conversation (i.e., topic initiation), changes to a new topic, and ends a conversation. For example, most English speakers learn to use conversational openers, such as "Guess what?" or "You know what?" to initiate a conversation. They also learn to keep conversation going through the use of a sustained gaze, occasional verbal acknowledgments (e.g., "Yeah" and "Really?"), or both. In cases in which there has been a communication breakdown, persons must know the appropriate mechanism for clarifying vague or confusing information, and responding appropriately to requests for clarification. Good communicators in any speech community must also be aware of that community's rules for turn-taking. Finally, they must know how to share information from a perspective that the listener will understand, which is termed *listener presupposition*. One important aspect of listener presupposition includes being accurate and clear in the use of pronominal references, so that these terms accurately reflect the listener's perspective. This accuracy ensures that listeners understand who is being referred to with pronouns, such as *he*, *she*, and *they*, and deictic terms (i.e., terms with shifting reference), such as *here*, *there*, *this*, and *that*.

As with every other dimension of language, there is a great deal of cross-cultural variability in the rules for initiating, sustaining, and terminating conversations. For example, there are a number of speech communities in which sustained gaze is not used as a primary means for keeping conversation going and conveying attentiveness. The amount of pause time and overlap between the conversational turns of speakers may also differ. In the African-American speech community, for example, call and response (i.e., the frequent use of verbal acknowledgments) is an important conversational device for keeping the flow of conversation going. In addition, there is a greater tolerance for conversational overlap during turn-taking exchanges. It is, therefore, not uncommon for several persons to be speaking at the same time or for the length of pause between turns to appear much shorter than that seen between most Euro-American speakers. Differences in turn-taking or communicative style can also vary as a function of one's geographical residence. As one travels from the East Coast of the United States to the West Coast and from the North to the South, one is likely to find a range of turn-taking styles and differing rules for initiating, sustaining, and terminating conversations.

A final aspect of pragmatics has to do with the social conventions for adjusting one's communication to suit the needs and background of the listener. Understanding how to modify one's language in accordance with listener background characteristics (e.g., age, social status, gender, ethnicity, and language) constitutes another important part of listener presupposition. Every speech community has rules for how children are to talk to adults and how adults are to talk to children, as well as circumscribed conversational roles for children. In some communities, adults consider children to be conversational equals. As a result, the adults spend a great amount of time talking with children, children are allowed to initiate conversations with the adults, and children are encouraged to be elaborate in their responses to the adults' questions. There are many other communities, however, where adults direct fewer topics to children. In these communities, children are taught to speak only when spoken to and to respond minimally (Schieffelin and Eisenberg 1984). Children are also often not encouraged to initiate conversation with adults. Such differences can have important consequences in the speech and language testing situation, because children may respond to the clinician in a manner that is consistent with their community's communicative expectations but may differ from the communicative expectations of the clinician. Such differences can lead to a misdiagnosis of disorder in these children.

Theories of Language Learning

It should be clear by now that for children to become effective communicators, they must not only learn the rules for how sounds, words, and sentences are combined to produce meaningful and socially appropriate messages, but they must also learn to integrate all of these rules into a cohesive language system. This knowledge cannot be accomplished solely through formal language-teaching methods. It is something that children must learn informally through their interactions with mature speakers in their language community. Therefore, much of what children learn about language is intuitive and unconscious.

There are a number of differing views or theories as to how children acquire these basic building blocks of language. While every theory may not explain every part of a child's language acquisition process, each provides some degree of insight into children's language learning.

Cognitive Theories

Although there are a number of differing views on the relationship between language and cognitive development (i.e., thought), most researchers agree that these two aspects of development are somehow related and that cognition plays a key role in at least some aspects of the language acquisition process.

Most cognitive-based theories of language acquisition suggest that cognition serves as the base for later language development. Such theories support a cognitive determinism view of language learning (Owens 1996; Rice 1983). According to theories of cognitive determinism, advances in language development occur when children achieve certain cognitive prerequisites or milestones.

According to Piaget's (1952) model of child development, which has often been used to demonstrate the relationship between cognition and language, children progress through various stages of cognitive development during their early years. Each stage is associated with newly acquired knowledge and views of the world that result from biological and maturational changes that influence children's interactions with their surrounding environment. These changes ultimately impact how children store, organize, classify, and interpret information from their environment.

There are many child-language researchers who have discussed some of the cognitive developments addressed by Piaget that seem to parallel important language achievements (Cromer 1988; McCune-Nicolich 1981; Rice 1983). In a study examining the relationship between children's developing notions of object permanence (i.e., the recognition that an object still exists even when it is not present) and vocabulary development, McCune-Nicolich (1981) observed that at least 50% of words used by toddlers to discuss the nonexistence, disappearance, or recurrence of objects (e.g., *no, gone, away,* and *again*) emerged within 1 month of their entry into the object-permanence stage of cognitive development. McCune-Nicolich's results support the view that cognitive development and language development are intricately related processes.

In contrast to cognitive determinism models of language development, there are some theories that focus more on the role that language plays in the development of cognition (Whorf 1956). According to these theories, it is the structure of one's language that influences how one perceives and classifies the world. In other words, "language determines what we think" (Rice 1983). One of the best examples of such a model is that proposed by Whorf (1956), who suggested that the extensive snow vocabulary of Eskimo languages enables Eskimo children to see the distinctions between different types of snow that would not be discerned by children exposed to a language with a less rich snow vocabulary. Schlesinger (1982) also used linguistic determinism to explain how children eventually sort out the distinctive meanings of words like *a* (a nonspecified object from a given class of objects) and *the* (a specific object from a given class of objects) primarily on the basis of language input. Linguistic determinism models of language development are based on the view that children develop an understanding of key concepts from observing regularities in their language (Rice 1983).

Another cognitive model, known as the *interaction hypothesis,* focuses on the influence of cognition and language on each other (Rice 1983). According to this hypothesis, while cognition may initially serve as the basis for language development, at some point in development, the direction of this influence changes and language influences cognition. As support for this perspective, Blank (1974) points to the emergence of *how* and *why* questions in children's speech. According to Blank, there is insufficient information in children's surrounding environments for them to fully understand the appropriateness of how and why questions. Children must, therefore, try them out and determine from adult responses the full meaning of these question forms. This hypothesis can explain the why question stage that 3- to 4-year-old children go through, in which they seem to ask an endless stream of sometimes impossible-to-answer why questions. Take the following example from my 3½-year-old cousin Chenise. One day during a summer visit with Chenise and her family, Chenise overheard me say that I would only be staying one more night and I had to leave the next day. An ensuing stream of why questions followed, beginning with Chenise's initial query as to why I would only be staying one more night:

Chenise: Why just one more night?
Toya: Because I have to go to see my mommy.

Chenise: Why do you see your mommy?
Toya: Because she wants to see me.

Chenise: Why she wanna see you?
Toya: Because she misses me.

Chenise: Why she miss you?
Toya: Because she never gets to see me.

Chenise: Why she never gets to see you?
Toya: Because I live far away.

Chenise: Why it's far away?

Needless to say, Chenise's barrage of why questions eventually became exhausting. She seemed intrigued by my responses, which only spurred her on to more frequent queries. According to Blank, Chenise's relentless stream of why questions were not simply the result of requests for information but also for knowledge of how these question forms are to be used. According to cognitive theorists who subscribe to this theory, the use of such questions furthers children's knowledge of the causal relationship between real-world events and these question forms, which eventually leads to more appropriate use of these forms. With this scenario, cognition and language are viewed, therefore, as mutually influencing each other.

Social Theories

Another important set of theories frequently used to explain children's language development are social theories of language acquisition. In contrast to cognitive theories, which stress the importance of cognition on language acquisition, social theories stress the influence of caregiver-child social interactions on the language acquisition process. Under these theories, early caregiver-child nonverbal and verbal routines, including the giving and receiving of objects and verbal social games (e.g., patty-cake) are seen as crucial to the language-learning process, because they help teach important conversational skills (e.g., turn-taking). If children are to become effective communicators, it is important for them to understand their role as speakers and listeners and to understand how to time their conversational responses to others in a socially appropriate manner. Social theorists believe that the early social word games between caregivers and their infants help establish this skill.

Social theories of language development also focus on the natural adjustments that caregivers make to meet the language-learning needs and levels of their children. These adjustments, commonly referred to as *baby talk* (i.e., simplified speech and language directed toward infants) and *motherese* (i.e., a style of talking to toddlers), are often cited as two important verbal strategies used for accomplishing these goals. Both forms of caregiver-child discourse are considered to contain elements essential to the establishment of an optimal language-learning environment. This environment depends specifically on the ability to capture and maintain a child's attention during communicative exchanges and the use of language that promotes a child's understanding and participation (Owens 1996).

One of the primary weaknesses of social language learning theories is that they focus on language development from a mainstream, culture–based perspective, without necessarily taking into account some of the cross-cultural differences that occur in mother-child interactions. For example, as Schieffelin and Eisenberg (1984) point out, there are a number of different ways in which mothers teach their children to talk. Not every society believes in using baby talk with infants, and every community has its own norms for how children are taught language. In some cases, language behaviors that are considered to be important parts of the language teaching process (e.g., expansions) by many mainstream American parents are not found in the teaching practices of mothers from nonmainstream American backgrounds. Yet, children exposed to these differing language practices still manage to develop into normal communicators in their own communities.

Behavioral Theories

During the 1950s and 1960s, most speech and language professionals subscribed to behavior theories of language learning that viewed language learning from a more structured and less child-oriented view. According to behavior theories of language learning, language is a social behavior that can be learned, modified, and controlled through a process of behavioral conditioning.

The most common applications of behavioral theory have occurred in fields (e.g., psychology) in which behavioral conditioning techniques have been used to control the behavior of rats, dogs, and other animals during experimental studies. For example, anyone who has taken a basic psychology course is familiar with Pavlov's classic conditioning dog experiment and Skinner's operant conditioning study of rat lever-pressing behavior (Mowrer 1982). In both studies, researchers were able to change some aspect of their animal subjects' behaviors through the use of rewards (e.g., the presence of food in conjunction with or following a conditioned stimulus) and punishment (e.g., shock). Through their research, Pavlov and Skinner demonstrated how a desirable behavior can be developed or increased in frequency through the presentation of a rewarding consequence, and how undesirable behaviors can be decreased in frequency when they are ignored or punished.

These paradigms have also been used to explain the process of language learning. According to behavioral theories of language learning, children learn language through (1) modeling, imitation, practice, and the positive reinforcement of correctly produced language forms and (2) the correction or ignoring of incorrectly produced forms (Owens 1996). Adults take the primary responsibility in shaping children's language behavior by positively rewarding correct language behavior through the use of social rewards (e.g., verbal praise, attention, and smiling) and punishing inappropriate behavior through the use of parental correction, requests to repeat, or nonacknowledgment of incorrectly produced language forms.

According to Owens (1996), however, behavioral theories of language learning have come under attack because of questions about the importance of imitation in the language-learning processes. Researchers, such as Chomsky (1965), who view children as active participants in the language-learning process think that rewarded and punished imitation cannot account for some of the creative language errors often made by children during the early stages of language development. They also believe that it cannot explain the speed with which children master the basic grammatical forms of their language.

Biological Theories

A final set of theories proposed for explaining children's language learning are biologically based theories. In contrast to behavior and social theories, which emphasize the role of environment, biological theories of language learning emphasize the more innate, biological aspects of development. According to theories, such as that proposed by Chomsky (1965), children are born with an innate capacity for language learning and knowledge of the basic grammatical structure that exists in all human languages (i.e., universal grammar). They also possess the necessary skills for making hypotheses about the grammatical structure of the language(s) to which they are exposed by using incoming language input. The hypothesis-testing mechanism responsible for this accomplishment is commonly referred to as the *language acquisition device*.

Biological theorists have attempted to demonstrate support for this view of language learning by drawing attention to the amazing similarities between the language stages and language errors of children from diverse language backgrounds. Some linguists have determined that there are certain errors that children never seem to make and structures that they never seem to produce, regardless of the child's language background. It is believed that such errors and structures would violate important constraints in human language. As reported in the *Los Angeles Times* (TH Maugh. Deaf infants say "goo-goo" in sign language. March 22, 1991), biological views of language learning have been used to explain research findings that deaf infants of deaf parents who are exposed to American Sign Language as their first language go through a stage of manual (hand) babbling at the same age that hearing infants of hearing parents who are exposed to spoken language go through a stage of oral babbling. It has also been used to explain why deaf children begin to produce two-sign utterances at the same time that hearing children produce two-word utterances (i.e., around 18 months of age) (Meier 1991).

Summary of Language Theories

Although a number of different theories have been proposed to explain children's language development, it is difficult to state that any one theory is more accurate than another. Each theory has its own strengths and weaknesses. In addition, as Lahey (1988) notes, it is possible for one or more theories to be more appropriate when attempting to explain one aspect of language development and for another to be more appropriate when attempting to explain other aspects. For example, theories that emphasize the relationship between cognition and language can best explain how children develop the conceptual (semantic) bases of language. On the other hand, theories that emphasize the importance of caregiver-child interactions can be most useful for explaining the development of pragmatics. Correspondingly, theories that emphasize the biological aspects of language can best explain children's early syntactic development.

Schlesinger (1977) suggests that differing cognitive models of language acquisition can account for linguistic developments at different stages of the language acquisition process. For example, cognitive factors may play a bigger role during certain stages of language development, while linguistic factors may play a role in fostering cognitive development at other stages of development. In addition, some children may tend to display a more cognitively oriented approach to language learning, while others may display a more socially based approach. The possibilities are endless. In any event, each theory provides some contribution to the overall understanding of children's language learning.

References

American Speech-Language-Hearing Association. Definition of language. ASHA 1983;25:44.

Blank M. Cognitive functions of language in preschool years. Dev Psychol 1974;10:240–242.

Bloom L, Lahey M. Language Development and Language Disorders. New York: Macmillan, 1978;2–500.

Cheng LR. Asian-American Cultures. In D Battle (ed), Communication Disorders in Multicultural Populations. Boston: Andover Medical Publishers, 1993;45.

Chomsky N. Aspects of the Theory of Syntax. Cambridge, MA: MIT Press, 1965.

Cromer RF. The Cognition Hypothesis Revisited. In F Kessel (ed), The Development of Language and Language Researchers. Hillsdale, NJ: Erlbaum, 1988;239.

Heath SB. Sociocultural Contexts of Language Development. In Bilingual Education Office (ed), Beyond Language: Social and Cultural Factors in Schooling Language Minority Students. Los Angeles: Evaluation, Dissemination and Assessment Center of California State University, 1986;148–174.

Kochman T. Rappin' and Stylin' Out. Urbana, IL: University of Illinois Press, 1972.

Lahey M. Language Disorders and Language Development. New York: Macmillan, 1988;184–433.

Langdon HW. Hispanic Children and Adults with Communication Disorders. Gaithersburg, MD: Aspen Publishers, 1992;57–132.

McCune-Nicolich L. The cognitive bases of relational words in the single word period. J Child Lang 1981;8:15–34.

Meier RP. Language acquisition by deaf children. American Scientist 1991;79:62–64.

Mowrer DE. Methods of Modifying Speech Behaviors. Prospect Heights, IL: Waveland Press, 1982;12–19.

Owens RE. Language Development: An Introduction (4th ed). New York: Merrill, 1996;29–229.

Piaget J. The Origins of Intelligence in Children. New York: International Universities Press, 1952.

Rice ML. Contemporary accounts of the cognition/language relationship: implications for speech-language clinicians. J Speech Hear Disord 1983;48:347–359.

Schieffelin BB, Eisenberg AR. Cultural Variation in Children's Conversations. In R Schiefelbusch, J Pickar (eds), The Acquisition of Communicative Competence. Baltimore: University Park Press, 1984;384–414.

Schlesinger IM. The role of cognitive development and linguistic input in language acquisition. J Child Lang 1977;4:153–167.

Schlesinger IM. Steps to Language: Toward a Theory of Native Language Acquisition. Hillsdale, NJ: Erlbaum, 1982.

Whorf B. Language, Thought, and Reality. New York: Wiley, 1956.

Chapter 3   Study Questions

1. List and describe each of the five major components of language.
2. What are the primary differences between the cognitive, social, biological, and behavioral views of language learning?
3. List three defining characteristics of a language.
4. What is the relationship between a language and a dialect? How are languages and dialects similar?
5. List one way in which languages can differ from each other with respect to (a) phonology and (b) syntax.

4   Children's Language Development

Toya A. Wyatt

In addition to understanding what children learn about their language and how they learn language, it is also important to understand the stages that children go through in acquiring the basic elements of their language. This chapter describes some of the key language stages and milestones that characterize children's language development during the infant, toddler, preschool, and school-age years. Differences between the language development of children from monolingual versus bilingual backgrounds, as well as differences between the language development of children from nonstandard English–speaking versus Standard American English (SAE)–speaking backgrounds are also discussed.

While it is often difficult to pinpoint the exact ages at which children acquire various aspects of their language, there are common points during the developmental process at which all normally developing children, regardless of their cultural or language backgrounds, begin to acquire key language behaviors and structures. For example, all children, including those with hearing impairments, begin to produce two-word or two-sign utterances in their native language at around 18 months of age. In addition, according to "Deaf infants say 'goo-goo' in sign language" by T.H. Maugh in the *Los Angeles Times*, March 22, 1991, normally developing hearing children begin to say their first words at approximately 1 year of age, which corresponds to the age at which normally developing deaf children begin to produce their first signs.

It is also important to understand, however, that there is a degree of individual variation in how children progress through the various stages of language development. Every child develops at his or her own pace. Therefore, no two children display the same pattern of language development. As a result, developmental profiles that provide normative data on when children acquire certain behaviors and structures should only be used as a general guide to children's development (Owens 1996).

Language Development of Infants

Language development begins before children say their first words. During the first few months of life, infants are beginning to use the earliest form of communication (i.e., crying) to signal that they are, for example, hungry, distressed, or fatigued. However, these cries serve as an indication of their internal states (e.g., the fact that they are hungry) and not as intentionally conveyed requests to be fed. This is because infants are not yet aware of the communicative impact that their vocalizations have or can have on their listener. They do not yet know how to use their early vocalizations to control the behavior of others. This period of development is, therefore, commonly referred to as the *perlocutionary stage of development*. Most parents, however, often ascribe meaning to their infant's coos and cries at this stage of development. They are also convinced that their infants are using these coos and cries in a meaningful manner.

During the first month of life, infants are also beginning to produce a limited number of noncrying vowel-like sounds called *quasi-resonant nuclei* (Oller 1978; Owens 1996). These sounds lack the full resonance of adult vowel productions, because they are produced with more restricted mouth opening and nasality than those produced by adults. The lack of full resonance can be attributed to the fact that the speech mechanism of infants is still immature and developing.

In addition to producing sound, infants are beginning to respond to sound in their environments. They are beginning to visually search for the source of sounds and demonstrate a growing interest and attention to objects and people in their surrounding environment. At this stage of development, infants are also beginning to explore their environment using their limited physical abilities (e.g., crawling, grasping, reaching, or mouthing objects). Each of these developments is important to later language development, because each provides infants with incoming information from the environment that is key to the later development of important language concepts.

At around 2–3 months of age, infants begin to go through a cooing or gooing stage, in which vowels and consonant-like sounds produced in the back of the mouth make up the majority of their speech sound productions. Between 4 and 6 months of age, normally developing infants go though a babbling stage, in which they are starting to produce repetitive consonant-vowel syllable sequences of increasing lengths. All infants, including deaf infants, generally go though these stages, if they are developing normally. However, over time, the babbling behavior of deaf infants has been noted to decrease. Some scholars (Bernstein and Tiegerman 1993) have attributed this decrease to the fact that deaf infants are not receiving the same reinforcing auditory feedback from their productions as hearing infants. This feedback is considered to be crucial to the speech development process.

Language Development of Toddlers

One-Word Stage of Development

At about 10 months of age, infants are beginning to use nonverbal gestures (e.g., pointing) with or without accompanying vocalizations to achieve a number of different language goals (e.g., attracting the listener's attention, requesting objects, or rejecting requests). Children are also learning that they can use the same vocalization to express a variety of different language meanings, simply by varying the pitch and tone of their productions. The stage of development at which children begin to realize that their verbal messages have an impact on the listener and that speech can be used for affecting the behaviors of others is known as the *illocutionary stage of development.*

At about 12 months of age, children begin to move into a locutionary stage of language development. This stage is marked by the appearance of a child's first words. Many parents believe that their children produce their first words at 6 months of age, when children are beginning to produce babbling strings that sound like "dada" and "mama." In reality, such vocalizations cannot be characterized as true words until they are used consistently to refer to the same referent. Most of the babbling strings that are produced by children before 1 year of age do not fit this criteria, because they are often produced indiscriminately in response to a wide variety of different visual stimuli or events.

By 18 months of age, most children have approximately 50 words in their expressive vocabulary. Their receptive vocabulary, however, appears to be larger since children generally comprehend more words than they can express. Nouns generally constitute the majority of children's first words, although there are a number of children who have been characterized as "noun leavers" rather than "noun lovers." Such children tend to use more social words, such as *hi* and *bye* (Nelson 1973; Owens 1996). According to Clark (1978), children's first words involve terms from the following categories: food (e.g., *juice*), clothing items (e.g., *hat*), body parts (e.g., *eye*), animals (e.g., *dog*), toys (e.g., *ball*), household items (e.g., *key*), and people (e.g., *dada*).

The most important development during this stage, however, is the fact that children are learning to express their various wants, needs, and desires using a conventional linguistic code that is understood and used by a community of speakers. The code(s) that children acquire is the one to which they have had the most exposure. Codes can represent a spoken language, such as English, or a nonspoken language, such as American Sign Language. Children are also beginning to use

TABLE 4.1   Dore's Primitive Speech Acts

Speech Act Category	Example
Labeling	Monique touches her doll's eyes and utters "eyes," then she touches its nose and utters "nose."
Repeating	Monique, while playing with a puzzle, overhears her mother say "doctor" (while in conversation with the teacher) and utters, "doc." Her mother responds, "Yes, that's right honey, doctor," then continues her conversation. Monique resumes her play with the puzzle.
Answering	His mother points to a picture of a dog and asks Jason, "What's this?" Jason responds, "Bow-wow."
Requesting action	Jason tries to push a peg through a hole and, when he cannot succeed, looks up at his mother, keeping his finger on the peg, and utters, "push" (with constant contours and minimal pause between syllables). His mother then helps him push the peg, saying, "Okay."
Requesting answer	Monique picks up a book, looks at her mother, and utters, "Book?" Her mother responds, "Right, it's a book."
Calling	Jason, whose mother is across the room, shouts, "Mama" loudly. His mother turns to him and says, "I'm getting a cup of coffee. I'll be right there."
Greeting	Jason utters, "Hi" when the teacher enters the room. The teacher responds, "Hello."
Protesting	Jason, when his mother attempts to put on his shoe, utters an extended scream of varying contours while resisting her. Monique, in the same circumstance, utters, "No."
Practicing	Monique utters, "Daddy" when he is not present.

Source: Adapted from J Dore. Holophrases, speech acts and language universals. J Child Lang 1975;2:21.

words by the end of their first year of life to accomplish an even wider range of language functions. Some of the more commonly expressed language functions during this period of development, referred to by Dore (1975) as *primitive speech acts,* can be found in Table 4.1. These language functions can be expressed through the use of single words or vocalizations used in conjunction with related nonverbal gestures (e.g., pointing and reaching).

Children are also beginning to use their one-word utterances by 12 months of age to express a common core of language meanings. Bloom and Lahey (1978) stated that as early as the first year of life, all children are beginning to talk about universal topics, such as the existence of objects, the relationships between objects, the relationships between objects and events, and the relationships between objects and their environment. Based on their longitudinal study of children's emerging meanings, Bloom and Lahey developed a taxonomy of semantic categories that attempts to capture the range of meanings generally expressed by children between the ages of 16 and 36 months (Table 4.2).

TABLE 4.2   Bloom and Lahey's Content Categories

Content Category	Category Description	Example
Existence	Utterances that point out the existence of objects or persons in the immediate environment. Frequently coded with the demonstratives *this* and *that*.	Child, while touching a swing set, says, "This a swing set."
Recurrence	Reference to the reappearance of an object or event, additional instances or occurrences of an object or event, or both. Frequently coded with the words *more* and *again*.	Child who holds up a cup and says, "More juice" to request a refill.
Nonexistence or disappearance	Reference to the absence or disappearance of an expected or anticipated object or event. Frequently coded with words such as *all gone*, *no more*, and *no*.	Child looking at empty cup of milk says, "All gone."
Rejection	Reflects opposition or refusal of an object or action. Frequently coded with the word *no* or *don't*.	Child who says, "No bed," when mother states that it is time for bed.
Denial	Denial of some previous statement, proposition, or assertion. Frequently coded with the word *no* or *not*.	Child who says, "That not a doggy," when father points out a dog different from the one at home.
Attribution	Reference to the properties (i.e., color, shape, size, or condition) of objects.	Child who says, "Green," in response to parent's question, "What color is that comb?"
Possession	Reference to the possessive relationship between an object and person. Frequently coded with the use of possessive pronouns, such as *his* and *her*, or the possessive *-s* marker.	Child who takes doll from another and says, "My dolly."
Locative action	Reference to the movement and subsequent placement of an object or person that involves some change in location. Can be used to refer to the direction of the movement, nature of movement, or end-goal of the movement.	Child who says, "She lays down," while putting her doll in the bed.
Action	Reference to the movement of an object or person without any reference to location of the action.	Child who says, "I mixing," while using a spoon to stir in a cup.
Locative state	Reference to the static location or placement of an object or person without any reference to currently occurring movement.	Child who says, "He in a chair," while placing boy doll in a chair.
State	References to the internal state, external state, attribute state, or possessive state (condition) of an object or event.	Child who says, "It's dark," when talking about a haunted house.
Quantity	Reference to the number of objects. Used to code the concept of more than one and frequently involves use of number terms (e.g., *two* or *three*), the plural *-s* marker, and other terms such as *some* and *many*.	Child who says, "Two puppy," when looking at a picture of two dogs.

TABLE 4.2   continued

Content Category	Category Description	Example
Notice	Shows attention to a person, object, or event. Frequently coded by words such as *look*, *watch*, and *see*.	Child who points and says, "Look, Mickey," in reference to Mickey Mouse doll on shelf.
Dative	Designates the recipient of an object or action.	Child who says, "This for Daddy," while drawing a picture.
Additive	Contains two independently expressed meanings conjoined within the same utterance. Frequently coded with the use of the conjunction *and*.	Child who says, "He goes here and she goes there," while placing boy and girl doll in separate cars.
Temporal	Reference to the temporal relationship between two different events. Often coded with temporal terms, such as *then* and *when*, or verbs marked for tense (e.g., *broke* or *played*).	Child who says, "Now it's fixed," after fixing the broken wheel of a train.
Causal	Reference to the cause-effect relationship between states, events, or both. Frequently coded with the conjunction *because*.	Child who says, "She has to go to bed because she's tired," while placing a doll in bed.
Adversative	Reference to an adversative or contrastive relationship between events, states, or both. Frequently coded with the conjunction *but*.	Child who says, "This is the mommy, but she's mean."
Epistemic	Reference to mental states. Frequently coded with forms of the mental verbs *to know*, *to think*, and *to wonder*.	Child who says, "I know how to do it."
Specification	Reference to a specific object, person, or event in contrast to other objects, persons, events. Generally coded with the use of the article *the* or demonstrative pronoun *this* or *that*.	Child who says, "This is the piece that goes right here," while putting together a puzzle.
Communication	Reference to the act of communication. Frequently coded with the use of verbs such as *say* and *tell*.	Child who says, "I'm gonna tell the teacher."

Source: Adapted from M Lahey. Appendix E: Definitions of Content Categories. In M Lahey (ed), Language Disorders and Development. New York: Macmillan, 1988;429–433.

Because of the biological constraints of a speech mechanism that is still quite immature, the speech-sound patterns of children's first words are still limited. As a result, the majority of children's first words represent only approximations of the adult versions. For example, instead of saying water, children might say "wawa." They also may say "tat" for cat, "goggie" for doggie, "nana" for banana, and so forth. In addition, it is common for children to avoid certain words due to factors such as word length, syllable complexity, or the nature of sounds used. Some children may also demonstrate a preference for certain word shapes (sound patterns). Such children are likely to modify words that do not conform to their preferred word-shape patterns to match their preferences. For example, a child who demonstrates a preference for two-syllable words that begin with labial sounds (i.e., /b/, /p/, and /m/) may produce the word *kitty* as "pipi." According to Owens (1996), the majority of children's first words at this stage of development conform to a consonant-vowel (e.g., go), vowel-consonant (e.g., up), consonant-vowel-consonant-vowel reduplicated (e.g., dada), or consonant-vowel-consonant-vowel nonreduplicated (e.g., doggie) shape.

It is also common for children to use their first words to mark meanings in a way that differs from how adults use the same words to mark meanings. For example, a child may use the word *dog* to refer only to his or her dog and not to other dogs. This type of word meaning error is commonly referred to as *underextension.* Another common type of word meaning error (i.e., overextension) occurs when children use a word to refer to a wider range of referents than appropriate. For example, the child who uses the word *dog* to refer to dogs as well as other four-legged animals (e.g., dogs, cows, sheep, cats) is engaging in the practice of overextension. Children often underextend or overextend their words on the basis of perceived differences or similarities in the physical characteristics (attributes) or the functional uses of objects.

Two-Word Stage of Language Development

At about 18 months of age, all normally developing children are beginning to produce their first two-word combinations. One of the key language developments during this period is the expansion of the semantic meanings and language functions that are expressed. Not only are children beginning to use two-word utterances to mark those semantic meanings and pragmatic functions expressed during the one-word stage of development, but they are also beginning to express new meanings and functions.

It is at the two-word stage of development that child-language researchers and clinicians begin to describe children's language developments in terms of language stages and mean length of utterance. One of the most commonly used language stage models is Brown's stages, which is used to profile the development of children's language. The stages are based on research conducted by Roger Brown (1973), who studied the language development of three children over an 18-month period. During his study, Brown followed all of the children as they moved from a single-word to a multiword stage of development. He found that the patterns of development among the three children were similar and the same language forms generally emerged at about the same maturational stage of development (i.e., age). Based on the findings of his study, Brown proposed a sequence of development for 14 key grammatical forms, as well as a stage model of language development composed of five different language stages. Each

TABLE 4.3   Brown's Stages of Language Development

Language Stage	Mean Length of Utterance Range	Approximate Age Range
Early stage I	1.01–1.49	16–27 months
Late stage I	1.50–1.99	19–32 months
Stage II	2.00–2.49	22–38 months
Stage III	2.50–2.99	25–42 months
Early stage IV	3.00–3.49	29–47 months
Late stage IV and early stage V	3.50–3.99	32–49 months
Late stage V	4.00–4.49	38–53 months
Post stage V	4.50 and above	41–67 months

Source: Adapted from J Miller. Procedures for Analyzing Free Speech Samples: Syntax and Semantics. In J Miller (ed), Assessing Language Production in Children. Austin, TX: PRO-ED, 1981;26.

TABLE 4.4   Brown's Fourteen Morphemes

Morpheme	Example	Language Stage
Present progressive -ing	"I mixing."	Stage II
Plural -s	"Puppies."	Stage II
In	"In here."	Stage II
On	"On table."	Stage III
Possessive -s	"Mommy's hat."	Stage III
Irregular past tense	Fell.	Stage V
Articles a and the	"A doggie."	Stage V
Regular past tense	Pushed.	Stage V
Third person singular -s	"This walks."	Stage V
Contractible copula be	"That's a big one."	Stage V
Contractible auxiliary be	"This is swimming."	Stage V and above
Irregular third person singular	"It goes here."	Stage V and above
Uncontractible auxiliary be	"Is he going home?"	Stage V and above
Uncontractible copula be	"Yes, she is."	Stage V and above

Source: Adapted from J Miller. Procedures for Analyzing Free Speech Samples: Syntax and Semantics. In J Miller (ed), Assessing Language Production in Children. Austin, TX: PRO-ED, 1981;32.

stage is associated with certain linguistic achievements and is marked by significant changes in grammatical growth, such as increased sentence length and complexity. A list of these 14 morphemes and five language stages can be found in Tables 4.3 and 4.4.

During Brown's first two stages of development, several morphologic forms, such as the prepositions *in* and *on*, the present progressive *-ing* marker, and the plural *-s* marker are beginning to appear in English-speaking children's speech. Although many of these forms are beginning to emerge at this stage of development, they are often inconsistently or incorrectly used. Most of these errors result from children's overuse of a certain language rule. For example, it is not uncommon to hear children use the plural *-s* marker not only with regular but also irregular plural nouns. As a result, one may hear a Standard

English–speaking child say "feets" instead of feet, because he or she has not yet recognized the difference between irregular and regular plurals. This type of overuse is often referred to as *overgeneralization.*

At this stage of development, children are also beginning to produce their earliest questions, which are characterized primarily by the simple use of rising intonation (e.g., "Daddy going?"). During the earliest stages of development, the majority of children's questions consist of simple yes or no (e.g., "Doggie bed?"), what (e.g., "What doing?"), and where (e.g., "Where daddy?") questions. The majority of children's what and where questions are produced with a missing subject or verb form.

Children are also beginning to produce simple negatives (e.g., *not, don't,* and *can't*) and early developing pronouns (e.g., *I, you, me, mine, my,* and *it*). It is still very common, however, for children to use earlier developing negatives, such as *no* and *not,* in place of later emerging negatives, such as *can't* and *don't.* Therefore, at this stage of development, it would not be unusual for a child to say "I not can do it" or "I no can do it" instead of "I can't do it." They may also place the negative outside instead of within the verb phrase, as in the case of the child who says, "No Daddy eating," for "Daddy is not eating."

By the age of 3 years, children are beginning to master sounds, such as /n/, /m/, /p/, and /h/ in at least two word positions (Sanders 1972). In most cases, these sounds are mastered in initial and final word positions before they become stabilized in medial word position. Children are still, however, continuing to modify the sound and syllable structure of words that contain difficult-to-produce sounds or sound patterns. In contrast to earlier stages of development, however, the pronunciation strategies employed by children at this age are fairly universal and rule governed. For example, it is common for all children at this stage of development to omit the last sounds of words, reduce consonant clusters to one sound (e.g., skate might be produced as "kate"), delete unstressed word syllables (e.g., elephant might be produced as "elfant"), and to substitute later developing sounds with earlier developing sounds. These rule-based patterns, which are referred to as *phonologic processes,* generally disappear by 3–4 years of age in normally developing children.

Preschool Stage of Language Development

Standard English–Speaking Children

As children move into the preschool years (3–5 years of age), their utterances become longer and more complex, and the structure of their sentences begins to resemble more closely the syntactic structure of the adult language to which they have been exposed. Their phonologic system is also becoming more stable, and they are continuing to refine their semantic and pragmatic skills.

They are also continuing to master key morphologic forms. Later emerging morphologic inflections (i.e., the irregular past tense marker, possessive -*s* marker, articles, regular past tense -*ed* marker, regular and irregular third person singular -*s*, and auxiliary and copula *be*) are finally beginning to stabilize. Children are, however, still producing some interesting word errors on more complex morphologic forms. Bowerman (1982) and Clark (1983) both provide excellent examples of the type of errors frequently made by children who are still trying to master derivational markers like -*er* and affixes like *un*-. Examples include using the word *mistaker* to refer to someone who makes mistakes and the term *storier* to refer to someone who tells stories. Other examples include the creative use of phrases like *unclothes her* to refer to the act of taking one's clothes off or *unshorten* to refer to the act of lengthening something.

As English-speaking children begin to produce their first three-word sentences, the majority of their sentences conform to either an agent (person or object conducting action) plus action plus object (person or object affected by action) or agent plus action plus location structure. Over time, children begin to expand the basic structure of their sentences by producing more elaborated noun-phrase and verb-phrase structures. Expansion of the noun phrase occurs through the addition of articles, possessive pronouns, and other modifiers. Expansion of the verb phrase occurs through the use of more morphologic inflections, such as the past tense -*ed*, present progressive -*ing*, and auxiliary verbs.

As children progress through the next few stages of development, more complex sentence forms, such as embedded and conjoined phrases and clauses, start to emerge (Owens 1996). Embedded clauses and phrases are those syntactic units that either modify or serve as the subject or object of a main clause and include structures such as prepositional phrases (e.g., "The cup is *on the table*"), gerunds (e.g., "*Rollerskating* is dangerous"), infinitives (e.g., "I want *to do that*"), indirect questions or embedded *wh*- questions (e.g., "I know *who did it*," and "She saw *where the kitty went*"), and relative clauses (e.g., "This is the one *that I want*," and "The boy *who lives in that house* is a brat"). Embedded clauses can either serve as the subject (e.g., "*For you to do that* was not nice") or the object (e.g., "I know *that you can do it*"). Embedded clauses are also referred to as *subordinate clauses*.

At this stage, children are also beginning to produce sentences containing two independent clauses that are conjoined. Conjoined clauses occur when two main, independent clauses in a sentence are joined through the use of words such as *and, but,* and *or*. Examples of conjoined clauses are the sentences "*I got a tricycle and my sister got a dolly*," and "*I have a basketball at home, but I can't play with it*." The emergence of these complex sentence structures is directly related to children's acquisition of conjunctions, which become more prevalent in the speech of children around the age of 4 years. *And* is usually the first conjunction to emerge, followed by the emergence of others such as *if*, *but*, and *because*. Until children master the later-developing conjunctions, however, it is not uncommon for them to overuse *and*.

During the preschool years, children are becoming much more sophisticated in their use of questions and negatives. For example, during the earliest stages of development, children primarily ask yes or no questions and what or where questions. As they move into the preschool years, however, children begin to ask when, how, and why questions. At the beginning of the preschool period, it is also common for children to place verbs, such as *is*, at the end rather than in the middle of utterances (e.g., "Where daddy *is*?" instead of "Where *is* daddy?") and to omit certain verb forms (e.g., "Where daddy going?" instead of "Where *is* daddy going?"). With age, these word-order differences and omissions become less common in the questions of children acquiring SAE. Subject-verb inversion occurs more often because the rules of standard English require that the verb precede the subject (e.g., "Where is Daddy going?" instead of "Where Daddy is going?"). Missing auxiliary verbs are also becoming less common at this point. Children acquiring other dialects may continue to persist in the production of questions with noninverted word order (e.g., "What *you would* say?") and missing auxiliaries (e.g., "What you doin'?"), however, if subject-verb inversion is not required to occur in the dialect to which they are exposed.

Toward the end of the preschool years, later-developing negative forms (e.g., *won't, isn't, aren't, didn't, wasn't, couldn't*, and *nobody*) and later-developing pronouns (e.g., *they, them, her, him, their, herself*, and *himself*) begin to emerge. Children are also beginning to master later-developing sounds (e.g., /s/, /z/, /l/, /r/, /ng/, /sh/, and /ch/). It is, however, still common for children to make errors, such as saying "wing" for ring or "bacuum" for vacuum. Most sounds are also acquired in the initial positions of words before they are acquired in the medial or final positions of words. See Figure 6.1 for a chart of children's speech-sound development.

Because their grammatical skills are still developing, preschoolers tend to have some difficulty with the comprehension of later-developing grammatical forms in the absence of environmental or contextual cues. Therefore, it would not be unusual for a normally developing child to respond to a why question as if it were a what or when question during the early preschool years. Younger preschoolers also tend to use a subject-verb-object strategy for interpreting sentences. Therefore, many passive-voice sentences are likely to be interpreted as if they were active-voice sentences. For example, a child might interpret the sentence, "*The cat was chased by the dog*," as meaning the cat was chasing the dog. He or she may also interpret the event in the first clause of a conjoined sentence as occurring first, regardless of the conjunction used. Therefore, each of the following sentences may be interpreted by preschoolers as if going to school occurred first:

"Before you go to school, stop at the store."
"Go to school before you stop at the store."
"After you go to school, stop at the store."
"Go to school after you stop at the store." (Owens 1996)

In addition to improving their speech and grammatical skills, preschoolers are beginning to refine their conversational and vocabulary skills. By 3 years of age, children are much better at providing their listener with the information necessary to understand their messages. Part of this can be attributed to their more accurate use of deictic terms, such as *here* and *there*, and articles, such as *a* and *the*.

Three-year-olds are also becoming much more sophisticated in their turn-taking skills. As toddlers, children are rarely able to sustain discourse beyond a few turns, they often interrupt at inappropriate times, and the majority of their utterances are not on topic. However, by 3 years of age, approximately 75% of children's utterances are on topic, although repetition of a previously made statement serves as the primary strategy for accomplishing this (Owens 1996). By 5 years of age, 50% of children are able to sustain topics for approximately 12 turns.

As they become more aware of the listener's perspective and more familiar with the social conventions of discourse in their speech community, children also become increasingly better in adapting their speech to fit the needs and social background of their listener. For example, by 4 years of age children are learning to use a different style of communication with adults as compared with younger children. In addition, they learn to use more polite forms (e.g., please, thank you, and excuse me) in conversation. In addition to becoming more responsive to the listener's perspective, children become more adept at responding to requests for clarification and repairing conversational breakdowns.

Language Development of Nonstandard English and Bilingual Child Speakers

African-American English–Speaking Children

Several researchers have found that it is often difficult to detect differences in the language development of African-American English (AAE) and SAE child speakers below the age of 3 years (Blake 1984; Steffensen 1974; Stockman 1986; Cole 1980). According to this research, the morphosyntactic development of AAE-speaking children differs little from that of children from other English language backgrounds up to the age of 3 years. This is partly attributed to the fact that many of the language forms commonly associated with nonstandard English dialects (e.g., the absence of the copula and morphologic markers, such as the past tense -*ed*) occur in the speech of all English-language child speakers during the earlier stages of language development. Between the ages of 3 and 5 years, however, there is a marked increase in the use of nonstandard English dialect grammatical forms by children acquiring AAE and, possibly, other nonstandard English dialects as their primary language code. This contrasts with children acquiring SAE as their primary code. These children tend to display a decrease in nonstandard-feature use beginning at around 3 years of age. Many of the nonstandard forms produced by AAE child speakers are considered to be characteristic features of AAE. Table 4.5 lists common AAE features.

In my study of preschool-aged AAE child speakers, I found that by 3 years of age the children were beginning to acquire knowledge of the AAE rules for when certain verb forms are to be used (Wyatt 1991; Wyatt 1996). For example, several AAE scholars have noted that there are certain grammatical environments that tend to favor or disfavor the use of the zero or absent copula verb form in adult AAE (Labov et al. 1968; Labov 1969; Wolfram 1969). Specifically, Labov and others observed that the zero copula rarely occurs in AAE in the following linguistic contexts: (1) past tense contexts (e.g., "They *were* sick," or "They *was* sick"), (2) at the ends of clauses (e.g., "Yes, he *is*"), (3) first person singular contexts (e.g., "I *am* sick"), and (4) in emphatic utterances (e.g., "Yes he *IS* sick!"). Labov (1969) also noted that the zero copula is more likely to occur (1) after personal pronoun subjects (e.g., "She sick") than noun phrase subjects (e.g., "Tameka *is* sick"), and (2) before adjectives and prepositions (e.g., "She sick," and "She over there") than before nouns (e.g., "She's a lady"). In addition, Wolfram (1969) noted more use of the zero copula within second person singular *are* (e.g., "You are") and plural *are* (e.g., "They are") contexts (e.g., "They sick") than third person singular *is* contexts (e.g., "She *is* sick"). I observed that the 3- to 5-year-old AAE child speakers displayed these same patterns of copula use (Wyatt 1991; Wyatt 1996).

Stockman and colleagues (1982) found similar knowledge of these variable rules in African-American children when they studied the production of final nasals. Just as had been found for adult AAE speakers, they noticed that by the age of 3 years, AAE child speakers omitted the final /n/ more often than final /m/, that final /ŋ/ was absent more often than final /m/ and /n/, and that final nasals were more likely to be absent before consonants than before vowels.

Studies of African-American children's phonologic development have, however, also documented similarities between the language development of AAE and SAE speakers. For example, Stockman and Settle (1991) found that up to the age of 3 years, African-American children produce the same minimal core of initial consonants as white children of the same age. Specifically, they found that 100% of the African-American subjects in their study, in addition to at least 90% of white children studied by Prather et al. (1975), produced the following 11 sounds in initial word position by 3 years of age: /m/, /n/, /p/, /k/, /g/, /h/, /j/, /t/, /d/, /b/, and /s/. Another study by Haynes and Moran (1989) found that African-American children go through the same

TABLE 4.5   Selected Features of African-American English

African-American English (AAE) Feature	Examples
Phonologic features of AAE	
Final consonant cluster reduction (absence of final consonant when both members of consonant cluster are either voiced or voiceless)	dɛsk (desk) → dɛs old (old) → ol
Use of -es plural marker with words ending in -sk, -st, or -sp (usually as the result of hypercorrection)	tɛsts (tests) → tɛsəz
Production of /d/ for /ð/ (initial word position)	ðɪs (this) → dɪs
Production of /f/ for /θ/ and /v/ for /ð/ (medial and final word positions)	brʌðə (brother) → brʌvə boθ (both) → bof
Dropping of postvocalic /r/ and /l/	moɵ (more) → mo:
Devoicing of final voiced consonants	pɪg (pig) → pɪg̊
Nasalization of vowels preceding deleted final nasals	mæn (man) → m̃~
Use of -in for -ing word endings	rʌnnɪʃ (running) → rʌnɪn
Deletion of initial unstressed syllables	abaʊt (about) → baʊt
Substitution of /k/ for /t/ in initial str- clusters	strit (street) → skrit
Grammatical features of AAE	
Absence of past-tense marker in regular verb forms (sometimes due to consonant cluster reduction)	mɪst (missed) → mɪs pleɪd (played) → pleɪ
Nonstandard productions of irregular verbs	"I had went there Monday," "He seen 'em before."
Use of habitual/aspectual be	"Sometimes she be here."
Use of remote time been	"I been had this."
Absence of auxiliary and copula be	"You a bigger one," "He kickin' all the things."
Nonstandard subject-verb agreement	"He sit right there everyday," "There was five of 'em," "It don't go like that."
Use of the word ain't for isn't, haven't, and don't	"She ain't tell her," "This ain't no Mickey Mouse," "He ain't seen her in a while."
Multiple negation	"He don't know nothin'," "Can't nobody beat him."
Absence of plural -s marker	"I got five cent."
Regularization of irregular plurals	"The mens are standin' up."
Absence of possessive -s marker	"That's John hat."
Regularization of possessive pronouns	"It's mines."
Pronominal differences	"He hurt hisself."
Use of nonstandard relative pronouns	"That's the one what I was tellin' you 'bout."

Source: Adapted from T Wyatt. Linguistic constraints on copula production in black English child speech, Ph.D. diss., University of Massachusetts, 1991.

TABLE 4.6   Pragmatic Categories in African-American English and Standard American English: Comparisons by Example

Pragmatic Category	African-American English Example	Standard American English Example
Comment	"We almost done."	"We are almost done."
Report and inform	"That's what my brother said. ... He said do she be on TV all the time?"	"... He said, 'Is she on TV all of the time?'"
Obtain response	"Ain't this a broom?"	"Isn't this a broom?"
Obtain information	"Where the bird at?"	"Where is the bird?"
Routine	"Here go Grover ... here go Bert ... here go his brother."	"Here's Grover ... here's Bert ... here's his brother."
Negate	"Ain't no baby bottle!"	"That's not a baby bottle!"
Pretend	"You be the daddy, and I'ma be the mommy."	"You be the daddy, and I'll be the mommy."
Direct action	"Don't be callin' nobody that!"	"Don't call anyone that!"
Protest	"Sheez, Candi not even doin' nothin'."	"Sheez, Candi's not doing anything."

phonologic process stages as other English-speaking children with one exception—final consonant deletion persisted longer in the speech of African-American children.

Another study by Seymour and Seymour (1981) revealed that the type of articulation errors made by preschool-aged African-American and white children are similar, although the frequency of errors differed. They found that African-American children are more likely than their white counterparts to substitute /f/ for /th/, /b/ for /v/, and /d/ for /th/ in certain word positions. In contrast, they found that white children are more likely to substitute /w/ for /r/, /t/ for /ch/, /s/ for /th/, and /s/ for /sh/.

Stockman and Vaughn-Cooke (1982) and Bridgeforth (1987) also found that African-American children go through the same stages of semantic and pragmatic development as other children. Specifically, these researchers found that African-American children acquire the same semantic and pragmatic categories at the same stages of development and in the same sequence as other children. The difference is that the linguistic code (i.e., AAE) used by AAE child speakers to express these meanings and speech acts differs from that used by SAE child speakers. See Tables 4.6 and 4.7 for examples of these differences.

In addition to developing uses of language considered to be universal to all speech communities, many African-American preschoolers also develop a very sophisticated knowledge of the sociocultural rules necessary for performing some of the speech acts generally associated with the African-American experiences (Wyatt 1991; Wyatt 1995). During a study of AAE preschooler's acquisition of the

TABLE 4.7 Semantic Categories in African-American English and Standard American English: Comparisons by Example

Semantic Category	African-American English Example	Standard American English Example
Existence	"This Minnie Mouse."	"This is Minnie Mouse."
Nonexistence	"Ain't no other feet."	"There aren't any other feet."
Locative state	"Where's the boy at?"	"Where is the boy?"
Locative action	"Why don't he be walkin' right here?"	"Why not put him walking right here?"
Attribution and possession	"Mine's big."	"Mine is big."
Rejection	"I 'ont want that one."	"I don't want that one."
Denial	"That don't go right there, boy!"	"That doesn't go right there."
Quantity	"Here go two cars."	"Here are two cars."
Recurrence	"Here go another one right here."	"Here's another one right here."
Notice	"See, lookit."	"See, look at this one."
Dative	"I'ma get me one of them big ones."	"I'm going to get one of those big ones."
Additive	"He a boy and she a girl."	"He's a boy and she's a girl."
Causal	"We don' s'pose to have none tonight cuz we goin' to a party."	"We aren't supposed to have any tonight because we're going to a party."
Temporal	"We seen that one already."	"We saw that one already."
Adversative	"That one's big, but it ain't big like this."	"That one's big, but it's not big like this."
Epistemic	"I know where he go."	"I know where he goes."
Specification	"That's the one what hit me."	"That's the one who hit me."
Communication	"Don't be tellin' me to shut up."	"Don't tell me to shut up."

copula, I observed preschoolers performing a variety of different traditionally African-American speech events, such as rapping and playing the dozens. In general, the children's verbal performances were similar to those produced by adult speakers in that they retained many of the discourse elements considered essential to the structure and organization of these speech events. However, the children's productions lacked some of the more sophisticated linguistic elements found in adult versions. For this reason, I labeled the children's performances as baby versions of the adult forms. See Table 4.8 for examples of the type of baby rap and baby dozens sequences produced by the children.

As early as the age of 5 years, some African-American children who are exposed to both AAE and SAE are already beginning to code-switch between the two dialects in response to changes in topic, listener, and communicative intent (Wyatt and Seymour 1990). Seymour and Ralabate (1985) found that these code-switching abilities continue with age and appear more deliberate as the child gets older.

TABLE 4.8   African-American Preschoolers' Speech Acts

"Baby dozens" transcript

??*:	Your mother don't have no mo-ther/
??:	(laugh)/
DN:	Your mother don't have no mo-tor and your mother .../
??:	(all three children over-rapping in unison) ... don't have no ... (unintelligible)/
DD:	Your daddy don't have no car/
DN:	Your mother have a car but she don't have no keys/
TW:	Oh! (laughing)/ Excuse me!/
DN:	No/ No. .../
JW:	My mother do drive/ She drive it with her hands/
TW:	She drives with her hands?/
DD:	(softly singing in background) Mo-tor ... mo-tor ... motor/
DN:	And that's why your mother don't have no mo-tor/
TW:	OK, fine. ... and what do you have to say to that John/
DN:	Wait ... wait ... wait ... wait ... wait ... ease up ... ease up ... ease up man ... ease up ... ease up ... ease up .../
JW:	(overlapping DN) Your mother don't have no car/
DN:	Ease up ... ease up ... ease up/

"Baby rap" transcript

DN:	(rap tempo) An' I love her!/
DD:	An' tell her I love her/ I love her!/
JM:	(overlapping DD, in background) I love her!/
DN:	I love her/ I'ma love her everytime/
JM:	(in background) I'ma love her everytime/
DD:	An' she can call me everytime/An' I answer the phone, I say "get off the phone, mom!"/
DN:	She's my girl and I'ma see her/
DD:	Everytime, she call me, I say "moms, get off the dag-gone phone/I wanna talk to the girl"/
DN:	(laughs)/ Everytime, I see her, I'm gonna kiss her/I'm gonna see her and I'm gonna kiss her/
DD:	Everytime she call me, I'ma kiss the phone/ I'ma say "Hello, who is it?"/ Ah, babes/ shut the heck up/ I'ma tell my brother, "get the heck off the phone/ It's my girlfriend, man!/ I'm not joking around with you man"/ [intervening dialogue]
DD:	(singing) An' I'ma say, "I got to get the woman/ I got to sing the woman"/
DN:	(singing) I gotta kiss the woman/
DD:	(singing) (unintelligible) the woman that look nice and coolin'/ I like the woman/
DN:	I like how she looks /I like her looks on her face cause she looks so pretty/ Cause I love her whole body though she doesn't know me/

*Unknown speaker.
Source: Videotaped samples collected as part of doctoral dissertation research. T Wyatt. Linguistic constraints on copula production in black English child speech. University of Massachusetts, 1991.

When considering these studies, it is important to remember that all African-American children are not classified as AAE speakers, even when they come from the same socioeconomic background. Therefore, research studies that generalize about the language skills of African-American children must be viewed with caution, and findings must be interpreted in light of the language diversity that exists within the African-American speech community.

Bilingual Children

Since the 1970s, child language researchers have also studied more carefully the differences between the language development of bilingual children (i.e., children who have been exposed to and speak or understand two or more languages) and monolingual children (i.e., children who speak one language). One key finding is that the language development of bilingual children varies as a function of several variables, such as age and degree of exposure to two (or more) different languages, as well as the conditions under which the languages are learned (Langdon and Merino 1992).

One of the most important variables is the age at which bilingual children are exposed to a second language. For example, scholars have noted that the language development of children exposed to more than one language before the age of 3 years (referred to as *simultaneous bilingualism*) differs slightly from that of children exposed to more than one language after the age of 3 years (referred to as *sequential bilingualism*) (Kessler 1984; Langdon and Marino 1992).

Common characteristics of simultaneous bilingualism, according to Kessler (1984), Langdon and Merino (1992), and Roseberry-McKibbin (1995), are as follows:

1. It is common to see an extended silent period (sometimes up to the age of 3 years) in which bilingual children do not use either language. Some researchers have speculated that this extended silent period occurs because children are taking more time to absorb and figure out the distinctive rules of the language systems to which they are being exposed.

2. It is common for children exposed to more than one language before the age of 3 years to frequently mix the two languages during the early stages of language development. Although code-mixing is a normal part of many bilingual speakers' communication styles and in some cases represents the typical language pattern exhibited by a community, it is generally more common in the early stages of bilingual development. A good example of code-mixing is the Spanish/English bilingual child who says "kitty-gato" for the word *kitty-cat*. (Kessler 1984).

3. By 2½ years of age, many children who have been exposed to two or more codes since birth are beginning to engage in code-switching (Kessler 1984). Code-switching can be defined as an alternation between two or more linguistic codes in response to social changes in the speaking situation (e.g., change in listener background, change in topic, and change in setting) and often occurs between speaking turns or between sentences within a turn.

4. It is common for one language to develop faster than another. In addition, children are usually more proficient in one language as com-

pared with the other. The more proficient language is often referred to as the *dominant language.*

There are, however, some key differences that, according to Hamayan and Damico (1991), Langdon and Cheng (1992), and McLaughlin (1984), distinguish sequential bilingualism from simultaneous bilingualism. Examples include:

1. Interference errors, which are errors resulting from influence of the first language on the second language, are more common. The type of error patterns produced can often (but not always) be predicted if one knows something about the grammatical and phonologic differences between a child's first and second language. Some of the common types of interference errors exhibited by children acquiring Spanish as a second language are found in Table 4.9.*

2. It is normal for children acquiring a second language to go through a period of language regression in which they lose proficiency in the use of their first language (Schiff-Myers 1992). Such children often become what is referred to as *passive bilinguals.* Passive bilinguals are able to comprehend in the first language but are often unable to produce utterances in the first language.

3. It is not uncommon for children to go through a period of language change in which their language dominance shifts, with the more dominant language becoming least dominant over time.

The following are two other common features of bilingual development for both simultaneous bilingual children and sequential bilingual children:

1. It is common for bilingual children to know the labels for items in one language but not the other. For example, many bilingual children know in their first language (which is usually their home language) the labels for objects found at home; however, they may know the labels for objects at school in their second language (which is usually the language used most often at school). In some cases, phonologic ease plays a role in determining whether objects are labeled with a word from the first or second language. For example, Celce-Murcia (1978), who studied the language development of her French-speaking daughter who had been exposed to both the French

---

*Although interference errors are common, it is important to know that they make up only a small portion of those errors produced by second-language child learners. The majority of the second language errors made by bilingual children are similar to those made by monolingual children at a similar stage of language development (McLaughin 1984; Kessler 1984).

TABLE 4.9 Examples of Common Speech Sound and Grammatical Productions Made by Native Spanish Speakers Acquiring English as a Second Language

Common forms of phonologic interference
  /s/ for /z/, as in "sebra" for "zebra"
  /ʃ/ for /tʃ/, as in "shair" for "chair"
  /tʃ/ for /ʃ/, as in "chip" for "ship"
  /d/ for /ð/, as in "den" for "then"
  /t/ for /θ/, as in "bat" for "bath"
  /f/ for /v/, as in "fan" for "van"
  /b/ for /v/, as in "berry" for "very"
  dentalization of /t/ and /d/, as in "t̪oday" for "today"
  /i/ for /ɪ/, as in "cheap" for "chip"
  /ʊ/ for /u/, as in "pull" for "pool"

Common forms of grammatical interference
  Absence of auxiliary verbs in statements and questions, as in, "He going," and "How the story helps?"
  Placement of negative before verb, as in, "He not can play anymore."
  Use of the word *no* for other negatives, as in, "No help him," for "Don't help him."
  Expression of possession using the word *of* instead of the possessive *-s* marker, as in, "The car of the boy," for "The boy's car."
  Gender confusion in use of pronouns, as in, "She is putting a towel on his head," instead of "… on her head."
  Use of the preposition *on* for *in* and confusion in the use of the preposition *of* versus *from*.
  Differing ordering of adjectives and nouns, as in, "The house red," instead of "The red house."
  Omission of subject pronouns, as in, "Then flew back," instead of "Then he flew back."
  Differing subject-verb agreement, as in, "The girl are playing," instead of "The girls are playing."
  Use of uninflected future and past tense verbs, as in, "I take one paper," instead of "I took one paper."

Sources: Adapted from HW Langdon, BJ Merino. Acquisition and Development of a Second Language in the Spanish Speaker. In HW Langdon, LL Cheng (eds), Hispanic Children and Adults with Communication Disorders. Gaithersburg, MD: Aspen Publications, 1992;154–155; and H Kayser. Speech and language assessment of Spanish-English speaking children. Lang Speech Hear Serv Schools 1989;20:242–244.

(*papillon*) and English (*butterfly*) terms for butterfly, found that her daughter tended to avoid the word *butterfly* and favor the word *papillon* because the latter was easier to pronounce. Professionals who work with Spanish bilingual children have probably also noticed the same type of avoidance when attempting to elicit the Spanish word for the color yellow. In such cases, professionals may find that even when children label the majority of their colors in Spanish, they will generally favor the English word *yellow* over the Spanish word *amarillo*, because of the length and phonologic complexity of the latter.

  2. Research on Spanish-speaking children also reveals that even when children from non-English–speaking backgrounds speak a language that contains the same sounds as English, the order in which the sounds are acquired and the stages at which they are acquired

can differ. For example, both Acevedo (1988) and Jimenez (1987) have found that Mexican-American Spanish-speaking children acquire the /t/ and /l/ sounds at a much earlier age than English-speaking children. Similarly, Kvaal et al. (1988) noted that Spanish-speaking children acquire the Spanish articles (i.e., *el*, *la*, *las*, *los*, *un*, *uno*, and *una*) and the Spanish form of the English word *be* at an earlier language stage than English-speaking children. Kvaal et al. also found, however, that regarding prepositions, Spanish-speaking children acquire the Spanish preposition *en*, which means both *in* and *on*, at a later stage of development than English-speaking children acquire *in* and *on*.

School-Age Language Development

School-age, English-speaking children are starting to master several later-developing morphosyntactic forms, such as the derivational -*er* ending (as in the word teach*er*), which change the grammatical status of the verb to a noun. As children move into the later stages of language development, they continue to refine several language skills. The average length of children's sentences continues to increase during the school years. Children are also expanding their receptive and expressive vocabulary and are becoming better at defining and understanding the meanings of words, including those with multiple meanings.

School-age children also develop the ability to distinguish language form from meaning. The ability to separate form from meaning is an important aspect of language knowledge referred to as *metalinguistic awareness*. Metalinguistic awareness involves being able to judge the grammaticality of a sentence (e.g., differentiating between a good and a bad sentence) and being able to detect what is bad or wrong about the grammatical structure of a sentence, regardless of its semantic content. During earlier stages of development, when asked to detect what is wrong with a sentence, many preschoolers are likely to judge a sentence, such as "My mother made a cake" as bad, because their mother does not bake cakes. In such a case, it does not matter that the sentence is grammatically well-formed. They may also have a difficult time explaining what is wrong or what needs to be changed in a sentence such as "I cut paper by scissors" (Gleitman et al. 1972; deVilliers and deVilliers 1972).

By the time they are in upper elementary grades, however, children should be able to do each of the above tasks. They should also know how to create rhyming words and count the number of syllables in a word. At this age, they are also developing the ability to construct puns, riddles, and other forms of humor (Owens 1996). Another key development is the ability to correctly interpret figurative language forms, such as idioms, metaphors, and proverbs.

Perhaps one of the greatest hallmarks of language development during the school-age years, however, is the ability to tell stories or narratives. Although children begin to tell stories during their preschool years, their stories are often incomplete and difficult to follow. Over time, however, children's narratives begin to increase in length and complexity, and the structure of their stories becomes more organized, adult-like in form, and easier to follow.

Child language researchers have also found that as children age, they tend to include more orientation information (e.g., information on who, where, and when) in their stories. They do this by sharing more details about the names of characters, settings of events, relationships between characters, and character traits. As children become older, they also tend to place more of the orientation information at the beginning of narratives, instead of scattering this information throughout the narratives, as is common in younger child narratives. Older children also tend to use more evaluations (i.e., expressed feelings about the events of a story) and state them more explicitly than younger children. Finally, older children tend to use a greater number of appendages (i.e., openings and closings) and are more creative and sophisticated in the type of appendages used. All of these developments are associated with later stages of language development.

Although, as Heath (1986) notes, narratives are universal to all speech communities, there are cross-cultural differences in how children organize their stories, what is emphasized in the stories, and how the stories begin and end. There are also differences in the degree to which detail and elaboration are used and the extent to which audience participation is involved or encouraged. For example, Scollon and Scollon (1989) found that Athabascan children tend to produce less-detailed narratives than their American counterparts. They also tend to highlight narrative events within their stories that are most pertinent and salient to their lives. Other studies cited by Gutierrez-Clellen and Quinn (1993) provide evidence that many Japanese children's narratives contain fewer narrative units (e.g., only a complication and a consequence) than American children's narratives, and that African-American children's narratives tend to contain fewer formulaic openings and more embedded or implied evaluations than the stories of their Euro-American counterparts. In addition, in some communities, such as Pacific Islander communities, storytelling is considered to be more collaborative than in mainstream American culture. As a result, it is more common for several persons to contribute to the sharing of stories.

A final skill that is considered to be an important part of school-age language development is the acquisition of written language. In the 1980s, there was a growing awareness of the relationship between the development of literacy (i.e., reading and writing) skills and oral language (Wallach and Butler 1994). Part of this awareness is based on changing perspectives of reading and writing, which view reading and writing as language-based and not a visually based activity. There has also been a great deal of research documenting a close relationship between the existence of oral-language disorders and reading problems in some children (Aram and Nation 1980; Gillam and Johnston 1992; Kamhi and Catts 1986; Snyder and Downey 1991). For example, there is research that suggests that reading-disordered children have a greater history of oral-language problems than good readers (Carrow-Woolfolk and Lynch 1981). The same research has shown that reading-disordered children demonstrate the same types of language problems observed among some children with oral-language disorders. These problems include difficulties with auditory memory and metalinguistic skills.

Society's changing views of literacy also hold that children begin to develop key literacy skills during the first year of life. Children display evidence of early developing literacy skills, for example, when they initially are exposed to books. Children also display evidence of developing literacy skills when they recognize the significance of everyday graphic symbols (e.g., recognize the golden arches as a sign of McDonald's), treat prewriting scribbles as meaningful text, talk about drawn pictures as if they tell a real story, use invented spellings to label pictures, and begin to hold books the correct way (Koppenhaver et al. 1991).

According to Koppenhaver and colleagues, children develop literacy skills by observing and participating in daily home literacy events, such as writing thank you notes, checking the *TV Guide*, and engaging in interactive exchanges with adults during book-reading activities. As children become older and move into their school-age years, these early exposures to written text serve as the base for later reading and writing activities.

Adolescent Language Development

In the past, there has been a general assumption that normally developing children have achieved all of the important language milestones by the end of their preschool years (Nippold 1993). However, as is demonstrated in *School-Age Language Development*, there are several important developmental changes that continue well into the elementary school years and beyond.

The most important language development that occurs during adolescence is that children continue to expand the average length of their sentences. They do this through the increased use of low-frequency syntactic structures, such as appositive constructions (e.g., "Margaret, *the attorney*, bought a town house"), post-noun modifiers, including prepositional phrases (e.g., "They knew the cyclist *in the lead* would win the race"), and modals (e.g., "We *should* have gone skating") (Nippold 1993).

According to Nippold (1993), the average length of sentences (measured by determining the number of words per communication [C-unit]) also begins to increase significantly during the later elementary and high school years. A C-unit consists of one independent clause plus any modifying dependent clauses. Research by Loban (1976) revealed that the average number of words per C-unit increases from 9.82 for sixth graders to 11.70 for twelfth graders. The mean number of subordinate clauses per C-unit also increases from 0.37 among sixth graders to 0.58 among twelfth graders in oral language. Similar increases occur in written language. Normally developing adolescents are also beginning to use a greater variety of different clause types. Although subordinate clauses first appear in the speech of preschoolers, there is a significant increase in the frequency and types of clauses produced by children in the sixth through the twelfth grades. Other important syntactic developments include the emerging use of more sophisticated adverbial conjuncts (e.g., *moreover, consequently*, and *furthermore*). Improved production and comprehension of these forms occurs in both spoken and written language.

Finally, in the areas of semantics and pragmatics, adolescents become more competent in the use of abstract vocabulary (e.g., literate verbs such as *interpret, concede,* and *predict*) and figurative expressions (i.e., idioms, metaphors, and proverbs). They also start to master the use of popular slang expressions, as well as several different interpersonal negotiation strategies considered important to the establishment of positive social relationships with peers (Nippold 1993). Interpersonal negotiation strategies include knowing how to use language to resolve conflicts in personal and work situations.

Conclusions

The acquisition of language is a very complex and involved process, in which several factors (i.e., social, environmental, biological, and cognitive) play a key role. It is imperative that the speech-language professional acknowledge all of the factors that contribute to the development of language, as well as those factors that can lead to differing patterns of normal development (i.e., cultural backgrounds, language backgrounds, or both). Speech-language professionals must also realize that language development does not end after preschool but continues well into adolescent and adult life. The process of language development involves the acquisition of written (i.e., reading and writing) as well as oral (i.e., speaking and listening) skills. As is demonstrated in the forthcoming chapters, understanding each of these issues is crucial for those professionals involved with the delivery of speech and language services to normal and disordered children from varied cultural and language backgrounds.

References

Acevedo MA. Development of Spanish Consonants in Three- to Five-Year Olds. Presented at the Annual Convention of the American Speech-Language-Hearing Association. Boston, November, 1988.

Aram D, Nation J. Patterns of language behavior in children with developmental language disorders. J Speech Hear Res 1980;18:220–241.

Bernstein DK, Tiegerman E. Language and Communication Disorders in Children (3rd ed). New York: Merrill, 1993;349–350.

Blake IJ. Language development in working class black children: an examination of form, content and use, Ph.D. diss., Columbia University Teachers College, 1984.

Bloom L, Lahey M. Language Development and Language Disorders. New York: Macmillan, 1978;13–200.

Bowerman M. Reorganizational Processes in Lexical and Syntactic Development. In E Wanner, LR Gleitman (eds), Language Acquisition: The State of the Art. London: Cambridge University Press, 1982;323–328.

Bridgeforth C. The identification and use of language functions in the speech of 3 and 4½ year-old black children from working class families, Ph.D. diss., Columbia Teachers College, 1987.

Brown R. A First Language: The Early Stages. Cambridge, MA: Harvard University Press, 1973;63.

Carrow-Woolfolk E, Lynch JI. An Integrative Approach to Language Disorders in Children. The Psychological Corporation 1981;321–322.

Celce-Murcia J. The Simultaneous Acquisition of English and French in a Two-Year-Old. In E Hatch (ed), Second Language Acquisition. Rowley, MA: Newbury House, 1978;50.

Clark EV. Discovering What Words Can Do. In D Farkas, WM Jacobson, KW Todrys (eds), Papers from the Parasession on the Lexicon. Chicago: Chicago Linguistic Society, 1978;34–35.

Clark EV. Meanings and Concepts. In P Mussen (ed), Handbook of Child Psychology (Vol 3). New York: Wiley, 1983;826.

Cole LT. A developmental analysis of social dialect features in the spontaneous language of preschool black children, Ph.D. diss., Northwestern University, 1980.

deVilliers JG, deVilliers PA. Early judgments of semantic and syntactic acceptability by children. J Psycholinguist Res 1972;1:299–310.

Dore J. Holophrases, speech acts and language universals. J Child Lang 1975;2:21–40.

Gillam RB, Johnston JR. Spoken and written language relationships in language learning impaired and normally achieving school age children. J Speech Hear Res 1992;35:1303–1315.

Gleitman L, Gleitman H, Shipley E. The emergence of the child as grammarian. Cognition 1972;1:137–164.

Gutierrez-Clellen VF, Quinn R. Assessing narratives of children from diverse cultural/linguistic groups. Lang Speech Hear Serv Schools 1993;24:2–9.

Hamayan EV, Damico JS. Limiting Bias in the Assessment of Bilingual Students. Austin, TX: PRO-ED, 1991.

Haynes WO, Moran MJ. A cross-sectional developmental study of final consonant production in southern black children from preschool through third grade. Lang Speech Hear Serv Schools 1989;20:400–406.

Heath SB. Sociocultural Contexts of Language Development. In Bilingual Education Office (ed), Beyond Language: Social and Cultural Factors in Schooling Language Minority Students. Los Angeles: Evaluation, Dissemination and Assessment Center, California State University, 1986;148–174.

Jimenez BC. Acquisition of Spanish consonants in children aged 3–5 years, 7 months. Lang Speech Hear Serv Schools 1987;18:357–361.

Kamhi AG, Catts HW. Toward an understanding of developmental and reading disorders. J Speech Hear Disord 1986;51:337–347.

Kessler C. Language Acquisition in Bilingual Children. In N Miller (ed), Bilingualism and Language Disability: Assessment and Remediation. San Diego: College-Hill Press, 1984;37–39.

Koppenhaver DA, Coleman PP, Kalman SL, Yoder DE. The implications of emergent literacy research for children with developmental disabilities. Am J Speech Lang Pathol 1991;1:38–40.

Kvaal J, Shipstead-Cox N, Nevitt S, et al. The acquisition of 10 Spanish morphemes by Spanish-speaking children. Lang Speech Hear Serv Schools 1988;19:384–394.

Labov W, Cohen P, Robins C, Lewis J. A Study of the Nonstandard English of Negro and Puerto Rican Speakers in New York City [final report, Cooperative Research Project No. 3288]. Washington, DC: U.S. Office of Education, 1968;174–218.

Labov W. Contraction, deletion, and inherent variability of the English copula. Language 1969;45:715–762.

Langdon HW, Cheng LL. Hispanic Children and Adults with Communication Disorders. Gaithersburg, MD: Aspen Publications, 1992.

Langdon HW, Merino BJ. Acquisition and Development of a Second Language in the Spanish Speaker. In HW Langdon, LL Cheng (eds), Hispanic Children and Adults with Communication Disorders. Gaithersburg, MD: Aspen Publications, 1992;135–159.

Loban W. Language Development: Kindergarten Through Grade Twelve [research report 18]. Urbana, IL: National Council of Teachers of English, 1976;35–37

McLaughlin B. Second Language Acquisition in Childhood. Preschool Children (Vol 1). Hillsdale, NJ: Lawrence Erlbaum, 1984;219–222.

Nelson K. Structure and strategy in learning to talk. Monogr Soc Res Child Dev 1973;38(1–2).

Nippold MA. Developmental markers in adolescent language: Syntax, semantics, and pragmatics. Lang Speech Hear Serv Schools 1993;24:21–28.

Oller D. Infant vocalization and the development of speech. Allied Health Behav Sci 1978;1:523–529.

Owens RE. Language Development: An Introduction (4th ed). New York: Merrill, 1996;68–371.

Prather EM, Hedrick DL, Kern CA. Articulation development in children aged 2 to 4 years. J Speech Hear Disabilities 1975;40:179–191.

Roseberry-McKibbin, C. Multicultural Students with Special Language: Practical Strategies for Assessment and Intervention. Oceanside, CA: Academic Communication Associates, 1995:31–47.

Sander EK. When are speech sounds learned? J Speech Hear Disord 1972;37:55–63.

Schiff-Myers NB. Considering arrested language development and language loss in the assessment of second language learners. Lang Speech Hear Serv Schools 1992;23:28–30.

Scollon R, Scollon SBK. Cooking It Up and Boiling It Down: Abstracts in Athabascan Children's Story Retellings. In D Tannen (ed), Coherence in Spoken and Written Discourse. Norwood, NJ: Ablex, 1984.

Seymour HN, Ralabate PK. The acquisition of a phonologic feature of black English. J Commun Disord 1985;18:139–148.

Seymour HN, Seymour CM. Black English and Standard American English contrasts in consonantal development of 4- and 5-year old children. J Speech Hear Disord 1981;46:274–280.

Snyder LS, Downey DM. The language-reading relationship in normal and reading disabled children. J Speech Hear Res 1991;34:129–140.

Steffensen MS. The acquisition of black English, Ph.D. diss., University of Illinois, 1974.

Stockman IJ, Settle S. Initial Consonants in Young Black Children's Conversational Speech. Presented at the Annual Convention of the American Speech-Language-Hearing Association. Atlanta, November, 1991.

Stockman IJ, Vaughn-Cooke FB, Wolfram WA. A Developmental Study of Black English—Phase I [Final Report, ERIC Document Reproduction Service No. ED 245 555]. Washington, DC: Center for Applied Linguistics, 1982;98–125.

Stockman IJ, Vaughn-Cooke FB. Semantic categories in the language of working class black children. Proceedings of the Second International Child Language Conference 1982;1:312–327.

Stockman IJ. Language Acquisition in Culturally Diverse Populations. The Black Child as a Case Study. In O Taylor (ed), Nature of Communication Disorders in Culturally and Linguistically Diverse Populations. San Diego: College Hill Press, 1986;133–149.

Wallach GP, Butler KG. Language Learning Disabilities in Adolescents: Some Principles and Applications. New York: Merrill, 1994.

Wolfram WA. A Sociolinguistic Description of Detroit Negro Speech. Washington, DC: Center for Applied Linguistics, 1969;173–174.

Wyatt TA. Linguistic constraints on copula production in black English child speech, Ph.D. diss., University of Massachusetts, 1991.

Wyatt TA, Seymour HN. The implications of code-switching in black English speakers. Equity and Excellence [Special Issue: Language and Discrimination] 1990;24:17–18.

Wyatt TA. Language development in African-American English child speech. Linguistics and Education 1995;7:13–15.

Wyatt, TA. Acquisition of the African-American English Copula. In AG Kamhi, KE Pollock, JL Harris (eds), Communication Development and Disorders in African-American English. Baltimore: Paul H. Brookes, 1996;95–115.

Chapter 4   Study Questions

1. Identify some of the common meanings and functions expressed in children's first words.
2. Describe at least three major stages of language development associated with preschoolers' acquisition of questions.
3. Describe one way in which the language development of the African-American English child speaker differs from that of the Standard American English child speaker. Then describe one way in which the language development of these two groups is similar.
4. Discuss some common characteristics of bilingual language development.
5. Discuss one major difference between the language development of sequential bilinguals and simultaneous bilinguals.
6. List three language accomplishments that occur during the school-age years of development.

III Speech-Language Pathology in Children and Adults

5 Language Intervention for Linguistically Different Learners

Harry N. Seymour and Luciano Valles

Chapters 3 and 4 provide a structural framework for viewing language and its course of development in children. This chapter's discussion of language assessment and treatment extends the description of language function and acquisition to a discussion of impairment. In keeping with the theme of this text, social complications and implications of child language disorders are discussed from two perspectives: (1) school status and (2) cultural and linguistic status. Because language is perhaps the most pervasive means for social interaction, its aberration has serious social consequences for children. These consequences are particularly serious within the school setting and among the participants of that setting who make up a multicultural context.

Throughout the United States, the public schools have numerous language groups comprised of both diverse dialects of English and learners of English as a second language. These groups represent large numbers of African Americans, Asians, Hispanics, and Native Americans, as well as other ethnic and racial groups. The population expansion of students of color has been so significant that in 25 major cities "minority" students now make up a majority of the student enrollment. It is estimated that by the year 2000, minority groups will comprise 28% of the overall United States population, and by the year 2020, they will comprise 38% of the overall population (Davis et al. 1983). Students of color will make up one-third of the public schools in the next decade. As a consequence, the context in which language disorders exist has become increasingly heterogeneous. Because of the increased diversity, there is a considerable challenge to provide assessment and treatment protocols that are culturally fair and effective for language disorders.

Because of the importance of the school setting and the fact that the clinical approach can be different for preschool-age and school-age children, the sections in this chapter discuss *Preschool-Age Language Assessment and Treatment* and *School-Age Language Assessment and Treatment* separately. School status refers to whether the child is of preschool or school age. The assessment and treatment of language can be different for these two groups. When a child enters school, it is expected that his or her language development has reached a maturational level approximating adult behavior and that this language state is adequate for learning school curricula. The requirements of the school curricula often reflect a child's problems and constitute the target goals for intervention. In contrast, the preschool child is evaluated against acquisitional milestones established as chronological age norms (Lahey 1990). These milestones are the indicators of disorder and the barometers for intervention.

Preschool-Age Language Assessment

Although the prelinguistic period is an important time for a child's growth and acquisition of precursory language skills, this discussion is limited to the period during which expressive language is clearly manifest. This period begins with the first word, which typically occurs sometime between 9 and 15 months of age. Within a period of about 3 years, the child develops an adult-like language system complete with phonology, syntax, semantics, and pragmatics. It is within and among these areas of language that pathologic entities can become evident.

What is most apparent in the form of symptoms is the delay of onset of some aspects of language. With the exception of serious retardation, multiple handicapping conditions, or both, obvious milestone events, such as a premature secession in babbling, delay of the first word (which is expected at about 1 year of age), or delay in joining of two words (which should occur at around 18 months), are typically noticed. The awareness of such delays can cause worry in parents, curious relatives, or concerned friends.

After a language problem is detected, the social complications and consequences for the child and family begin. There is obviously no single pattern of social complication. Each family constellation has its unique reactions and consequences. Typical reactions are anxiety by the parents about the seriousness of the problem and a sense of guilt about its cause. This anxiety and guilt can be transmitted in a variety of ways to the child, at a time when bonding, social interaction, and personality development are reliant on the quality of parent-child contact. In fact, much of what emerges as confidence in one's communicative skills has its onset in early interactions with family members.

In many respects, it is the aberrant language behavior itself that is the most serious social consequence both for the child and his or her family members. The inability to develop speech and language can prevent or impede the most fundamental of human qualities—that is, the capacity to share ideas within a social context. However, a parent is not only concerned with the consequence of language but also with etiologic factors and accompanying symptoms. The discovery of aberrant language can be preceded or followed by a diagnosis of hearing impairment, developmental disability, cerebral palsy, or autism, to name just a few of the possible problems associated with language impairment. Indeed, with few exceptions, language disorders have concomitant disabilities that may be etiologic, associative, or both.

Clearly, there are many possible causes of child language disorders. One cause can be a peripheral-sensory deficit, such as a hearing impairment. If, during the development of speech and language, a child has difficulty hearing surrounding speech and language, his or her development of language can be affected (see Chapter 11). Another serious impediment to language development occurs when a child has some degree of cognitive-intellectual deficit. A child who falls below the normal range of intelligence more than likely has an associated depression in language functioning. The lower the child's IQ, the poorer the child's language skills. Another culprit of language problems is damage to the central nervous system. Large numbers of young people are diagnosed as language and learning disabled because of some hidden neurologic problem that is difficult and, in most cases, impossible to specifically identify. Finally, when children experience extreme environmental abuse and deprivation, their psychoemotional growth can be retarded. A consequence of serious emotional problems can be an inability to acquire the important social and interpersonal requisites for effective language communication.

Language Impairment Diagnosis

Although the causes of language disorders are many and often undetermined, there is usually sufficient evidence from one or more symptoms to make a diagnosis of language impairment. In fact, a child identified as having a language problem is often described in terms of specific symptoms regardless of known and unknown etiologies. These symptoms can be specific to language, nonlinguistic symptoms that are presumed to be related to language, or both. Nonlinguistic symptoms include abilities having to do with memory, perception, auditory discrimination, visual discrimination, fine and gross motor skills, and so on. Nonlinguistic descriptors such as these are viewed as belonging to a point of view known as the *specific abilities orientation.* In a sense, according to this view, the child's deficits are defined by abilities thought to be critical to adequate language function.

Children may also be classified or grouped according to a cluster of syndromes that define categories such as developmentally disabled, hearing impairment, specific language impairment, and autism. This viewpoint constitutes a *categorical orientation* in which children are grouped according to some dominant etiology. For example, developmentally disabled children are defined by their cognitive-intellectual deficit, and deaf children are defined by their hearing impairment. When the dominant symptom is language aberration with no accompanying peripheral-sensory, cognitive-intellectual, or known neurologic difficulties, the category is described as *specific language impairment* (Stark and Tallal 1982).

Another orientation simply focuses on language alone. This orientation is defined by behavioral symptoms of phonology, syntax, semantics, pragmatics, or any combination of these. In recent years, the viewpoint known as *language orientation* has dominated the clinical focus in assessing and treating language disorders in children. There are several reasons that language orientation is favored. For example, categorical orientation is not particularly useful in defining the nature of a child's language problem, because language symptoms can and do occur across categories. By knowing the category, a speech-language pathologist does not necessarily know what language symptoms a child has. There are many variables (e.g., intelligence, personality, age of onset of problems, severity of problems, or other medical problems) that can determine the nature of a child's language difficulties. Indeed, it is possible for children with different etiologies to have similar language behaviors and for children with the same etiology to have different language behaviors. Consequently, it may be more important to know, as precisely as possible, the child's language characteristics than to know etiology, since clinical assessment and treatment are more likely to address language symptoms than causes.

In comparison to the language orientation approach, etiology is central to the specific abilities orientation. There is the presumption of a cause-and-effect relationship between some nonlinguistic ability and language symptoms. If a child demonstrates auditory discrimination problems and an accompanying language deficit, the speech-language pathologist may reach the conclusion that the auditory discrimination problem causes the language deficit. As a consequence, clinical intervention might focus on auditory discrimination and not language. The problem is that, more often than not, such a relationship cannot be proved, and the possibility exists that both the language problem and the discrimination difficulty are caused by a third unknown factor. Treatment of the auditory discrimination problem, therefore, may or may not influence language. The effect of language treatment on the auditory discrimination problem is similarly questionable. Because of uncertainty with respect to the relationship between language and specific abilities, there is a persuasive argument to emphasize language treatment as primary and specific abilities as secondary (if at all). For this reason, the remainder of this chapter focuses on the language orientation approach—that is, language symptoms.

Symptoms of Language Disorders

Symptoms of language disorders in preschool children can be quantitative, qualitative, or both. Quantitative symptoms involve a systematic delay in one or more of the areas of language with respect to developmental norms. All aspects of a child's language profile appear intact, except that the profile is characteristic of children of a younger age. In other words, the sequential pattern of acquisition is maintained, but the rate of acquisition is delayed. A qualitative problem, on the other hand, can violate developmental norms in both rate and sequence of acquisition. The child's behaviors may appear bizarre and unpredictable, or he or she may articulate clear and syntactically correct sentences that have no relation to the topic of conversation or produce apparent gibberish without content or purpose.

An important key to identifying both quantitative and qualitative language problems is the availability of developmental milestone data. Because of research efforts over the past several years, there is a relatively rich account of what language structures children acquire and when. However, these data have been acquired almost exclusively on Euro-American, middle-class children of Standard English backgrounds. Thus, the essential information for determining whether a child's acquisition of language is appropriate in terms of sequence and rate is seriously lacking for language groups other than English and for dialects other than Standard American. As pointed out in Chapter 3, there are efforts underway to address this problem, and limited developmental data exist for a few of the higher-profile groups such as African-Americans and Latino-Americans. The general paucity of information, however, remains a serious obstacle to effective assessment and treatment of language disorders among linguistically diverse groups (Seymour 1992). The nature of these obstacles is discussed further in this chapter within an overall context of assessment and treatment issues.

In the assessment of language disorders in children there are three important questions that must be answered: (1) is there a problem? (2) what is the nature of the problem? and (3) what should the intervention goals be? In general, the first question is answered by using norm-referenced standardized tests. The second question requires sampling language in naturalistic contexts and in-depth probing of language in controlled contexts. In many respects, this question is answered within a diagnostic-intervention framework that can take place over several weeks, while diagnosis and intervention occur simultaneously. By answering the second question, an answer to the third question, "What should the intervention goals be?" emerges directly from a determination of the nature of the problem. However, the implementation of intervention goals is moderated by several nonlinguistic factors, such as the child's physical and mental limitations, age, personality, school and home environments, and cultural and linguistic background.

Of the three questions raised above, the first, "Is there a problem?", is perhaps the most controversial and problematic with respect to serving linguistic and culturally diverse populations. This is because of the heavy reliance on standardized tests for answering this question. In keeping with the discussion of developmental norms in Chapter 3, standardized tests simply reflect those norms in various ways. These norm-referenced tests are almost always based on large numbers of children and are established for particular dimensions of language (i.e., syntax, phonology, and morphology). For each of these language dimensions, milestones for appropriate language behavior are determined for successive age levels. These milestones constitute the normative reference. This normative reference can be useful in identifying children who deviate far enough from the standardized mean to be suspected of a problem. However, as with developmental data in general, these tests have greater currency for Euro-American children of Standard American English (SAE) backgrounds than for language groups for whom SAE is not the most proficient language or dialect. Herein lies a major dilemma for speech-language pathologists who often must rely on such tests for making diagnostic decisions for all children regardless of their cultural and linguistic backgrounds.

Many school districts throughout the country require objective and standardized test results to classify children with special educational needs. However, to implement a truly valid and nonbiased approach would require a specialized group reference, relative to language and culture, that is indigenous to each language group. Such a tactic is a tall order in light of the fact that in some school districts there are as many as 80 different language groups represented. The notion that norm-referenced standardized tests can be developed for limited–English proficient speakers, who represent diverse groups such as Vietnamese, Cambodian, Puerto Rican, Chinese, Cuban, Haitian, Korean, and Mexican, may be unrealistic. Moreover, there are dialectal variations associated with each of these language groups. These dialectic variations also have to be captured in the normalization of any truly valid test.

Test developers have addressed this diversity issue to date by including a small percentage of minority populations in the sampling pool in accordance with their demographic representation in the population at large. Based on this broad inclusion, the argument is made that representation has been achieved within the standardization process of the tests. Such an argument is misleading and erroneous, because too few persons are sampled to be truly representative of the diverse languages and dialects found in these groups. For example, because of the bilingual language and dialect variation that is likely to exist among Spanish speakers from Cuba, Puerto Rico, and South America, a simple random representation within the sampling pool from each of these Latino-American groups cannot possibly address the diversity of language found among and within them. Clearly, the issue is not whether minority groups are included in the sampling pool, but whether there is sufficient representation of the language patterns typical of these groups.

Although the standardized testing issue is a serious one when assessing diverse language groups, there are some reasonable alternative approaches. Alternatives to norm-referenced tests suggested by Seymour and Bland (1991) include the following: (1) referral-source data, (2) direct observations, (3) standardized tests of non-speech and language behaviors, and (4) language sampling and probing. Information obtained by referral sources (i.e., parents, teachers, and others familiar with the child) can be immensely important in determining whether a child is behaving in a way that warrants further diagnosis. It is important to keep in mind that the first step in a diagnosis typically leads only to a strong suspicion about the pathologic causes. This suspicion must be verified through more in-depth diagnosis such as the diagnostic-intervention process discussed above. Reports from those most familiar with the child combined with clinician observations can result in an appropriate decision to admit a child for therapy.

After the therapy decision is made, the next step is to attempt to determine the nature of the child's problem. More often than not, a decision to admit a child for therapy also includes some notion about the child's problem area(s), which is derived from the various sources of diagnostic input. It is this notion that can constitute hypotheses for further testing. A common and accepted practice for testing a clinical hypothesis is to sample language in various settings and to probe comprehension and production of language for information that confirms or refutes the diagnostic hypothesis. If a clinician suspects a child of having difficulty with morphologic inflections, for example, that clinician would attempt to determine, through sampling of language and probing, the extent of the child's strengths and weaknesses in using numerous and varied inflections. After the profile of strengths and weaknesses has been established, the intervention goals would be to strengthen those inflectional markers that are weak.

The aspect of diagnosis that leads to intervention strategies can be particularly difficult when working with minority children. It can be difficult because too often either speech-language pathologists lack knowledge and training in multicultural issues (American Speech-Hearing-Language Association 1985), or there is insufficient normative information about the particular language or dialect of the child. As more research is performed, these problems will undoubtedly be resolved. The level of sophistication surrounding the assessment of language has improved considerably since the 1980s. No longer are speech-language pathologists trained to rely solely on standardized tests for making clinical judgments. They are encouraged to supplement test data with naturalistic language samples and language probes, which can provide a far richer and more representative indication of a child's language competence.

Notwithstanding these efforts, Vaughn-Cooke (1983) aptly pointed out that the obvious diagnostic merits of a rich and meaningful language sample soon diminish in light of a lack of normative reference on which to make clinical judgments about a child who does not speak English or speaks a nonstandard variety of English. On the other hand, Seymour (1986) argued that despite the major limitation of inadequate normative data, reliance on what is known about those aspects of language functioning and acquisition that vary little across language groups can provide clinical options for effective diagnosis of language disorders among children of nonstandard English backgrounds such as African-American English (AAE).

The merit of Seymour's position is, in part, evident from the work of Stockman and Vaughn-Cooke (1982). They showed that the acquisition of semantic-content categories are no different between African-American children acquiring AAE and Euro-American children acquiring SAE. Semantic-content categories refer to the interaction of meaningful content and linguistic forms to express some language function. For example, the linguistic form *eat* expresses the semantic-content category action. *Two* is in the attributional semantic-content category, and *apple* is in the existence semantic-content category. In the course of language development, children are likely to utter "eat" before joining it with "apples" and sometime later will produce "eat two apples." By the time they have joined all three words, the SAE-speaking child more than likely includes the plural -*s* marker on the word *apples*. This plural marker may not be present, however, for the AAE-speaking child, because the plural -*s* marker absence can be a dialect feature of AAE. This absence of the -*s* marker indicates a difference in form between the two dialects, despite the fact that the semantic content categories of existence, attribution, and action are the same. Seymour (1986) would argue that the semantic content category data may be more diagnostic than the absence of the plural -*s*. One possible key to nonbiased assessment of language disorders is to focus on aspects of language that do not vary as a function of linguistic and cultural factors.

School-Age Language Assessment

Many of the issues discussed previously also apply to the school-age child. However, the communication and social difficulties a child experiences in preschool become exacerbated in the school environment. In this environment, language skills are needed for academic success and to establish peer relationships. It is not uncommon for children with language disabilities to feel isolated and even ostracized by their peers. Also, the academic performance of children with language disabilities tends to lag behind classmates well into high-school years and adulthood.

Clearly, the school environment and the academic curriculum demands create unique circumstances in treating the language-impaired student. These circumstances are undergoing considerable change. One trend has been the adoption of the classroom collaborative model by many school systems throughout the country (see Chapter 2). This collaborative model requires the speech-language pathologist to work closely with other school personnel and parents in identifying and remediating language problem areas for the ultimate purpose of promoting school success. An additional trend, the inclusion model, advocates having children with disabilities included in the regular classroom as opposed to the traditional pull-out model. The focus of inclusion is on school success, with language intervention objectives somewhat subjugated to and driven by academic curriculum demands.

Although the areas of language discussed for the preschool child are germane for the older child, there is, at this age, an academic dimension to them. According to Nelson (1993), students with language disorders have difficulty in school as a function of specific problems in one or more of the following language areas: (1) morphosyntactic knowledge (morphologic and grammatical structure); (2) semantic knowledge (word meaning); (3) graphophonemic knowledge (sound-symbol association for reading words and word production); (4) phonologic knowledge (speech sound production); (5) world knowledge (inferring about events in the world); (6) classroom discourse; and (7) pragmatic knowledge (communication rules and strategies, topic management, story grammar and oral narrative, and language comprehension).

To appropriately address students' language needs in the classroom setting, various factors must be considered that influence learning. These factors include (1) individual learner needs and differences, (2) cultural and linguistic background, (3) socioeconomic status, (4) motivation and cognitive skills, (5) social and academic strengths, and (6) the academic instructional practices to which the student is exposed (Wang et al. 1990; Wallach and Butler 1994). Because these factors are so numerous and interactive, there is considerable variation among students. This variability creates a complex and challenging clinical context for practicing speech-language pathologists. Therefore, to assure a valid diagnosis leading to appropriate and effective intervention, it is critically important that student performance be interpreted appropriately and in a nonbiased manner.

With this objective in mind, this chapter uses a case study to demonstrate the nature of the assessment and intervention process within a classroom context. The case study is referred to throughout the remainder of this chapter in discussing a language assessment and intervention process in the classroom within the framework of three factors: (1) the classroom collaboration and inclusion movement; (2) cultural and linguistic diversity; and (3) the observational lens model, an ethnographic approach.

Case Study: Language Background and Bilingual Classroom

Arturo is an 11-year, 5-month-old boy who was born and raised in Arecibo, Puerto Rico, where he learned Spanish as his first language. Arturo has been living in Boston, Massachusetts, since he was 8 years old and is currently learning English as a second language. He has one brother and one sister who are also learning English as a second language and are doing well in school. Arturo's parents speak only Spanish at home, and his mother volunteers as a classroom assistant in Arturo's bilingual fifth grade classroom on Monday and Wednesday mornings.

Arturo's classroom is located in an inner-city public school in Boston. The classroom contains 27 students whose socioeconomic backgrounds range from low to high. The classroom is taught by a bilingual Spanish-English teacher, Ms. Rios. The students' and their community's ethnic composition is comprised of Latino-American, African-American, and Euro-American heritage. Each student speaks one or more of the following languages: Puerto Rican Spanish, Standard English, and AAE.

Continuous language assessment and intervention measures by a bilingual speech-language pathologist indicate that Arturo demonstrates significant problems with the comprehension and production of language in Spanish. Arturo has a history of multiple ear infections and a mild bilateral conductive hearing loss. Arturo's language problems adversely influence his ability to learn English as a second language. Arturo receives individual and group therapy from the bilingual clinician during the classroom lessons. The teacher and the speech-language pathologist work jointly to heighten Arturo's language-learning potential in the classroom.

Classroom Collaboration and Inclusion

The purpose of a language assessment and intervention is to help a student learn and use the communication rules and strategies needed to succeed socially and academically in the classroom and in the world (Lidz 1991; Nelson 1993; Wallach and Butler 1994; Wang 1992). To be effective, assessment procedures should drive the intervention and meet the communication and learning needs of students. From this perspective, the reasons for conducting a language assessment are threefold: (1) to provide instructional feedback to students, which in turn promotes language learning and motivation; (2) to improve instruction and teaching, which in turn promotes students' metacognitive (higher order thinking) and metalinguistic skills (thinking about the appropriate use of language for social and academic purposes); and (3) to evaluate the interactional sequences (types of teacher-student and peer-peer interactions) to determine their influences on a student's metacognitive and metalinguistic growth. Recent practices in carrying out the above procedures and objectives have been dominated by the collaborative-inclusion movement.

Classroom collaboration is an intervention process for language-impaired and other special-needs children. It has developed as a result of the classroom inclusion movement in schools (Silliman and Wilkinson 1991; Rosenfield 1987). Classroom collaboration is also a problem-solving process involving an intervention team composed of some or all of the following members: teacher, speech-language pathologist, special education personnel, and others. Depending on the student's learning, academic, and communication needs, the team works together to provide the student with the necessary guided participation to succeed socially and academically in the classroom. Classroom collaboration is composed of various formats: (1) team teaching in a regular classroom with the classroom teacher, other resource specialists, or both (Wang 1992); (2) providing one-to-one or small-group intervention in the classroom, outside of the classroom, or both (Nelson 1993; Wallach and Butler 1994); (3) providing collaborative consultation with regular or special-education teachers and other staff (Despain and Simon 1987); and (4) providing in-services related to curriculum or program development (Nelson 1989). Through the varied use of these formats, the speech-language pathologist determines whether communicatively impaired students' communication opportunities in the classroom are optimal in maximizing those students' social and academic language-learning potentials.

Classroom inclusion means that all children, regardless of their disability, are taught in the regular classroom. The inclusion practice was instigated as a result of Public Law (PL) 94-142, which was reauthorized in 1990 as the Individuals with Disabilities Education Act (see Chapter 2). This act requires state education departments to assure that

> to the maximum extent appropriate, children with disabilities, including children in public or private institutions or other care facilities, are educated with children who are not disabled, and that special classes, separate schooling or other removal of children with disabilities from the regular education environment occurs only when the nature or severity of the disability is such that education in regular classes with the use of supplementary aids and services cannot be achieved satisfactorily (National Association of State Boards of Education 1992).

The reauthorization of PL 94-142 has resulted in the complete restructuring of the education system. This restructuring requires that all team members learn to work together to provide communicatively impaired and other special-needs children with optimal learning opportunities in the regular classroom.

Cultural and Linguistic Diversity

Given the diversity of the student population in the United States, children begin school with different language- and literacy-based experiences and skills (Battle 1993; Heath 1986; Iglesias 1985; Vygotsky 1978; Wong and Wang 1994). These differences need to be addressed appropriately within the classroom collaboration and inclusion model. Students from culturally and linguistically diverse backgrounds who are suspected of having language disorders need appropriate and culturally unbiased diagnostic intervention, which guides and promotes their social and academic success. The language assessment and intervention procedures used should distinguish those language differences related to social and cultural factors from differences that result from language impairments.

The diagnostic-intervention process can involve the combined use of the following procedures if used appropriately to reduce cultural bias: (1) standardized tests, criterion-referenced language tests, and curriculum-based language tests (McCauley and Swisher 1984; Haynes et al. 1992); (2) naturalistic language assessment methods (Retherford 1993); (3) dynamic language assessment; (4) ethnographic observational procedures; and (5) observational lens model within classroom discourse activities (teacher-student and peer-peer interactions) (Haynes et al. 1992; Nelson 1993; Pena et al. 1992; Silliman and Wilkinson 1991).

As stated earlier, standardized language tests are designed to measure a student's score on a particular language area (e.g., semantics, phonology, and syntax). The score is then compared to a large group of normally developing students on whom the test was normed. The appropriateness of standardized tests greatly depends on the extent to which they are free of cultural and linguistic bias. Criterion-referenced tests and curriculum-based language assessment procedures are designed to measure a student's development of particular skills. For example, one might assess a student's ability to answer specific questions regarding stories taken from grade-specific basal readers. Naturalistic language assessment procedures involve analyses of the student's spontaneous language used during social and academic interactions with peers, teachers, clinicians, parents, and others. Dynamic language assessment is a process whereby the student's modifiability (i.e., ability to learn a language task) is measured during mediation (i.e., teaching). Through mediation, the student learns how to apply specific strategies, which in turn facilitate the student's abilities to complete a language task on his or her own. After mediation, the student's modifiability is measured. The measurements can include selective attention, the ability to plan and use materials, the ability to apply learned strategies to a new task, and the ability to show enthusiasm for the new task. The information gained from all of the testing sets a precedence for an intervention plan to maximize the student's language-learning potential for social and academic success.

The results of Arturo's performances on a series of standardized and criterion-referenced language tests, naturalistic language analysis, and dynamic language assessment measures revealed that he had difficulty in several areas in Spanish. Arturo had some difficulty understanding grammatical morphemes (e.g., past tense, future tense, and irregular past tense) and had trouble understanding cohesive devices (e.g., *so*, *while*, and *because*). He demonstrated difficulties related to the sequence of events and causal coherence in oral narratives and had difficulty generating *if* statements and embedded sentences. Problem areas were also noted in word retrieval, subject-verb agreement, and the production of multisyllabic words.

An examination of oral mechanism revealed intact structures and adequate functions for speech maintenance. Overall, his conversational speech production was judged as good. Dynamic language assessment revealed that his language-learning ability regarding the specified problem areas of language was modifiable during individualized and small-group instruction conducted by the speech-language pathologist in and outside of the classroom.

Observational Lens Model: An Ethnographic Approach

The observational lens model is an ethnographic (i.e., the study of human interaction in naturally occurring situations) approach involving a systematic framework of interactive assessment and intervention applied to communication in the classroom (Silliman and Wilkinson 1991). By using this model, the speech-language pathologist can identify specific communication strengths, weaknesses, and breakdowns involving communicatively impaired students and their peers and teacher. The identification of these strengths, weaknesses, and breakdowns facilitates the speech-language pathologist's ability to develop and apply language-learning strategies for the target students within the classroom setting. These strategies promote essential social and academic skills of the target students within a variety of communicative situations involving peers, teachers, and other school personnel.

The components of the observational lens model include the classroom sketch map, the wide-angle lens, the regular lens, the close-up lens, and the micro–close-up lens (Silliman and Wilkinson 1991). The classroom sketch map is illustrated in the work of Wong-Fillmore and colleagues (1983). As shown in the appendix, the classroom sketch map includes a description of the contextual aspects in which learning of language takes place. These aspects are physical, cognitive and tasks, language, and social. The following is a general description of Arturo's bilingual classroom using the observational lens model components.

Classroom Sketch Map

The physical arrangement of Arturo's classroom consists of small-group cluster seating arrangements (with 4–5 students per group) and five learning centers. The student group clusters are arranged according to the students' ability to work well together and not according to special education categories or ethnic groups. The five learning centers (i.e., games, writing, listening, leisure reading, and social studies) are situated along three of the four walls of the classroom and are used by the students according to their self-schedules and individualized prescription sheets (Wang 1992). The self-schedules delineate the assigned dates of a student's participation in learning activities within different learning centers. They are negotiated between the students and the teacher and are based on the student's performance on completed academic assignments. The prescription sheets are individualized in that they specify each student's academic assignments and general progress. The classroom is decorated with multicultural education posters representing famous athletes, politicians, poets, celebrities, and musicians from African-American, Latino-American, Asian-American, and Euro-American backgrounds.

Ms. Rios' teaching schedule and philosophy is such that both English and Spanish are used to teach all of the students by encouraging the students to take an active conversational role during the classroom lessons. Spanish is used to teach math, science, and language arts, and English is used to teach reading, social studies, and language arts. Small group, whole class, and individualized lessons transcend language arts and the content areas, such as math, science, and social studies. This teaching schedule and philosophy is consistent with developmental bilingual education and guided participation (Fradd and Tikunoff 1987; Iglesias 1994; Reynolds 1991; Rogoff 1990; Trueba 1987). According to the bilingual education and guided participation philosophy, students become academically successful through two languages, if they receive comprehensible input through interactive instructional methods. Ms. Rios ascribes to this teaching philosophy, which is supported by the best-practice literature in bilingual and adaptive education.

Wide-Angle Lens

Using the wide-angle lens, the bilingual speech-language pathologist noted that the communication demands (i.e., linguistic analogies, linguistic associations, and information processing and inferring) imposed on Arturo during the classroom lessons were above his language ability in both languages. The wide-angle lens involves the observational use of categorical tools (e.g., checklists and rating scales) regarding general communication and academic behaviors expected in students during classroom lessons. Teachers' written descriptions of target students' communication and academic skills during classroom lessons are also used. These categorical and descriptive tools are used to determine if a student demonstrates communication and language-learning problems. To use categorical tools appropriately, the speech-language pathologist should (1) have a sufficient level of training before the observational use of the tools, (2) be aware that there must be a focus on what students can do (i.e., the social contexts of ability) rather than on what students fail to do (i.e., the social contexts of disability), and (3) be aware that the items listed on the tools may not necessarily represent the communication opportunities in the classroom.

To facilitate Arturo's language learning in the classroom, the teacher and clinician worked jointly to modify their language in ways that promoted and challenged Arturo's language-learning potential.

Regular Observational Lens

The regular observational lens allowed the clinician to describe Arturo's communication behaviors and the communicative context during classroom lessons. Using this lens, the clinician is able to determine the types of communication opportunities afforded to students during teacher-student, peer-peer, and clinician-student interactions. In Arturo's case, he was cooperative and talkative during individualized and small group (e.g., two to three students) instruction. He also enjoyed working in the games and reading centers with certain peers. During whole-class instruction, however, he withdrew and became frustrated when he did not receive guidance that facilitated his language comprehension and task completion.

Close-Up Lens

The close-up lens permits the clinician to more specifically describe particular types of communication, such as requests for information, used by particular students. For example, Arturo received support from his bilingual peer, Jose, during small-group reading lessons. During reading lessons, Jose provided instructional directives in Spanish and English (e.g., look at the first sentence to find the answer), which in turn helped Arturo understand language concepts to complete classroom assignments. The instructional directives, provided by the teacher and Jose, enabled Arturo to formulate questions in English and Spanish that promoted his conversational participation, reading comprehension, and task completion.

Micro–Close-Up Lens

The micro–close-up lens allows the clinician to examine and describe communicative breakdowns during classroom lessons. Using the micro–close-up lens, the clinician noted that Arturo had tremendous difficulty answering the teacher's process questions (i.e., why or how questions) because of his difficulty with syntax and language processing. As a result, Arturo shied away and lost interest in the lesson as his frustration level escalated. To promote Arturo's language comprehension, the speech-language pathologist and the teacher used product questions (i.e., what and when questions) and choice yes and no questions (Cazden 1988; Valles 1995). The plan was to gradually introduce him to process questions as his competence developed in answering product and choice yes and no questions.

Application of the Diagnostic-Intervention Process

The application of the diagnostic-intervention process facilitates the speech-language pathologist's ability to identify a student's strengths and weaknesses and maximizes the student's social and academic learning potential. Consequently, along with the collaboration-intervention team (comprised of parents, teachers, special educators, psychologists, and so on), the speech-language pathologist is best prepared to address the communication and cognitive needs of students on an individual basis.

In Arturo's case study, the bilingual clinician, the teacher, and some of Arturo's peers worked closely with Arturo to facilitate and promote his language-learning potential. Specifically, they used mediation strategies such as (1) sustaining attention and planning through the use of materials via visual and auditory cues (e.g., sound-symbol association, prescription sheets, and self-schedules); (2) self-talk for problem solving during individual work; (3) applying learned strategies to new tasks; and (4) using a continuum of simple to complex language as the medium of instruction to promote his comprehension and self-monitoring of his academic progress. These mediation strategies served to promote his metacognitive and metalinguistic skills while circumventing his language needs in the following areas: auditory retention, language processing, word retrieval problems, syntax, and oral narratives.

Summary

In summary, the speech-language pathologist conducts language assessments and interventions geared to foster communicative competence and academic success in language-disordered students. To maximize these students' communication and academic learning potential, the speech-language pathologist devises and uses specific language-learning strategies. He or she uses metalinguistic strategies to foster the student's ability to think about language (e.g., semantics, phonology, syntax, morphology, and pragmatics) to use it more effectively for learning purposes. In addition, he or she uses metacognitive strategies to promote higher-order thinking for problem solving and analysis. These language-learning strategies are individualized based on the student's communication needs and on the communicative demands imposed on students in the classroom (Goldenberg 1991;

Tharp and Gallimore 1991; Trueba 1987; Wallach and Butler 1994; Wang 1992). By learning to apply these strategies in the classroom, as guided by the speech-language pathologist and the teacher, the students learn to monitor their own learning for social and academic success during small-group, whole-class, or individualized lessons and interventions.

Conclusion

The assessment and treatment of language disorders in children is greatly influenced by several factors, such as the nature of the problem, the age group, the setting in which clinical treatment takes place, and the linguistic and cultural background of the children being served. These factors determine a clinician's perspective toward treatment. Clinical perspectives in the treatment of language disorders can be different regarding preschoolers and school-age children. Preschoolers require a norm-referenced treatment perspective. On the other hand, with school-age children, the curriculum demands greatly influence clinical strategies. Moreover, a multicultural perspective must be considered for both groups, because speech-language pathologists in the United States are faced with more linguistically and culturally diverse children than at any time in history (Battle 1993). These clinical perspectives converge and are exemplified in the case study of Arturo, a bilingual child whose treatment plan highlights various strategies for simultaneously enhancing both language skills and academic skills.

References

American Speech-Hearing-Language Association. Clinical Management of Communicatively Handicapped Minority Language Populations. ASHA 1985;27.

Battle DE. Communication Disorders in Multicultural Populations. Boston: Andover Medical Publishers, 1993.

Cazden CB. Classroom Discourse: The Language of Teaching and Learning. Portsmouth, NH: Heinemann Educational Books, 1988.

Davis C, Haub C, Wilette JA. U.S. Hispanics: Changing the Face of America. Washington, DC: Population Reference Bureau, 1983.

Despain AD, Simon CS. Alternative to failure: a junior high school language development-based curriculum. J Childhood Commun Disord 1987;11:139–179.

Fradd SH, Tikunoff WJ. Bilingual Education and Bilingual Special Education: A Guide for Administrators. Boston: College Hill Press, 1987.

Goldenberg C. Instructional Conversations and Their Classroom Application. Santa Cruz, CA: National Center for Research on Cultural Diversity and Second-Language Learning, University of California, 1991.

Haynes W, Pindzola RH, Emerick LL. Diagnosis and Evaluation in Speech Pathology. Englewood Cliffs, NJ: Prentice-Hall, 1992.

Heath SB. Sociocultural Contexts of Language Development. In Bilingual Education Office (ed), Beyond Language: Social and Cultural Factors in Schooling Language Minority Students. Los Angeles: Evaluation, Dissemination and Assessment Center, California State University, 1986;143–186.

Iglesias A. Cultural Conflict in the Classroom: The Communicatively Different Child. In DN Ripich, FM Spinelli (eds), School Discourse Problems. San Diego: College Hill Press, 1985.

Iglesias A. Programs for Children with Limited English Proficiency. In KK Wong, MC Wang (eds), Rethinking Policy for At-Risk Students. Berkeley, CA: McCutchan Publishing, 1994.

Lahey M. Who shall be called language disordered? Some reflections and one perspective. J Speech Hear Disord 1990;55:612–620.

Lidz CS. Practitioner's Guide to Dynamic Assessment. New York: Guilford Press, 1991.

McCauley RJ, Swisher L. Use and misuse of norm-referenced tests in clinical assessment. J Speech Hear Disord 1984;49:338–348.

National Association of State Boards of Education. Winners All: A Call for Inclusive Schools. The Report of the NASBE Study Group on Special Education. Alexandria, VA: National Association of State Boards of Education, 1992.

Nelson N. Childhood Language Disorders in Context: Infancy Through Adolescence. New York: Macmillan, 1993.

Nelson NW. Curriculum-based language assessment and intervention. LSHSS 1989;20:170–184.

Peña E, Quinn R, Iglesias A. The application of dynamic methods to language assessment. J Special Edu 1992;26:269–280.

Retherford KS. Guide to Analysis of Language Transcripts. Eau Claire, WI: Thinking Publications, 1993.

Reynolds AG. Bilingualism, Multiculturalism, and Second-Language Learning. Hillsdale, NJ: Lawrence Erlbaum, 1991.

Rogoff B. Apprenticeship in Thinking: Cognitive Development in Social Context. New York: Oxford University Press, 1990.

Rosenfield S. Instructional Consultation. Hillsdale, NJ: Lawrence Erlbaum, 1987.

Seymour H. Clinical Intervention for Language Disorders Among Nonstandard Speakers of English. In O Taylor (ed), Treatment of Communication Disorders in Culturally and Linguistically Diverse Populations. San Diego: College Hill Press, 1986;135–152.

Seymour HN, Bland L. A minority perspective in diagnosis of child language disorders. Clin Commun Disord 1991;1:25–38.

Seymour HN. The invisible children: a reply to Lahey's perspective. J Speech Hear Res 1992;35:640–641.

Silliman ER, Wilkinson LC. Communicating for Learning: Classroom Observation and Collaboration. Gaithersburg, MD: Aspen, 1991.

Stark R, Tallal P. Specific language impairment in children. Adv Dev Behav Pediatr 1982;3:257–271.

Stockman I, Vaughn-Cooke F. Semantic Categories in the Language of Working-Class Black Children. In CE Johnson, CL Thew (eds),

Proceedings of the Second International Child Language Conference. 1982;312–327.

Tharp RG, Gallimore R. Rousing Minds to Life: Teaching, Learning, and Schooling in Social Context. New York: Cambridge University, 1991.

Trueba HT. Success or Failure? Learning and the Language Minority Student. New York: Newbury House, 1987.

Valles L. Teaching as guided participation during small group and whole class reading lessons [manuscript]. 1995.

Vaughn-Cooke, FB. Improving language assessment in minority children. ASHA 1983;25:29–34.

Vygotsky LS. In M Cole, V John-Steiner, S Sribner, E Souberman (eds), Mind in Society: The Development of Higher Psychological Processes. Cambridge, MA: Harvard University Press, 1978.

Wallach GP, Butler KG. Language Learning Disabilities in School-Age Children and Adolescents: Some Principles and Applications. New York: Merrill, 1994.

Wang MC, Haertel GD, Walberg HJ. What influences learning? A content analysis of review literature. J Educational Res 1990;84:30–43.

Wang MC, Reynolds MC, Walberg HJ. Special Education Research and Practice: Synthesis of Findings. New York: Pergamon Press, 1990.

Wang MC. Adaptive Education Strategies: Building on Diversity. Baltimore: Paul H. Brookes, 1992.

Wong KK, Wang MC. Rethinking Policy for At-Risk Students. Berkeley, CA: McCutchan Publishing, 1994.

Wong-Fillmore L, Ammon P, Ammon MS, et al. Learning English Through Bilingual Instruction: Second-Year Report [contract 400-80-0030]. Washington, DC: National Institute of Education, 1983.

Chapter 5   Study Questions

1. Which language areas would a speech-language clinician evaluate and address when working with communicatively impaired students to promote these students' academic performances?

2. How can familiarity with the classroom collaboration model and cultural and linguistic diversity issues aid the speech-language clinician in appropriately evaluating students' communication skills?

3. How can a speech-language clinician use the observational lens or ethnographic model to promote a communicatively impaired student's social and academic communication skills in a bilingual classroom? (Your response should address the classroom sketch map, the wide-angle lens, the regular lens, the close-up lens, and the micro–close-up lens.)

4. Discuss some possible causes of language disorders in children and how these causes may be categorized.

5. What are some of the possible consequences of relying on developmental norms when assessing the language of minority children?

Appendix

Classroom Sketch Map

Name of activity:_____

Date:_____

Physical aspects:

1. Draw a map of the classroom.
2. Describe the location (indicate the location of various activities on the map).
3. Describe the daily schedule (indicate activity and time).
4. Describe the materials used (e.g., pencils, books, or blackboard).

Cognitive and task aspects:

1. Describe the content of the material to be learned during this activity. Is it appropriate for this age or grade level?
2. Describe the curriculum materials involved in this activity (give specific description). Do all the materials seem to be appropriate for the age or grade level?
3. Are the goals for the activity clearly stated? How?
4. What written products are to result from this activity? How will they be evaluated? What feedback on these will be given to the students and when? If possible, attach copies of the curriculum materials.

Language aspects:

1. Describe the language used during this activity (indicate whether oral or written).
2. How are language directions given for the activity? Are there any restrictions on the use of language (e.g., only speak English)?
3. If there are students who speak more than one language in this activity, describe their language usage.

Social aspects:

1. Provide names of participants and indicate where they are located during the activity. Describe the students (e.g., age, languages spoken, grade, and gender).
2. Describe the activity structure (e.g., large group, small group, individual, or pairs). If groups or pairs are used, describe (a) how the students were assigned (e.g., ability and achievement, friendship, age, grade, language, homogeneous or heteroge-

neous); (b) the stability of assignment; (c) whether the group or pair is directed by the teacher or by a student; and (d) if directed by a student, how the student was selected (e.g., by teacher or by students) and on what basis.

3. Describe the management of the activity. Does the teacher provide discipline? How does the teacher deal with interruptions and discipline during the activity?

Source: Reprinted with permission from L Wong-Fillmore, P Ammon, MS Ammon, et al. Learning English Through Bilingual Instruction: Second-Year Report [contract 400-80-0030]. Washington, DC: National Institute of Education, 1983.

6 Articulation and Phonologic Disorders

Ruth Huntley Bahr

Clinicians and researchers recognize that there are both motor and linguistic aspects to speech production. The term *articulation* is used frequently to refer to the physical act of talking. The term *phonology* refers to the linguistic rules that govern how the speaker puts sounds together to form words. These combined elements form the basis for the motor and linguistic aspects of speech production. This chapter provides the reader with a foundation in the development of speech sounds and the potential causes of speech sound disorders (i.e., misarticulations), as well as considers how to evaluate and remediate these difficulties.

Phonologic Development

Children pass through two major periods of speech sound development. The first stage is known as the *phonetic period*. It occurs from birth to about 18 months. At this time, the child learns the sensorimotor movements necessary for sound production. When the child produces a truly meaningful word, he or she enters the stage known as the *phonemic period*. At this point, sounds are used to make a difference in word meaning. This stage occurs sometime between 1 and 2 years of age. A child, therefore, learns much about sound production during the first 2 years of life.

The Phonetic Period

Utterances of the phonetic period are characterized as reflexive or nonreflexive. Reflexive utterances are seemingly automatic responses that indicate pleasure and discomfort. Nonreflexive utterances include vocal play and squealing (Stark 1978). Both types of sounds appear to be influenced most by the form and size of the infant's vocal tract. As such, the variety of sounds that can be produced is limited. To be specific, an infant's tongue is large relative to the oral cavity, and the larynx rides high in the pharynx. Furthermore, the slope of the back wall of the pharynx is gradual, as compared with the right-angle shape noted in adults. In infants, this configuration moves the epiglottis closer to the velum, which results in restricted tongue movement. As the infant grows, and the oral cavity becomes more adult-like, the number of sounds that can be produced increases. The sounds produced during this phase are produced with little or no planning on the infant's part. These sounds reflect the size and shape of the oral cavity and may serve as precursors to later developing sounds.

During the latter part of the phonetic period, first cooing and then babbling begin to appear. Oller (1980) distinguishes cooing from babbling by its phonetic content. Cooing consists largely of back sounds and vowels, especially lip-rounded vowels. It is believed that these vocalizations reflect the process of gaining control over voicing; however, these utterances lack regularity of timing among syllables and the syllable reduplication characteristic of babbling. At 6–9 months, these vocalizations become more speech-like due to the presence of reduplicated syllables. Babbling tends to be consonant-vowel sequences, but vowel-consonant and consonant-vowel-consonant syllables also occur. At this time, parents often report hearing their child say "mama" or "dada." However, these early attempts at words should be considered only as sound play until the child demonstrates that he or she is actually naming someone.

At 10–12 months, the syllable patterns are composed of different consonants and vowels within a series. In addition, the child begins using adult-like intonation patterns. At times, one may feel as though he or she should understand what the toddler is saying. The child, however, does not intend a meaning: He or she is just trying out new phonetic and suprasegmental patterns. It is at this point in the developmental sequence that the child is ready to utter his or her first word. The relationship between sound play or babbling and the true onset of speech is unclear and the reader is referred to more advanced treatments of this topic (Wood 1976; Vihman et al. 1986). Nevertheless, the prevailing view is that children tend to babble (or practice) sounds that they will later include in their sound systems or phonologies.

The Phonemic Period

The transition from babbling to speech occurs during the period from 9 to 18 months. It is difficult to mark the exact point at which the child moves into the phonemic period; however, a landmark is the use of 50 words consistently. At this point, word use appears to become dominant over babbling, and the child demonstrates comprehension of the adult language and has mastered the production of several speech ges-

TABLE 6.1   Phoneme List by Manner of Production*

Manner of Production	Phonemes Included
Nasals	/m/, /n/, /ŋ/
Plosives	/b/, /p/, /t/, /d/, /k/, /g/
Glides	/j/, /w/
Fricatives	/f/,/ v/, /θ/, /ð/, /s/, /z/, /ʃ/, /ʒ/, /h/
Affricates	/tʃ/, /dʒ/

These sounds can occur at various points in the production of a syllable or a word. Below is the example for the phoneme /p/.

Word Position	Word	Syllable	Linguistic Form
Initial position	pat	pa	CV
Medial position	keeper	apa	VCV
Final position	dip	ap	VC

*These groupings refer to the type of obstruction(s) produced within the mouth to create the desired sound. CV = consonant-vowel; VCV = vowel-consonant-vowel; VC = vowel-consonant.

tures. In terms of articulatory development, the child is beginning to use sounds to make a difference in word meanings.

While there is considerable variability in the acquisition of individual speech sounds, phonemes, as a whole, appear in the following developmental sequence (Table 6.1): (1) vowels, (2) nasals, (3) plosives, (4) glides, (5) fricatives, and (6) affricates (Wellman et al. 1931; Poole 1934; Templin 1957). While there is little disagreement that phonologic acquisition is mastered by the age of 7 or 8 years, there is considerable controversy as to when a particular sound should be produced correctly in single words. This type of information is particularly important for the speech-language pathologist in determining who is in need of treatment.

One of the biggest problems in the area of phoneme acquisition appears to be the idea of mastery, or the ability to produce a target sound correctly over a prescribed number of trials. The term *mastery* was coined by Sander (1972), who believed that the earlier studies on phonologic acquisition were too stringent in their definition of mastery. Earlier studies defined mastery as the correct production of the sound in all three word positions: initial, medial, and final (see Table 6.1). Sander argued that these ages of acquisition actually reflect the upper age limits for all children and not the average sound usage for most children. In contrast to this idea, he introduced the concept of *customary production*, or the age at which children produced the sound correctly more often than incorrectly in two of three word positions. In Sander's system, mastery becomes the point at which 90% of children produced the sound correctly in all word positions. Sander reanalyzed the data of Templin (1957) and Wellman and colleagues (1931) and arrived at age ranges that represent the period of customary production to mastery for all consonants tested. His results are depicted in Figure 6.1.

Age Level (years)

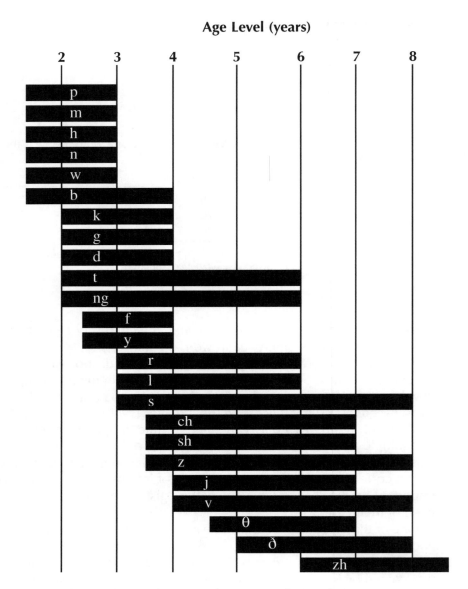

FIGURE 6.1 *Average age estimates and upper age limits of customary consonant production. The solid bar corresponding to each sound starts at the median age of customary articulation. The bar stops at an age level at which 90% of all children are customarily producing the sound. (Reprinted from EK Sander. When are speech sounds learned? J Speech Hear Disord 1972;37:62. Copyright, 1972, by the American Speech-Language-Hearing Association, Rockville, MD. Reprinted by permission.)*

In a similar fashion, Prather and colleagues (1975) also gathered normative data. They examined consonants in the initial and final positions only and vowels in only one context, using 75% accuracy in the initial and final positions as their criterion for mastery. Naturally, their procedures lowered the age norms a little more. As such, these investigators demonstrated that most children develop /p/, /b/, /m/, /w/, /t/,

/d/, /n/, /k/, /g/, and /h/ by age 3 years and should gain proficiency in the production of "th", /z/, /v/, /ʃ/, /ʒ/, /tʃ/, and /j/ at around 4 years of age. Therefore, these changes in the definition of sound mastery suggest that children should be intelligible by 3 years of age and should have learned to adequately produce most sounds by 6 years of age, which is the time at which most children enter the first grade.

Phonologic Process Development

The preceding discussion focused on the acquisition of individual phonemes. However, children learn both the movements associated with speech production and the rules regarding sound combinations (i.e., phonologic processes). These rules govern how a child produces a word. While many of these rules reflect the adult phonologic forms, several phonologic processes emerge during the early stages of sound development that appear to be simplifications of the adult forms (Grunwell 1982). As the child matures, these phonologic processes are modified and suppressed until the target form is achieved (Figure 6.2).

Ingram (1976) classified these developmental processes into three basic categories: syllable structure processes, assimilation processes, and substitution processes. The function of the syllable structure processes is to simplify the structure of a syllable. The basic function is to reduce any syllable to a consonant-vowel combination. This process can take several forms. The first is final consonant deletion. In this case, the child will delete the final consonant from most word productions. For example, the words *bat* and *back* would be reduced to /bæ/. When this process is used, different words would sound the same (i.e., become homophones). While homophones do occur in most languages and can be easily interpreted by the use of context, the use of final consonant deletion results in an excessive use of homonyms and a severe decline in speech intelligibility. However, final consonant deletion is commonly used by young children as they learn to speak, and its use usually subsides by the age of 3 years (see Figure 6.2). Only persistent use of final consonant deletion is considered a disorder.

Other syllable structure processes include weak syllable deletion, consonant cluster reduction, and reduplication (Table 6.2) (Ingram 1976). Again, all of these processes reflect simplification strategies used by most children during early phonologic development. Continued use of these processes results in speech unintelligibility.

The other two groups of phonologic rules include assimilation (or consonant harmony) and substitution processes (see Table 6.2). Assimilation refers to a process whereby one sound segment affects or influences the production of another. In other words, one phoneme becomes so dominant in a word that it affects the production of another phoneme in that word. Assimilation is easy to note, if one asks the child to produce a word without the dominant phoneme. For

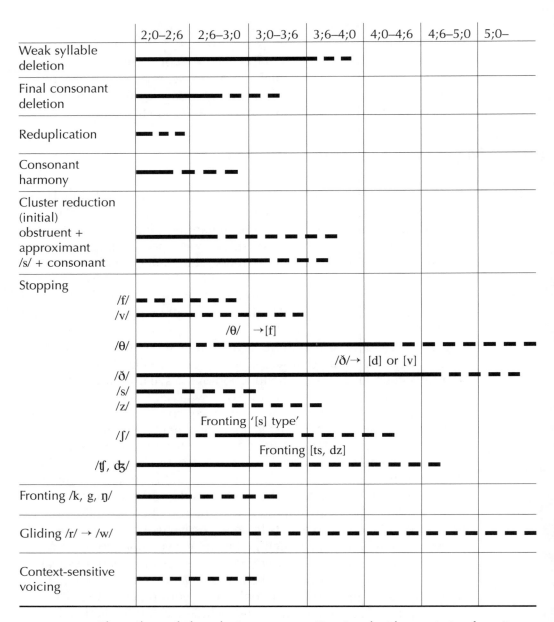

FIGURE 6.2 *Chronology of phonologic processes. (Reprinted with permission from P Grunwell. Clinical Phonology. Rockville, MD: Aspen Systems Corporation, 1982;183.)*

instance, a child may say "goggie" for *doggie*, but be able to correctly produce /d/ in the words *daddy* and *door*. Substitution processes, on the other hand, uniformly affect a particular phoneme or phoneme class (see Table 6.2). In this case, the child is presumed to be unable to produce the target sound and thereby chooses to simplify its production. Alternatively, the child may be able to produce the target, but he or she may not know how to use the phoneme appropriately. Many of

TABLE 6.2 An Adapted Illustration of Ingram's Classification System of Phonologic Processes

Process	Examples
Syllable structure	
Final consonant deletion	bat → /bæ/ pronounced as "baa"
Weak syllable deletion	elephant → /ɛfʌnt/ pronounced as "efunt"
Consonant cluster reduction	black → /bæk/ pronounced as "back"
Reduplication	water → /wɔwɔ/ pronounced as "wawa"
Assimilation processes	
Final consonant devoicing*	pig → /pɪk/ pronounced as "pick"
Velar assimilation	dog → /gɔg/ pronounced as "gog"
Alveolar assimilation	cat → /tæt/ pronounced as "tat"
Labial assimilation	stop → /bap/ pronounced as "bop"
Prevocalic voicing*	pig → /bɪg/ pronounced as "big"
Substitution processes	
Stopping	sun → /tʌn/ pronounced as "ton"
Fronting	cab → /tæb/ pronounced as "tab"
Backing	bad → /bæg/ pronounced as "bag"
Denasalization	room → /rub/ pronounced as "roob"
Gliding of liquids	rug → /wʌg/ pronounced as "wug"
Gliding of fricatives	zoo → /wu/ pronounced as "woo"
Affrication	shoe → /ʃu/ pronounced as "chew"

*These two processes also are known as *context-sensitive voicing* (Grunwell 1982).
Source: Adapted from D Ingram. Phonological Disability in Children. New York: Elsevier, 1976.

these phonologic rules occur early in the developmental sequence of phonemes. At some point, however, the child's phonemic system must mature by adopting more adult-like rules.

Phonologic process use in children between the ages of 2.5–8.0 years has been studied in an attempt to identify processes associated with unintelligible speech (Hodson and Paden 1981; Dunn and Davis 1983; Haelsig and Madison 1986; Roberts et al. 1990). Although these investigators use different phonologic rule classification systems, they agree that the processes of final consonant deletion, consonant cluster reduction, weak syllable deletion, glottal replacement (i.e., substitution of a glottal stop for another phoneme, usually a plosive), labial assimilation, velar fronting, and gliding of liquids occur frequently in the speech of children under 4 years of age. If these processes are noted in the speech patterns of older children, phonologic intervention may be warranted. Furthermore, these researchers indicate that use of any or a combination of the following processes is indicative of a delayed or disordered phonologic system: velar assimilation, prevocalic voicing, gliding of fricatives, affrication, and denasalization (see Table 6.2 for definitions). Hence, children with deviant phonologic systems use many of the same phonologic processes as children who are developing normally; however, they may differ significantly in the frequency with which they use any particular process. Lastly, children with phonologic disorders also use processes that are unique and never found in normal usage.

In conclusion, Stoel-Gammon (1991) suggested that the following types of errors in young children are suggestive of the need for a speech evaluation:

- Inaccurate vowel productions at 24 months
- Considerable deletion of consonants in the initial word position at 24 months
- Substitution of consonants with a glottal stop or /h/
- Substitution of front consonants for back consonants
- Deletion of final consonants at 36 months

Considerations with Dialects

The issue of speech sound acquisition is made more complex when one considers that all languages are learned within the context of a specific culture. As such, the developmental norms may not readily apply. While there is some information available that outlines the differences between certain dialects (particularly African-American English [AAE] vernacular) and Standard American English (SAE), there is a paucity of information describing the process of speech sound acquisition in the nonstandard English–speaking child.

Seymour and Seymour (1981) studied the influence of AAE on the phonologic development of African-American children. They compared the number, type, and pattern of errors made by white and African-American children on the *Goldman-Fristoe Test of Articulation* and found that the difference between these groups was largely in the number of errors and not the type of error. Phonemic development, therefore, appears to be determined more by standard English than the particular dialect spoken. It is important to remember that such results only apply to dialects that are derived from SAE and cannot be generalized to English dialects that are the result of learning English as a second language.

Another area of concern has been the identification of children who may not be developing speech adequately within their own dialect or native language (other than American English). To this end, Bleile and Wallach (1992) asked Head Start teachers of the same race and community to judge the speech patterns of children enrolled in their school programs. The goal was to identify children who had trouble speaking, independent of features that could be attributed to AAE vernacular. The following misarticulations were found to be useful in identifying children in need of speech sound remediation: (1) one or more stop errors, especially in the initial and medial positions of words; (2) more than three fricative errors, other than "th"; (3) affricate errors, other than final /dʒ/; (4) nasal and glide errors in children older than 4 years of age, especially difficulty with /r/ in the initial and medial positions; and (5) five or more errors on clusters, especially /s/ clusters. While the frequency of error type may differ among these children, these types of misarticulations were not related to the use of AAE vernacular. Additional studies like this would assist the speech-language pathologist in determining which dialect-speaking children are in need of treatment.

More information is becoming available on the development of Spanish in young children. This area of study is particularly difficult because of the presence of numerous Spanish dialects with significant phonologic differences. Goldstein and Iglesias (1996) presented an excellent description of phonologic patterns used by normal children who speak a Puerto Rican dialect of Spanish. They found that cluster reduction and gliding were the two processes used most often. In addition, they reported that these children also acquired the sounds of their language early. They attributed this finding to the phonologic characteristics of Spanish, with its emphasis on consonant-vowel syllable shapes and the infrequent use of the more difficult English phonemes (e.g., /r/, /s/ and "th"). Because their report is specific to the presence of certain phonologic characteristics, it would be possible to extrapolate the results to possibly identify children who may not be developing Spanish properly—at least if they speak with a Puerto Rican dialect. Nevertheless, more research is needed in the area of bilingual speech development.

Potential Causes of an Articulation or Phonologic Disorder

Winitz (1969) suggested that the articulatory process is a multivariate phenomenon, meaning that a number of variables can act simultaneously to influence speech production. For example, when one refers to a speaker's age, he or she also suggests a particular physical size, level of coordination, and degree of linguistic maturity. It is difficult to control one variable experimentally without influencing several other known or possibly unknown components. It is, therefore, important to carefully consider any research results that declare a causal relationship between any two variables. Actually, one can only state that such factors are related to one another, meaning that they are correlative. When the correlation is very high ($r \geq 0.90$), one can sometimes predict the status of one variable from knowledge of the status of another variable. However, it must be stressed that this relationship is not causal.

While there are many influences on speech production, many of the articulation problems that clinicians see can only be attributed to faulty learning. These types of disorders are often known as *functional articulation problems*. However, there are a few organic (i.e., medical) or structural factors that can impede the speech process (Table 6.3).

TABLE 6.3   Potential Causes of an Articulation or Phonologic Disorder

Area	Findings
Hearing and auditory perception	Auditory feedback is essential for the development of speech.
Middle ear involvement	Evidence is divided. Otitis media is probably associated with the articulation errors noted in the school-age years.
Speech-sound discrimination	Many persons have difficulty recognizing the production of sounds they produce in error. Speech discrimination is a complex issue.
Speech mechanism factors	
Lips	Difficulty with this articulator has little effect on intelligibility.
Teeth	Missing incisors or an open bite may contribute to a lisp.
Tongue	Large tongue size may negatively impact speech intelligibility.
	Few children are diagnosed with a restricted lingual frenum (i.e., tongue-tied).
	If the tongue is absent, one can develop good compensatory articulations.
	Tongue thrust is predominantly a swallowing dysfunction.
Hard and soft palate	Defects are corrected with surgery. Hard palate repair usually results in fewer speech difficulties than soft palate repair.
Oral sensory perception	
Oral tactile sensitivity	The tongue is quite sensitive and may play a role in monitoring speech production.
Oral stereognosis	It is possible to have poor oral stereognosis and still have good articulation.
Oral deprivation	Speech intelligibility is maintained despite lack of oral sensation.
Motor abilities	
General motor skills	No significant retardation in general motor skills has been noted.
Oral motor skills	Oral motor skills may be impaired without a resultant loss in speech intelligibility.

The following discussion of causes is not an exhaustive list of factors that influence speech production abilities. For example, it does not include articulation disorders that occur as the result of a neurologic insult or as part of a larger syndrome or language problem.

Hearing and Auditory Perception

Research conducted by Oller and Eilers (1988) suggested that auditory feedback is essential for the development of speech. From this conclusion it could be deduced that any defect in hearing negatively impacts articulation. The literature, however, is divided on this issue. Even so, the role of hearing loss due to fluid in the middle ear and speech-sound discrimination seems to be pertinent in any discussion of articulation disorders.

Middle Ear Involvement

Researchers have been unable to establish a strong relationship between early otitis media with effusion (OME) and later speech difficulties. The problems with the research are due, in large part, to the methods of research design, timing of data collection, and OME documentation procedures (Roberts and Medley 1995). Furthermore, the studies tend to be retrospective in that they use recall of past events by caregivers or review medical records to gather data. It would be better if these studies were conducted longitudinally from early infancy, or if children were tested for OME at specified intervals (i.e., a prospective study).

Despite these difficulties, a few studies are worth mentioning. The first group of researchers found no relationship between the number of days a child suffered with OME during the first 3 years of life and the number of common phonologic processes or consonants in error observed during the preschool years. These researchers went on to suggest that early OME can be associated with articulation errors noted in the school-age years. However, they were unable to carefully test this hypothesis and exclude the possible influence of socioeconomic status on the speech development of the children in question (Roberts et al. 1988).

Paden and colleagues (1987) also reported that OME was not the primary factor that contributed to phonologic delay at age 3 years. Nevertheless, they did suggest that children with a history of OME should be considered for phonologic treatment or at least have their speech patterns closely monitored if they have (1) an unusually large percentage of errors for their age on velars (i.e., /k/, /g/, and "ng"); (2) a large number of errors on plosives, fricatives, and affricates that occur after vowels; and (3) some errors with liquids (i.e., /l/ and /r/). In a second study, Paden and colleagues (1989) found that of the children they tested with OME only about one-fourth did not catch up with their peers by the age of 3 years. They attributed this finding to early aggressive treatment of OME and concluded that some children were bound to be phonologically delayed and it is possible that such delay is not related to OME.

While the above studies suggest little or no relationship between OME and later speech development, Roberts and Medley (1995) believed that there was evidence to link an early history of OME with later language and learning difficulties. They were quick to point out that there were multiple risk factors (e.g., child rearing practices, quality of day care, innate abilities) that also influence a child's development. As such, they suggested monitoring hearing loss and educating caregivers about providing optimal health and learning environments.

Speech-Sound Discrimination

Speech-sound discrimination refers to the listener's and speaker's abilities to distinguish perceptually between two sounds in a language. Clinically, this process refers to the difference between error sounds and their targets. While this skill seems to be essential to speech production, the relationship between articulation and speech discrimination is not well understood. Previous research has suggested that normal speakers can discriminate between error sounds and correct productions better than articulatory defective speakers (Sherman and Geith 1967). Furthermore, there is a positive correlation between performance on an articulation test and on a test of speech-sound discrimination (Sherman and Geith 1967). However, several other studies suggest that there is no difference between normal and articulatory defective children on speech-sound discrimination tasks (Winitz and Bellerose 1963; Schwartz and Goldman 1974). For example, Winitz and Bellerose demonstrated that with (enough) pretraining, articulatory defective children did as well as normal children on tests of speech-sound discrimination. In fact, many children can correctly discriminate the sounds they make in error. Schwartz and Goldman demonstrated that discrimination improved when words were presented in a carrier phrase rather than in a paired comparison context (e.g., goat-coat). Therefore, linguistic context plays a role in auditory discrimination. It also may be possible that discrimination difficulties are phoneme-specific (i.e., only present for certain error sounds). In like fashion, one may be able to identify an error in someone else's speech (i.e., external monitoring) but be unable to detect it in his or her own attempts (i.e., internal monitoring). In an attempt to make sense of these apparent contradictions, Weiner (1967) concluded that auditory discrimination is a developmental skill with a ceiling that occurs at 8 years of age. As such, he hypothesized that there is a positive relationship between poor auditory discrimination and severe articulation problems below the age of 9 years.

Speech Mechanism Factors

Lips

The lips are important in the production of several vowels and consonants. Difficulty with this articulator, however, has little effect on speech intelligibility, because only the /b/, /p/, and /m/ phonemes are affected. Further support for this notion comes from the assessment of articulatory skill in persons with cleft lip, who are able to achieve good compensatory articulation after surgical repair of the lip.

Teeth

Research on the effect of teeth on sound production has focused on the influence of malocclusion, or the imperfect or irregular positioning of the teeth when the jaws are closed. It is generally accepted that only missing incisors or an open bite may possibly influence articulation. Once again, only a few phonemes are affected, /s/ and /z/ in particular.

Tongue

The tongue is the most mobile of the articulators and plays a significant role in speech production. However, there is substantial controversy as to the role the tongue plays in maintaining speech intelligibility

(McEnery and Gaines 1941). For example, it has been proposed that the macroglossia (or enlarged tongue) noted in many Down syndrome children negatively affects their articulatory skill. Yet, Lynch (1990) proposed that tongue size may not be the issue but instead attributed the tongue mobility difficulties to the smaller than normal oral cavity that accompanies this genetic disorder. Due to this vocal tract difference, these children tend to protrude their tongue. Tongue reduction surgery has been recommended; however, this procedure remains controversial and may not deal with the issue of vocal tract shape. Furthermore, many Down syndrome patients develop adequate speech intelligibility despite these structural deviations.

In the past, articulation disorders frequently were associated with a condition known as *tongue-tied*, or ankyloglossia, or a restricted lingual frenum. In other words, the tongue appeared to be attached to the floor of the patient's mouth so that lingual movement was severely restricted. The treatment was to clip the short piece of skin limiting the tongue to allow greater lingual movement. However, researchers demonstrated that only 4 out of 1,000 persons had a frenum that was too short (McEnery and Gaines 1941). Therefore, in most instances, this surgical treatment was unnecessary.

It is also possible to either be born without a tongue (i.e., aglossia) or have the tongue removed for medical reasons (i.e., glossectomy). Many persons without tongues are able to develop compensatory articulations and achieve remarkably intelligible speech.

Finally, there is the issue of tongue thrust. This condition refers to a swallowing pattern characterized by an anterior tongue placement during chewing or swallowing. Tongue thrust is often associated with dental problems (e.g., malocclusions) and speech defects (e.g., frontal lisps). Many orthodontists request speech pathology services for this disorder; however, not all of these persons have a speech problem. Therefore, most clinicians treat the swallowing pattern while remaining aware of the possibility of articulatory disturbance.

Hard and Soft Palates

The majority of the problems with hard and soft palates are corrected with surgery or prostheses. While alterations in the hard palate are easier to correct, the muscular nature of the velum presents a challenge to any surgeon. If soft-palate surgery is not totally successful, speech production difficulties result. These difficulties focus on the competence of the velopharyngeal mechanism and most likely result in a hypernasal resonance, nasal emission noted on pressure consonants (i.e., plosives, fricatives, and affricates), or both. To compensate for the loss of intraoral pressure, persons often develop an articulatory pattern characterized by pharyngeal fricatives and glottal stops instead of the expected pressure consonants (Warren et al. 1989). These misarticulations often disappear when the oral cavity is able to maintain adequate intraoral pressure. Any residual misarticulations are most likely due to patient habit.

Oral Sensory Perception

Oral touch and kinesthetic cues play some role in monitoring articulation. (See Ringel [1970] for a review.) The importance of these cues has been demonstrated with tasks designed to assess oral tactile sensitivity. Use of two-point discrimination and texture discrimination tasks has revealed that the tongue (especially the tongue tip) is more sensitive than the lips (Putnam and Ringel 1972). This finding suggests that the tongue is more responsive to articulatory movements. Other experiments were designed to assess oral form recognition or oral stereognosis (Ringel 1970). In these experiments, participants were asked to identify small plastic forms. To do this, one must be able to receive sensation, recognize its position (kinesthesia), and process this information into a meaningful message. While the results of these studies were inconclusive, it was noted that a person could have poor oral stereognosis and good articulation. Finally, the researchers turned to oral deprivation studies (Borden et al. 1973a; Borden et al. 1973b; Horii et al. 1973). Participants underwent some form of anesthesia so that the normal channels of oral feedback were disturbed. Surprisingly, the participants were able to maintain their speech intelligibility despite the lack of oral feedback. Taken together, these studies suggest that oral feedback is important to speech production, but one is able to compensate adequately (i.e., maintain speech intelligibility) when it is impaired.

Motor Abilities

While speech is a complex fine motor activity, a person with an articulation problem does not necessarily present with significant retardation in general motor skills. However, one might suspect difficulties with oral-facial motor skills. To test these abilities, the clinician asks the client to rapidly repeat certain syllables (i.e., diadochokinesis). While children and persons with neurologic impairment may demonstrate difficulty with this task, clinical experience has revealed that many of these same persons remain completely intelligible in conversational speech. Therefore, measurement of the diadochokinetic rate may not be testing the aspects of speech production necessary for intelligible speech. Exactly what the diadochokinetic rate tells us about speech motor abilities remains to be tested.

Assessment and Treatment Considerations

Adequate diagnoses and treatment of articulation and phonologic disorders depends on a knowledge of the motor and linguistic aspects of speech production. In fact, problems with speech sound production can be divided into two areas: phonetic and phonemic disorders. Phonetic disorders include errors that result from the child's inability to plan or execute the proper motoric movements or gestures involved in sound production. Phonemic disorders, on the other hand, describe errors in which the child is able to execute the motor movements involved in a particular sound production but does not use this sound correctly in some linguistic contexts. While it is easy to describe these two categories of phonologic disturbance, it is not always easy to classify a child's error patterns neatly into one or the other category. If the child displays a few errors, the classification system works well. However, as speech intelligibility declines and the number of misarticulated phonemes increases, this distinction is more difficult to make. Therefore, one should expect both motor and cognitive-linguistic difficulties in any speech-sound production problem (Hoffman et al. 1989).

Assessment of Articulation Skills

When determining the need for treatment, one must consider the intelligibility of the person's connected speech. There are formal measures of intelligibility (Kent et al. 1994). This task, however, frequently is accomplished with a category rating (i.e., mild, moderate, or severe) that is determined as the patient converses with the clinician. The assessment of intelligibility largely relies on the subjective opinion of the examiner, whose ratings can be influenced by the number of sounds in error, the consistency of the misarticulation, and the frequency at which error sound occurs in the language. Shriberg and Kwiatkowski (1980) found that error type (i.e., deletions of sounds and manner of production changes) correlated more highly with intelligibility ratings than did the total number of errors. Therefore, it appears that judgments of intelligibility are influenced by error type and the number of errors present. The role of prosody in these assessments has received little attention and is worthy of continued research.

After intelligibility has been assessed, most articulation evaluations proceed with a speech-sound inventory, often referred to as an *articulation test*. The goal of this technique is to identify sounds that appear to be particularly troublesome for the patient. In this assessment procedure, each phoneme and most of the consonant clusters of the language are tested in each word position (i.e., initial, medial, and final). Some of these tests also evaluate vowel productions.

There are several problems with traditional articulation tests. The first obstacle is how to elicit the desired phoneme. Since children are variable in their production of sounds, they may be able to produce the sound correctly at the end of words or occasionally in the initial position of words. This type of variability can be attributed to differences in phonetic context. This context can facilitate the production of a sound when it occurs in a particular sound sequence. It would be possible, therefore, on a standardized test to ask a child to produce a target sound in the one word in which he or she consistently mispronounces a sound. Another problem in eliciting a target sound involves using words that most children mispronounce (e.g., *valentine*). While *valentine* may be one of the only words that a child knows that begins with /v/, it typically is pronounced as "balentime," even when the young child can produce an adequate /v/. Lastly, differences in testing procedures also produce discrepancies in phoneme productions. In this case, children may be able to produce a sound after a clinician's model that they may not be able to make in spontaneous conversation (Paynter and Bumpas 1977). Therefore, a clinician should never rely solely on the results of speech-sound inventories when making a diagnosis and determining the need for treatment.

The results of the intelligibility assessment and single-word articulation test determine the direction of the rest of the assessment procedure. A complete evaluation includes stimulability and contextual testing, which assess the consistency of the misarticulation. If numerous sounds are in error and the child's speech is difficult to understand, the clinician also considers a pattern analysis to identify any deviant phonologic rules that may be in operation.

Stimulability testing assesses one's ability to produce a particular phoneme in isolation and syllables. This type of test provides insight into the ease and stability with which a target sound can be elicited from the patient. Highly stimulable sounds should be considered first for remediation (Bernthal and Bankson 1993). Contextual or deep testing (as introduced by McDonald [1964]), on the other hand, analyzes articulatory skill in different phonetic contexts. Deep testing is useful in identifying one or more contexts in which the child is able to produce an error sound correctly. In this manner, it capitalizes on the inconsistent nature of most misarticulations by relying on the facilitating effects of coarticulation. For example, Hoffman et al. (1977) reported that certain vowels and consonants actually facilitated the production of /r/ in persons who typically mispronounce /r/. Therefore, stimulability and contextual testing can provide valuable information when the clinician is determining which sound(s) to treat.

The goal of pattern analysis (or the phonologic process test) is to identify the presence of phonologic rules or the absence of particular distinctive features that may be interfering with speech intelligibility. Some of the protocols devised for this type of testing are modeled after the single-word inventories, while others use a sample of the child's spontaneous speech. The goal is to identify the components of the child's phonetic and phonemic inventories (i.e., an independent analysis) and then to compare the child's word productions to the desired adult form (i.e., a relational analysis). The intent is to identify groups of sounds that are misarticulated in the same way. This type of testing identifies phonologic processes that are in need of remediation as opposed to individual phonemes. Taken together, the results of all of these tests provide the examiner with a fairly thorough appraisal of the child's production capabilities.

TABLE 6.4 Selected Phonologic and Grammatical Characteristics of African-American English (AAE), Southern English (S), and Southern White Nonstandard English (SWNS)

Features	Descriptions	Examples	AAE	S	SWNS
Consonant cluster reduction (general)	Deletion of second of two consonants in word final position belonging to the same base word	"tes" (test)	X	—	X
	Deletion of past tense -ed morpheme from a base word, resulting in a consonant cluster that is subsequently reduced	"rub" (rubbed)	X	—	X
	Plural formations of reduced consonant cluster assume phonetic representations of sibilants and affricatives	"desses" (desks)	X	—	X
/θ/ phoneme	/f/ for /θ/ between vowels and in word final position	"nofin" (nothing)	X	—	—
/ð/ phoneme	/d/ for /ð/ in word initial position	"dis" (this)	X	—	—
	/v/ for /ð/ between vowels and in word final positions	"bavin" (bathing) "bave" (bath)	X	—	—
Vowel nasalization	No contrast between vowels /ɪ/ and /ɛ/ before nasals	"pin" (pin or pen)	—	X	—
The /r/ and /ɪ/ phonemes	Deletion preceding a consonant	"ba game" (ball game)	X	X	—

Source: O Taylor. Language and Communication Differences. In GH Shames, EH Wiig (eds), Human Communication Disorders: An Introduction. Columbus, OH: Merrill, 1990.

It is also essential to consider dialect patterns in any assessment procedure. As mentioned earlier, a dialect is a consistent variation of a language, reflected in pronunciation, grammar, or vocabulary, that is used by a particular subgroup of the general population (Taylor 1994). These speech-language patterns are usually associated with sociocultural or ethnic identifications and are often influenced by socioeconomic status. Some examples of dialects include AAE vernacular, Hispanic English vernacular, Mandarin Chinese vernacular, Southern dialect, Appalachian dialect, and Boston dialect. Clinicians must remember that these dialects are not deviant forms of SAE but, instead, represent language differences and should not be considered for treatment unless performance lies outside the cultural norm for the region or group. Tables 6.4, 6.5, and 6.6 are included as illustrations of how native language and culture can

TABLE 6.5   Examples of Spanish-Language Influence on English Phonology

Features	Environments	Examples
/z/ phoneme	/s/ for /z/ in all positions	"sip" (zip); "racer" (razor)
/g/ phoneme	/n/ for /ŋ/ in the word final position	"sin" (sing)
/θ/ phoneme	/t/ or /s/ for /θ/ in all positions	"tin" or "sin" (thin)
/ð/ phoneme	/d/ for /ð/ in all positions	"den" (then); "ladder" (lather)
/i/ phoneme	/iy/ for /i/ in all positions	"cheap" (chip)

Source: LRL Cheng. Cross cultural and linguistic considerations in working with Asian populations. ASHA 1987;29:35.

TABLE 6.6   Phonologic Patterns of Interference in Three Chinese Languages

Mandarin

Substitutions	/s/ for /θ/; /z/ for /ð/; /f/ for /v/
Confusions	/r/ for /l/ and /l/ for /r/
Omissions	Final consonants
Additions	/ə/ in blends, i.e., "belue" (blue) and "gooda" (good)
Approximations	/tç/ for /tʃ/; /ç/ for /s/
Shortening or lengthening of vowels	"seat" (sit) and "it" (eat)

Cantonese

Substitutions	/s/ for /θ/; /s/ for /z/; /f/ for /v/; /w/ for /v/; /s/ for /ʃ/; /l/ for /r/; /e/ for /i/
Omissions	Final consonants
Additions	/ə/ in blends
Vowels	/ɪ/, /ʌ/, and /ɔ/ are difficult for Cantonese speakers

Vietnamese

Substitutions	/s/ for /θ/; /ʃ/ for /tʃ/; /b/ for /p/; /z/ for /dz/; /d/ for /ð/; /d/ for /dʒ/
Omissions	Final consonants and consonant blends: /t/, /æ/, /ʊ/, and /ə/
Vowels	May be difficult at times

Source: LRL Cheng. Cross cultural and linguistic considerations in working with Asian populations. ASHA 1987;29:35.

influence the articulatory patterns of a particular group. Nevertheless, one should not generalize features of a particular dialect to all the members of a particular subculture, since many members may not have the same linguistic patterns (Wolfram 1986).

Some researchers suggest that speech-evaluation procedures should be adapted to include local norms for the interpretation of test results (Taylor and Payne 1983; Haynes and Moran 1989). Washington and Craig (1992) tested this assumption with African-American children in the Detroit area. They found that adjusting the scores of the *Arizona Articulation Proficiency Scale* did not provide any clinically significant results. In other words, the original Arizona Articulation Proficiency Scale scoring procedures did not penalize these children for using AAE productions. Washington and Craig suggested that the need for such scoring adjustments may be dictated by certain regional or cultural dialects. These findings are in opposition to previous research (Cole and Taylor 1990), which advocated the use of scoring adjustments. More research is needed in this area and on other dialects of English.

Finally, it is important to assess the patient's attitude toward his or her speech. It may be that the patient is not too bothered by his or her lisp or that a small child is extremely anxious about being teased about his or her unintelligibility. Experience has indicated that the latter patient can be motivated to alter his or her speech patterns because of the reward of increased socialization. Other persons get the attention they desire because of the articulation impairment. A case in point is television commercials. Some children are selected for certain acting roles because they lisp or substitute /w/ for /r/. These types of speech patterns are considered cute and are believed to assist the television viewer in remembering the advertised product. In a more frequently encountered situation, some children maintain a childlike speech pattern because parents or primary caregivers encourage its use. The use of baby talk might be acceptable at home, but rarely will it be accepted by the child's peers or educators. On the other hand, it is possible that a parent may be too tough on a child who is having difficulty speaking. As a consequence, this child may withdraw and choose not to interact with others. For the above reasons, it would appear important to consider social and emotional factors in the maintenance of a speech-sound disorder.

Sometimes patients desire to alter their articulatory patterns due to vocational concerns. They may feel as though a misarticulation, such as a lisp, negatively influences their interactions at the workplace. If the person is bilingual or bidialectal, he or she may request accent-reduction therapy to obtain a promotion or to pursue a certain career. It is therefore apparent that good speech production has many socio-cultural advantages.

Selection of the Treatment Target

Several factors must be considered in the selection of which sounds to train. As mentioned earlier, the stimulability and contextual testing results can be used to identify sounds and contexts for treatment. It is a good idea to determine the highest linguistic level at which the child is stimulable and then start treatment at that level. For instance, if the child is stimulable at the word level, then training should begin there. If the child needs more work at the syllable level, then training should start there. Other factors to consider in sound selection include: ease of production, frequency of occurrence in the native language, and the age of phoneme acquisition. These considerations help the clinician select a target that the child can produce so he or she will experience success early in the treatment process. If one is interested in pursuing a phonologic approach to treatment, these same influences need to be considered. (See Dyson and Robinson

[1987] for a more complete discussion of this idea.) The goal is always to achieve maximum intelligibility (i.e., reduce the number of misarticulations) in the shortest period of time.

Approaches to Remediation

There are two basic strategies in the treatment of articulation disorders. In the motor approach, production errors are presumed to arise from the person's inability to perform the complex motor skills required for the articulation of speech sounds. The idea is to train correct sound productions and practice these motor movements at increasing levels of linguistic complexity. The cognitive-linguistic approach, on the other hand, is based on the idea that patients produce phonologic errors because they have not learned to use the sounds contrastively (i.e., to make a difference in meaning). This form of treatment involves training critical contrasts through minimal pairs (i.e., using words that differ only in the contrast to be trained), such as *beg* and *bed*, and activities requiring the application of the appropriate phonologic rule. It may be necessary to treat both motor and cognitive-linguistic impairments in one person; however, treatment focuses on one aspect more than the other.

Stages of the Treatment Continuum

Perceptual Training

Many treatment protocols begin with some form of speech-sound discrimination. Such activities involve making same/different judgments about speech stimuli. These discriminations are trained initially using distinctions produced by another talker and then move on to self-discrimination activities. This approach assumes that perception of differences between sounds (i.e., between the error sound and the intended sound) is a prerequisite to production. While this form of training can be beneficial, more research is needed to establish a clear relationship between perception and production.

Another form of perceptual training is known as *conceptualization training* or *minimal contrast training*. With these models, the child is trained to divide words or syllables into classes or categories. In this way, the child develops an awareness of patterns of similarity or difference between the error and target sounds. This type of approach is commonly used when attempting to add new features or phonemes to the child's phonetic inventory.

Production Training

During production training, the clinician attempts to elicit a target behavior from the patient and then to stabilize it at a voluntary level. Four basic techniques are used: imitation, contextual influences, phonetic placement, and successive approximation. Once a target sound is selected, the clinician attempts to establish the patient's ability to produce that sound. Since most error productions are inconsistent in nature, the clinician begins by assessing the person's ability to produce the sound on his or her own.

If the person is unable to imitate the target sound, the next step is to identify a phonetic environment in which the error sound is produced correctly. While it seems that consonant-vowel or vowel-consonant sequences are easier because they are presumed to be less complex linguistically, Gallagher and Shriner (1975) found consonant blends (consonant-consonant environment) to work better. Therefore, the clinician should consider the use of consonant clusters in the training of some phonetic distinctions.

The last two techniques, phonetic placement and successive approximation, should be used only when the first two strategies are unsuccessful. The phonetic placement technique involves verbal descriptions, accompanied by visual and tactile cues (when needed), that tell the patient where to place the articulators. Successive approximation, on the other hand, breaks complex behavioral responses down into a series of successive steps. This process is similar to that of shaping: The clinician proceeds with a response that the patient can make and then progresses through small steps that move closer and closer to the target, until the desired behavior is elicited. Once the patient is able to produce correctly or at least approximate the error sound, the clinician selects a treatment strategy.

Treatment Approaches

The Traditional Approach

The assumption underlying the traditional approach to treatment is that the perception or discrimination of the difference between the target and the error sound is faulty (Van Riper 1939). After the person is able to perceive the target sound, correction of the error involves practice of increasingly complex motor skills, usually in terms of increasingly complex linguistic structures. Treatment begins with sensory-perceptual training, in which the patient learns to distinguish the error sound from the target sound in other's productions and eventually his or her own productions. Once the target sound is accurately perceived, production training is initiated. The clinician helps the patient acquire and stabilize the target sound at increasingly complex linguistic levels (e.g., syllable, word position, and sentences). After the patient is able to produce the target correctly, the focus of treatment moves toward transfer of this correct production to other environments (i.e., generalization). This form of treatment is most useful when there are few sounds in error.

Sensory-Motor Treatment

The sensory-motor treatment protocol emphasizes production over discrimination. McDonald (1964) proposed that learning to articulate properly is based on motor practice in different phonetic contexts. This motor practice occurs in syllables, because it is presumed to heighten the auditory, tactile, and proprioceptive awareness of the speaker. The goal of the treatment is to train correct production of the error sound in all phonetic contexts. As such, the patient practices the target sound in bisyllables and trisyllables that vary the vowels, consonants, and stress patterns between the syllables in a systematic and increasingly more complex fashion. The intent is to heighten the patient's awareness of motor productions. After this type of strict motor practice, the focus of treatment shifts to finding facilitating contexts for that sound production at the word level. Eventually, the treatment moves on to short sentences with the facilitating context in them. Finally, the phonetic context is manipulated so as to provide more difficult contextual productions for the patient. At this point, the patient's production of the target sound should be stabilized in conversation.

Linguistic Approaches

In the linguistic approaches (Shriberg and Kwiatkowski 1980; Hodson and Paden 1983; Gierut 1989), the clinician looks for classes of sounds that have like error patterns, hereafter referred to as *phonologic rules*. For example, the clinician may note that the child tends to omit final consonants. Instead of teaching each phoneme individually in all word positions, he or she would target the concept of final consonants and teach the child to put a sound on the end of words that differ by final consonant. One way to do this is through contrast training (Gierut 1989). With this method, the client is asked to identify and later produce the target sounds when placed in contexts that differ by only the sound or phonetic feature to be trained (i.e., minimal pairs). In other techniques, a particular contrast is selected and the entire treatment session focuses on the perception and production of that rule using a few representative words (Hodson and Paden 1983). The goal of this form of treatment is to train the linguistic concept that underlies the production of several sounds and then look for generalization to untrained environments.

Conclusion

The process of articulation is complex, and a disorder in speech production can result from a number of physical, cognitive, and linguistic influences. Only after a clinician has carefully considered each of these areas can an effective treatment program be developed. There are several different ways to manage a speech sound production problem, and most patients will respond quite favorably to treatment.

References

Bernthal JE, Bankson NW. Articulation and Phonological Disorders. Englewood Cliffs, NJ: Prentice-Hall, 1993.

Bleile KM, Wallach H. A sociolinguistic investigation of the speech of African-American preschoolers. Am J Speech Lang Pathol 1992;1:54–62.

Borden GJ, Harris KS, Catena L. Oral feedback II. An electromyographic study of speech under nerve-block anesthesia. J Phon 1973a;1:297–308.

Borden GJ, Harris KS, Oliver W. Oral feedback I. Variability of the effect of nerve-block anesthesia upon speech. J Phon 1973b;1:289–295.

Cole P, Taylor O. Performance of working class African-American children on three tests of articulation. Lang Speech Hear Serv Schools 1990;21:171–176.

Dunn C, Davis B. Phonological process occurrence in phonologically disordered children. Appl Psycholing 1983;4:187–207.

Dyson A, Robinson T. The effect of phonologic analysis procedures on the selection of potential remediation targets. Lang Speech Hear Serv Schools 1987;18:364–377.

Gallagher T, Shriner T. Contextual variables related to inconsistent /s/ and /z/ production in the spontaneous speech of children. J Speech Hear Res 1975;18:623–633.

Gierut J. Maximal opposition approach to phonologic treatment. J Speech Hear Disord 1989;54:9–19.

Goldstein BA, Iglesias A. Phonological patterns in normally developing Spanish-speaking 3- and 4-year-olds of Puerto Rican descent. Lang Speech Hear Serv Schools 1996;27:82–90.

Grunwell P. Clinical Phonology. Rockville, MD: Aspen Systems Corporation, 1982.

Haelsig P, Madison C. A study of phonologic processes exhibited by 3-, 4- and 5-year-old children. Lang Speech Hear Serv Schools 1986;17:107–114.

Haynes W, Moran M. A cross-sectional developmental study of final consonant production in southern black children from preschool through third grade. Lang Speech Hear Serv Schools 1989;20:400–406.

Hodson B, Paden E. Phonological processes which characterize unintelligible and intelligible speech in early childhood. J Speech Hear Disord 1981;46:369–373.

Hodson B, Paden E. Targeting Intelligible Speech. San Diego: College Hill Press, 1983.

Hoffman P, Schuckers G, Daniloff R. Children's Phonetic Disorders: Theory and Treatment. Boston: College Hill Press, 1989.

Hoffman P, Schuckers G, Ratusnik D. Contextual coarticulatory inconsistencies of /r/ misarticulation. J Speech Hear Res 1977;20:631–643.

Horii Y, House AS, Li K-P, Ringel RL. Acoustic characteristics of speech produced without oral sensation. J Speech Hear Res 1973;16:67–77.

Ingram D. Phonological Disability in Children. New York: Elsevier, 1976.

Kent R, Miolo G, Bloedel S. The intelligibility of children's speech: a review of evaluation procedures. Am J Speech Lang Pathol 1994;3:81–95.

Lynch J. Tongue reduction surgery: efficacy and relevance to the profession. ASHA 1990;1:59–61.

McDonald E. Articulation Testing and Treatment: A Sensory-Motor Approach. Pittsburgh: Stanwix House, 1964.

McEnery E, Gaines F. Tongue-tie in infants and children. J Pediatr 1941;18:252–255.

Oller D, Eilers R. The role of audition in infant babbling. Child Dev 1988;59:441–449.

Oller D. The Emergence of the Sounds of Speech in Infancy. In G Yeni-Komshian, J Kavanaugh, C Ferguson (eds), Child Phonology. Production (Vol. I). New York: Academic, 1980.

Paden E, Matthies M, Novak M. Recovery from OME-related phonologic delay following tube placement. J Speech Hear Disord 1989;54:94–100.

Paden E, Novak M, Beiter A. Predictors of phonologic inadequacy in young children prone to otitis media. J Speech Hear Disord 1987;52:232–242.

Paynter E, Bumpas T. Imitative and spontaneous articulatory assessment of three-year-old children. J Speech Hear Disord 1977;42:119–125.

Poole E. Genetic development of articulation of consonant sounds in speech. Elementary Eng Rev 1934;11:159–161.

Prather E, Hedrick D, Kern C. Articulation development in children aged two to four years. J Speech Hear Res 1975;40:179–191.

Putnam AHB, Ringel RL. Some observations of articulation during labial sensory deprivation. J Speech Hear Res 1972;15:529–542.

Ringel RL. Oral sensation and perception: a selective review. ASHA 1970;5:188–206.

Roberts J, Burchinal M, Footo M. Phonological process decline from 2.5 to 8 years. J Commun Disord 1990;23:205–217.

Roberts J, Burchinal M, Koch M, et al. Otitis media in early childhood and its relationship to later phonologic development. J Speech Hear Disord 1988;53:424–432.

Roberts J, Medley L. Otitis media and speech-language sequelae in young children: current issues in management. Am J Speech-Lang Pathol 1995;4:15–24.

Sander E. When are speech sounds learned? J Speech Hear Disord 1972;37:55–63.

Schwartz A, Goldman R. Variables influencing performance on speech sound discrimination tests. J Speech Hear Res 1974;17:25–32.

Seymour H, Seymour C. Black English and Standard American English contrasts in consonantal development of four- and five-year-old children. J Speech Hear Disord 1981;46:274–280.

Sherman D, Geith A. Speech sound discrimination and articulation skill. J Speech Hear Disord 1967;10:277–280.

Shriberg L, Kwiatkowski J. Natural Process Analysis. New York: Wiley, 1980.

Stark R. Features of infant sounds: the emergence of cooing. J Child Lang 1978;5:379–390.

Stoel-Gammon C. Normal and disordered phonology in two-year-olds. Top Lang Disord 1991;11:21–32.

Taylor O, Payne K. Culturally valid testing: a proactive approach. Top Lang Disord 1983;3:8–20.

Taylor O. Communication and Communication Disorders in a Multicultural Society. In F Minifie (ed), Introduction to Communication Sciences and Disorders. San Diego: Singular Publishing Group, 1994.

Templin M. Certain Language Skills in Children: Their Development and Interrelationships [Institute of Child Welfare, Monograph 26]. Minneapolis: University of Minnesota Press, 1957.

Van Riper C. Speech Correction: Principles and Methods. New York: Prentice-Hall, 1939.

Vihman M, Ferguson C, Elbert M. Phonological development from babbling to speech: common tendencies and individual differences. Appl Psycholing 1986;7:3–40.

Warren D, Dalston R, Morr K, et al. The speech regulating system: temporal and aerodynamic responses to velopharyngeal inadequacy. J Speech Hear Res 1989;32:566–575.

Washington J, Craig H. Articulation test performances of low-income, African-American preschoolers with communication impairments. Lang Speech Hear Serv Schools 1992;23:203–207.

Weiner P. Auditory discrimination and articulation. J Speech Hear Disord 1967;32:19–28.

Wellman B, Case I, Mengurt I, Bradbury D. Speech sounds of young children. University of Iowa Studies in Child Welfare 1931;5.

Winitz H, Bellerose B. Effects of pretraining on sound discrimination learning. J Speech Hear Res 1963;6:171–180.

Winitz H. Articulatory Acquisition and Behavior. Englewood Cliffs, NJ: Prentice-Hall, 1969.

Wolfram W. Language Variation in the United States. In O Taylor (ed), Nature of Communication Disorders in Culturally and Linguistically Diverse Populations. San Diego: College Hill Press, 1986.

Wood B. Children and Communication: Verbal and Nonverbal Language Development. Englewood Cliffs, NJ: Prentice-Hall, 1976.

Chapter 6   Study Questions

1. Describe the two major periods of speech-sound development. In general, which types of speech sounds do children acquire first? Which do they acquire last?
2. What are some of the factors that contribute to the development of a speech-sound disorder?
3. What is the difference between a motor disturbance (i.e., articulation disorder) and a cognitive-linguistic disorder (i.e., a phonologic disorder)? Give examples.
4. What are some phonologic processes that describe the speech-sound errors typically produced by children? Give an example of each process.
5. How would a treatment approach focusing on articulatory movements differ from a cognitive-linguistic approach?

7   Voice and Voice Disorders

Mary V. Andrianopoulos

Our voices reveal who we are and how we feel, giving considerable insight into the structures and function of certain parts of the body.

—I.E. Titze

Oral communication involves an intricate interplay between the brain and the vocal system. That is, the ability to communicate requires the integration of several intellectual and physical processes: cognition, resonation, articulation, phonation, and respiration. The foundation of verbal communication is phonation, which is the physical act of sound production by means of vocal fold interaction with the exhaled air stream. Resonation and respiration, in addition to phonation, are aspects of voice production. Clinical voice disorders are a family of voice disorders. The specific components that are affected involve the processes of phonation and resonation. Each voice disorder, or dysphonia, can vary according to the set of symptoms, psychosocial manifestations, and etiology. Vocal symptoms can indicate the mechanism or pathophysiology of a particular voice disorder and, thus, assist the examiner and clinician in the differential diagnosis of the dysphonia.

To understand voice production and the discipline of clinical voice disorders, one must first acknowledge the structures and function of the vocal mechanism. This chapter acquaints the reader with the anatomy, physiology, and neurology of the vocal system. The acoustic perceptual features of phonation are presented as clinical correlates of normal voice production and abnormal vocal characteristics suggestive of a voice disorder. Voice disorders are explained in terms of organic and inorganic etiologies. Moreover, some clinical considerations are provided to address psychosocial and cultural aspects of voice disorders.

Phonation: Normal Versus Abnormal Voice

Thoughts, emotions, and feelings are transformed into verbal messages through a series of complex neuromuscular and musculoskeletal processes. Several sensorimotor systems activate the respiratory, articulatory, phonatory, and resonatory systems with precise timing, precision, and intensity to generate an acoustic signal. Malfunction of any one or all of these systems, regardless of the cause, results in a dysphonia.

A voice is like a blueprint. People are identified with a particular voice and vocal quality, regardless of how pleasant or unpleasant it sounds. Typically, a voice is perceived as sounding normal if it meets certain expectations associated with a person's community, society, culture, age, gender, and profession. The criteria for judging a voice as normal, as opposed to abnormal, are broad and poorly defined. According to Aronson (1990), the definition of a given voice as normal or abnormal depends on the orientation of the person making the judgment. The following are general standards for normal voice (Johnson 1965):

- Vocal quality is pleasant when marked by musical quality and the absence of noise.
- Pitch level is adequate and socially appropriate to the age and gender of the speaker.
- Loudness is appropriate to transmit the speaker's message under ordinary speaking conditions without drawing undesirable attention to the speaker.
- Vocal quality is flexible in that pitch, loudness, and paralinguistic features aid in the expression of emotions, attitudes, and feelings.

A voice disorder exists when the quality, pitch, loudness, and flexibility of a person's voice differs from the voices of others of a similar age, gender, and cultural group (Aronson 1990). Although in general people may pay little attention to the specific acoustical properties of voice, clinicians and research scientists are able to make clinical judgments based on acoustics that aid in the differential diagnosis of voice disorders. How the voice sounds and the manner in which one is perceived by the listener are referred to as the *acoustic perceptual qualities of voice*. A person's voice is subjectively judged as being too high or low in pitch, too loud or soft, rough or smooth, and strained-strangled or breathy. All of these symptoms have physiologic, neurologic, psychological, and cognitive-linguistic bases.

Perkins (1971) suggested that the following information can be extracted from the voice: (1) physical health, (2) emotional health, (3) personality, (4) identity, and (5) aesthetic orientation. Speech-language pathologists and lay persons frequently make subjective judgments about the speaker's personality, emotional state, culture, mental health, and attitude on the basis of his or her vocal quality. A speaker lacking volume or intensity in the voice may be perceived by the listener as being insecure, shy, or lacking confidence. A loud, low-pitched voice may signify confidence, power, and assertiveness. Strained phonation may be perceived as emotional or physical stress and tension manifested in the speaker's voice. A person with a quivering voice may be judged as nervous. The sound of a person's voice may, on occasion, be misleading to both the clinician and the listener, in that the paralinguistic features of the voice can be inaccurately diagnosed and subjectively misinterpreted.

Recognition and identification of an abnormal voice is important to the speech-language pathologist. An abnormal voice may signify illness, disease, or a communication disorder. Aberrant vocal qualities are symptoms of a voice problem or voice disorder. The etiology or the cause of an abnormal voice should be investigated with the help of medical practitioners and clinical specialists in general medicine, speech-language pathology, otolaryngology, neurology, psychology, and psychiatry (depending on the nature and scope of the problem). Determining the cause of the voice problem assists the speech-language pathologist in selecting the most appropriate course of action for treatment.

Anatomy and Physiology of the Vocal Mechanism

The Larynx

One of the most important structures of the vocal mechanism is the larynx. The larynx is a tube-like structure that is attached inferiorly to the trachea and superiorly to the pharynx. The larynx is positioned anteriorly to the third and sixth cervical vertebrae of the spinal column. The larynx serves many functions. Biologically, the larynx prevents foreign substances, such as food, liquids, and secretions, from entering the lungs. The larynx, which is composed of cartilage, membranes, and muscles, generates voice for communication purposes. The body of the larynx is composed of nine cartilages: three paired (arytenoids, corniculates, and cuneiforms) and three unpaired (thyroid, cricoid, and epiglottis) (Figure 7.1).

Cartilages

The thyroid cartilage is the largest of the laryngeal structures. Anteriorly, the thyroid cartilage has a large protuberance known as the Adam's apple, which is particularly pronounced in men. The thyroid cartilage forms the anterior and lateral walls of the larynx. Inferiorly, the thyroid cartilage articulates with the cricoid cartilage via the

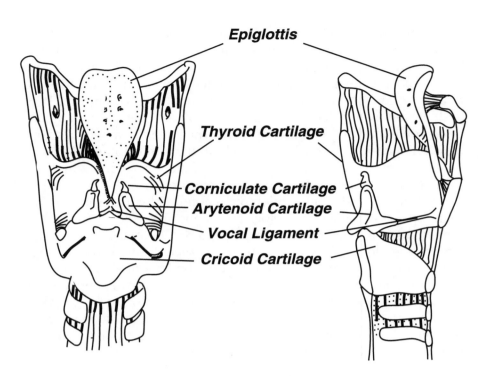

FIGURE 7.1 *The larynx and laryngeal cartilages.*

cricothyroid joint. The primary movement of the thyroid on the cricoid is rotation; however, some sliding is possible. The rotation is important to the pitch-changing mechanism of phonation.

The cricoid cartilage, located below the thyroid cartilage, is a round structure shaped like a signet ring. On the posterior-superior border of the cricoid cartilage rest the paired arytenoid cartilages. The arytenoid cartilages are two small, pyramid-shaped structures that articulate with the cricoid cartilage via the cricoarytenoid joint. The cricoarytenoid joint permits gliding and rocking movement of the arytenoid cartilages in medial and lateral directions, as well as forward and backward. These movements are crucial for phonation and voice production.

The cuneiform cartilages are embedded in the mucous membrane of the aryepiglottic folds extending from the sides of the epiglottis to the apexes of the arytenoid cartilages. The cuneiform cartilages are paired, elongated rods of elastic cartilage located anterior and lateral to the corniculate cartilages. The cuneiform cartilages are believed to lend support to the aryepiglottic folds in that they help maintain the opening of the larynx. The epiglottis is a long, broad structure that is flat and attaches to the thyroid cartilage via the thyroepiglottic ligament. The anterior surface of the epiglottis is connected to the body of the hyoid bone by an elastic ligament, which is the hyoepiglottic ligament. The superior portion of the epiglottis projects upward toward the base of the tongue. In humans, the epiglottis is believed to func-

TABLE 7.1 Extrinsic and Intrinsic Laryngeal Muscles

Muscles	Function
Extrinsic	
Infrahyoid	
Sternohyoid	Depresses hyoid
Sternothyroid	Depresses thyroid
Thyrohyoid	Decreases thyroid to hyoid distance
	With hyoid fixed, raises larynx
	With larynx fixed, depresses larynx
Omohyoid	Depresses hyoid
Suprahyoid	
Stylohyoid	Elevates hyoid
Mylohyoid	Elevates hyoid and tongue
	Depresses the jaw
Geniohyoid	Elevates and draws hyoid forward
	Depresses jaw
Digastric	
Anterior belly	Depresses jaw
	Raises hyoid
Posterior belly	Elevates and retracts hyoid
Stylopharyngeus	Elevates pharynx
Intrinsic	
Cricothyroid	
Pars recta	Rotates thyroid downward
Pars oblique	Pulls thyroid forward
Lateral cricoarytenoid	Adducts vocal folds
Posterior cricoarytenoid	Abducts vocal folds
	Dilates glottis
Oblique arytenoid	Approximates arytenoids
Transverse arytenoid	Approximates arytenoids
Thyroarytenoid	
Thyrovocalis	Tenses vocal folds
Thyromuscularis	Relaxes vocal folds
Aryepiglottis	Pulls epiglottis downward

tion as a protective device that prevents food from entering the larynx during swallow.

The hyoid bone is not part of the larynx; however, this bony structure is important to the physiologic functions of the larynx. The hyoid bone is located superiorly to the thyroid cartilage and resembles a horseshoe. The hyoid bone is suspended in the neck region by several muscles and ligaments. This structure serves as a surface for attachment of specific laryngeal muscle groups.

Laryngeal Musculature

The laryngeal musculature is comprised of two sets of muscle groups: the extrinsic laryngeal muscles and the intrinsic laryngeal muscles (Table 7.1). The extrinsic laryngeal muscles attach to one of the laryngeal cartilages at one end and to a bony structure outside the larynx on the other end. The name of each muscle is indicative of the structures to which they attach on each end. The extrinsic laryngeal muscles, in general, function to move the larynx as a total unit. The extrinsic muscles are subdivided into two groups: the suprahyoid and the infrahyoid. As the names suggest, the infrahyoid muscles attach below the hyoid bone and pull the hyoid bone and larynx downward to a lower position in the neck. The suprahyoid muscles attach above the hyoid bone and pull the hyoid bone forward, backward, and upward.

Laryngeal Mechanics of Phonation

The intrinsic laryngeal muscles change the shape of the glottis and modify the vibration of the vocal folds. These actions are largely dependent on contraction of specific laryngeal muscles and movement of particular cartilages in the larynx. The laryngeal musculature can be categorized according to the effect they have on the vocal folds: abduction, adduction, tension, and relaxation. The sound and vocal quality of a person's voice is shaped, modified, and altered on the basis of the laryngeal movements and mechanisms.

The bodies of the two vocal folds are composed of thyroarytenoid muscle, which attach posteriorly to the vocal processes of the arytenoid cartilages and anteriorly to the thyroid cartilage. The glottis is the space that exists between the vocal folds in either adducted (movement of the vocal folds medially) or abducted (movement of the vocal folds laterally) positions. During phonation, the vocal folds must be drawn together to vibrate. Movements between the cricoid and arytenoid cartilages on the cricoarytenoid joint permit the vocal folds to either adduct or abduct. Contraction of the lateral cricoarytenoid muscle permits the arytenoid cartilages to be brought together toward the midline, and thus the vocal folds are adducted. In contrast, the vocal folds abduct as the arytenoids move away from the midline on contraction of the posterior cricoarytenoid muscle.

The movements between the cricoid and thyroid cartilages on the cricothyroid joint are also important for phonation, in that their actions modify tension and length of the vocal folds. Contraction of the cricothyroid muscle functions to stretch and elongate the vocal folds. Such actions cause the vocal folds to become tense. Contraction of the thyroarytenoid muscle primarily relaxes the vocal folds. Although some controversy exists between the exact function of the thyromuscularis and the thyrovocalis muscles, the thyroarytenoid muscle as a whole is a relaxor of the vocal folds. The tension and relaxation mechanisms of the vocal folds are important to phonation because they modify pitch (Figure 7.2).

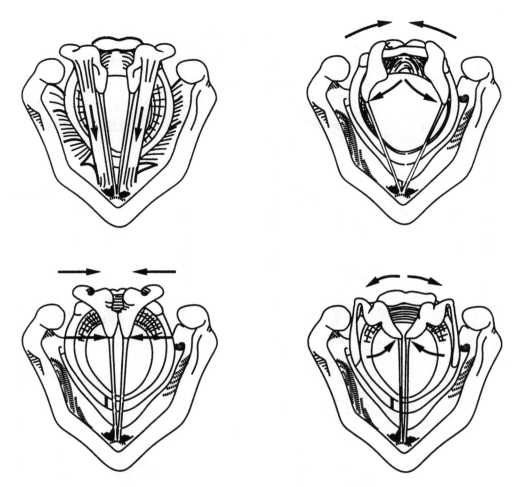

FIGURE 7.2 *Various movements of the laryngeal cartilages. (Adapted from AE Aronson. Clinical Voice Disorders [3rd ed]. New York: Thieme, 1990.)*

Neurology of Phonation and Resonation

Motor innervation to the muscles in the larynx and pharynx is provided by the tenth cranial nerve, the vagus. This nerve is significant to phonation and resonation. Damage to any part of this nerve modifies the integrity and neuromuscular coordination of the vocal mechanism. The effects are observed clinically in terms of weakness, paralysis, asymmetry, imprecision, and slow or reduced range of movement of the vocal folds and soft palate (bilaterally or unilaterally depending on the extent of damage). Acoustically, the speaker's voice sounds abnormal and unpleasant. The constellation of motor speech and vocal

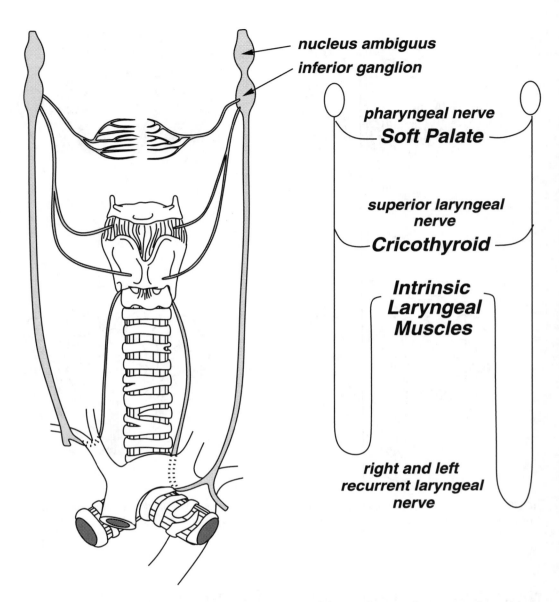

FIGURE 7.3 *Anatomic and schematic illustrations of the tenth cranial nerve. (Adapted from AE Aronson. Clinical Voice Disorders [3rd ed]. New York: Thieme, 1990.)*

symptoms can be generalized to the location of breakdown within or surrounding the vagus nerve.

The vagus nerve originates in the nucleus ambiguus, which is located intracranially deep within the medulla on the right and left sides of the brainstem. Each pair of nerves converge into a single trunk before exiting the cranium via the jugular foramen, which are paired openings located at the base of the skull. As this point, each vagus nerve divides into three branches: the pharyngeal nerve, superior laryngeal nerve, and recurrent laryngeal nerve (Figure 7.3).

The pharyngeal nerve emerges from the inferior or nodose ganglion and descends inferiorly to form the pharyngeal plexus. Fibers from the pharyngeal nerve project into the pharynx and to all muscles of the soft palate, except for the tensor vela palatini. Contraction of these muscle groups modifies the velopharyngeal port and resonation of sound in that the nasal cavity is either opened or closed from the oral and pharyngeal cavities.

The superior laryngeal nerve also emerges from the interior (nodose) ganglion and descends inferiorly adjacent to the pharynx. At this point, the superior laryngeal nerve subdivides into two additional branches: the internal laryngeal nerve and the external laryngeal nerve. The internal laryngeal nerve projects into the thyroid membrane and again subdivides into an upper branch and lower branch. Both the upper and lower branches of the internal laryngeal nerve supply sensory innervation to the mucous membrane lining the epiglottis, larynx, aryepiglottic folds, vallecula, and base of the arytenoid cartilages. The external laryngeal branch of the superior laryngeal nerve descends into the sternothyroid muscles and provides motor innervation to the cricothyroid muscle.

The right and left recurrent laryngeal nerves descend into the lower neck and chest regions; however, unlike the other branches, their pathways are not bilaterally symmetric. The right recurrent laryngeal nerve descends to the subclavian artery, loops around it front to back, and begins to ascend adjacent to the trachea and esophagus. It pierces into the posterior portion of the larynx between the thyroid and cricoid cartilages. In contrast, the left recurrent laryngeal nerve descends inferiorly to the arch of the aorta, loops around it front to back, and, similarly, enters the larynx between the thyroid and cricoid cartilages. The right and left recurrent laryngeal nerves provide motor innervation to all the intrinsic laryngeal muscles with exception of the cricothyroid. These nerves also supply some sensory innervation to the intrinsic laryngeal muscles.

Phonation and the Acoustic Signal

During quiet breathing, the vocal folds are apart or abducted, and the glottis is open. During phonation, the vocal folds must be adducted or come together to vibrate. Adduction of the vocal folds compresses the air stream and increases the air pressure below the glottis. As subglottic air pressure significantly increases, puffs of air are released until the adducted vocal folds are blown apart. The air stream moves out of the vocal tract with some velocity via oral and nasal cavities. The vocal folds are set into vibration and acoustic energy is generated and modified as rapidly moving air molecules exit the resonating chambers of the vocal tract. The acoustic energy created is perceived as an acoustic signal or sound distinguished on the basis of its fundamental frequency, intensity, and tone.

The air pressure below the glottis immediately drops and a vacuum effect (i.e., Bernoulli's effect) is produced in the vocal tract. The vocal folds return back to their adducted position in part due to their elastic properties and Bernoulli's effect. This process is repeated as series of vibrations and sound waves are produced. These principles are based on the myoelastic-aerodynamic theory.

Vocal Parameters: Pitch, Loudness, and Quality

The vocal parameters that distinguish a voice are pitch, loudness, and quality. The acoustic perceptual qualities of voice are based on the physical properties of the acoustic signal. Pitch is the perceptual correlate of fundamental frequency measured in cycles per second, or hertz (Hz). The vocal folds, which are set into vibration by the air stream, produce sound-wave patterns. The pitch or the musical scale of a person's voice is largely dependent on the frequency with which the vocal folds vibrate. The opening and closing of the vocal folds constitutes one cycle, whereas repetitive patterns of vocal fold movement produce a series of cycles. Under normal conditions, the vibrations or sound-wave patterns repeat themselves in regular and evenly spaced intervals between cycles. Subjectively, such periodic vibrations of physical sound are perceived by the listener as pleasant or normal. In contrast, vibrations that are irregular and aperiodic lack tone or a specific fundamental frequency. Aperiodic wave forms are subjectively perceived as noise and create the impression of a voice that sounds unpleasant or abnormal.

Pitch

Variables that affect the rate of vocal fold vibration are mass, tension, and elasticity. Vocal folds of greater mass and length vibrate at a slower rate and, therefore, at a lower fundamental frequency. A voice produced with low fundamental frequency is perceived as low pitch. Men's vocal folds vibrate on average approximately 125–130 Hz. The vocal folds of women are usually less massive and, therefore, vibrate at a faster rate. Women's vocal folds on average vibrate approximately 200 Hz and acoustically are perceived as high pitch. Vocal folds that are tense vibrate at a faster rate compared to relaxed ones. As tension of the vocal folds increases, the rate of vibration increases, and the fundamental frequency of the voice is perceived as high pitch. Elasticity, which is the relative speed of return of the vocal folds to their rest position after they have been displaced, is closely related to tension. Elongation or stretching of the vocal folds reduces mass, increases tension, and increases the rate of vibration, and as a result pitch is raised to a higher frequency. The effects of these variables can be observed clinically. An anxious and nervous person tends to speak with a high-pitched voice due to the psychological and physiologic effects of these emotions on increased vocal fold tension and vibration.

Vocal Loudness

In addition to pitch, a speaker's voice can be judged as too loud or too soft. Loudness is the perceptual correlate of intensity measured in decibels. Loudness is largely based on the intensity of the acoustic signal or sound wave. When a sound wave is generated, air molecules move forward and backward usually causing displacement of a structure or membrane (e.g., the speaker's vocal folds and the tympanic membrane of the listener's ear). The extent of movement is measured as amplitude; therefore, the greater the amplitude, the louder the voice is perceived. Variations in amplitude are generated by two sources: air pressure below the glottis and the degree of adduction of the vocal folds. To produce a loud voice, a significant amount of subglottic air pressure is created below the vocal folds by increasing the tension of the muscles responsible for adduction of the vocal folds. To control loudness of the voice, a fine balance must be maintained between the amount of subglottic air pressure and the degree of tension of the laryngeal adductor muscles.

Vocal Quality

Vocal quality is related to the complexity of the sound wave and other factors that are associated with the resonating properties of the vocal tract and the manner in which the vocal folds vibrate. The vocal tract above the level of the vocal folds contains a series of resonating cavities that reinforce or modify the frequency and amplitude of the acoustic signal. Structures that function as resonators include the larynx, the pharynx, and the oral and nasal cavities. Acoustically, vocal quality is subjectively perceived as breathiness, harshness, hoarseness, vocal tremor, or hyper- and hyponasality.

From a clinical perspective, a harsh voice is associated with excessive muscular tension and effort in that the vocal folds are overadducted and subglottic air pressure is released abruptly. Breathiness is related to incomplete adduction of the vocal folds, which allows air to escape during phonation. Failure of the vocal folds to adduct optimally, due to either overadduction or incomplete approximation of the vocal folds, results in hoarseness. Vocal tremor results when alternating contractions of the adductors and abductors of the vocal folds are of equal strength (Aronson 1990). Voice tremor is perceived as quavering intonation that is rhythmic and vibrates at a rate ranging from 4 to 7 Hz. Hypernasality is perceived as excessive nasal resonance due to incomplete closure of the nasal cavity at the level of the velopharynx. Similarly, too little nasal resonance for production of nasal sounds results in hyponasality, usually associated with obstruction in the nasal cavity.

Clinical Voice Disorders

Voice disorders can be explained in terms of organic or inorganic etiology. Particular voice disorders can be classified according to cause or etiology, the set of clinical symptoms and vocal characteristics, and psychosocial manifestations. Voice disorders may be explained on the basis of etiology, clinical symptoms, and clinical correlates associated with vocal quality.

Organic Etiologies

Voice disorders identified as having physiologic, neurologic, biological, and anatomic-structural bases are organic problems. That is, the resulting voice disorder is the product, manifestation, or symptom of a condition, disease process, or illness. The pathophysiology of an organic voice disorder is supported with physical evidence obtained from medical, neurologic, otolaryngologic, and other clinical findings. In the absence of physical findings, the etiology of the voice problem is conservatively referred to as being indeterminate in origin. A differential diagnosis is of significant importance in establishing an accurate cause-and-effect relationship underlying the voice disorder. Organic voice disorders include congenital conditions, inflammatory responses, cancerous lesions, hormonal disturbances, physical trauma due to accidents or surgery, and neurologic problems. As a result, one or all of the vocal processes (i.e., phonation, resonation, and respiration) are affected. Conditions that produce mass lesions or tissue changes of the vocal folds and larynx have the following effects: increasing size and shape of the vocal folds and surrounding regions, restricting vocal folds from adducting and abducting, obstructing the glottic airway, and changing the tension and vibration of the vocal folds (Table 7.2).

Congenital Conditions

Laryngeal Web
At birth, a small web of tissue may be present that extends across the glottis from one vocal fold to the other in the anterior portion of the larynx. This web of tissue is referred to as a *laryngeal web*. Webs can be congenital or the result of injury to the larynx. Asphyxiation and possible death of the infant can result if the laryngeal web is not identified and removed surgically. If the laryngeal web is small and asymptomatic, the condition can go undiagnosed. Depending on the size and extent of the web, the infant's cry and vocalizations can range from normal, to hoarse, to aphonic. A noisy vocal quality (inhalatory stridor)

TABLE 7.2   Disorders of Phonation and Resonation due to Organic Etiologies

Etiology	Specific Condition
Congenital disorders	Laryngeal web
	Cysts
	Papilloma
	Cri du chat
	Laryngomalacia
Inflammation	Viral
	Acute
	Chronic
Cancer	Cancer of the larynx
	Tumors
Endocrine related	Thyroid gland problems
	Pituitary gland problems
	Menopause
Trauma	Injury
	Improper vocal technique
Neurologic disorders	Dysarthria
	Spastic
	Flaccid
	Hyperkinetic
	Voice tremor
	Myoclonus
	Hypokinetic
	Ataxic
	Mixed
Anatomic-structural problems	Cleft palate
	Velopharyngeal insufficiency
Arthritis	Ankylosis

Source: Adapted from AE Aronson. Clinical Voice Disorders (3rd ed). New York: Thieme, 1990.

can accompany respiration. This condition is treated through surgical removal of the web.

Cysts

Congenital cysts are small, fluid-filled projections that can arise in the tissues of the larynx. If the cysts are sufficiently large, they can obstruct the glottal opening and prevent the vocal folds from adducting, causing the infant's vocalization to sound weak or aphonic. Congenital cysts are treated by physicians with various medical or surgical interventions.

Papilloma

Laryngeal papillomas occur more frequently in children than adults. They are most common between the ages of 4 and 6 years (Aronson 1990). This condition tends to subside with age. Papillomas are believed to be benign lesions caused by viruses. The lesions resemble small cauliflower-like masses that extend from the vocal folds to other regions above and below the larynx. Vocal quality can include hoarseness, aphonia, or inhalatory stridor during respiration. Asphyxiation and possible death can result if the lesions obstruct the airway. Despite laser surgery, lesions have a tendency to reoccur. Scarring or a web effect can result from repeated surgical interventions.

Cri du Chat

Cri du chat is due to a genetic defect that prevents several anatomic structures and physiologic processes from developing normally. Other symptoms and conditions associated with this problem include abnormal larynx, small jaw (micrognathia), small head (microcephaly), hypotonia, visual problems, low-set ears, midline clefts of the palate, and intellectual impairments (mental retardation). One of the most significant characteristics of Cri du chat is the vocal quality and pitch range of the infant's cry. Pitch level is high and resembles the cry of a cat. Inhalatory stridor (an involuntary sound made during inhalation) and strained phonation are also common.

Laryngomalacia

Laryngomalacia, also known as *congenital laryngeal stridor*, can be present at birth and tends to resolve by 2 years of age. The physical appearance of the larynx is unique: The epiglottis is low and narrow with curled edges, the aryepiglottic folds are adducted and sucked in and out of the glottis during inhalation and exhalation, and the tissue over the arytenoid is redundant (Aronson 1990). The predominant feature in this condition is inhalatory stridor. In severe cases, breathing problems may be present.

Inflammation

Acute

Inflammatory responses to occasional viral illnesses, upper respiratory infections, bronchitis, croup, allergies, and bacterial and toxic irritants result in acute inflammation of the larynx and surrounding tissues. The vocal folds and laryngeal tissues can exhibit erythema (redness due to congested capillaries) and edema (swelling) until the viral infection or irritants subside. These conditions produce what is known as *laryngitis*. Vocal symptoms include temporary hoarseness and inhalatory stridor during the course of the illness. In severe cases, the voice may be aphonic (an absence of a definable laryngeal tone in that the voice is severely breathy or whispered).

Chronic

Inflammatory conditions that are chronic can result in permanent tissue changes. Examples of conditions that can change the integrity of the vocal folds and laryngeal tissues include excessive smoking and chronic alcohol consumption. The tissue lining the larynx and vocal folds may atrophy or become permanently hypertrophied (thickened). If tissue changes are evident, vocal quality is permanently altered and sounds hoarse.

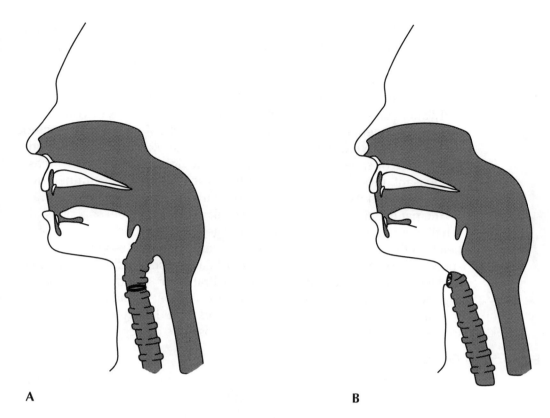

A **B**

FIGURE 7.4 *A. Normal anatomy. B. Anatomy after laryngectomy.*

Lesions due to Cancer

Chronic irritation to the tissue lining of the larynx due to smoking, alcoholism, and other irritants can produce cancerous lesions. The most common malignant cancer is squamous cell carcinoma. Most malignant cancers in the larynx occur at the level of the vocal folds; however, the cancer can spread to surrounding regions. Hoarseness is usually the first vocal symptom. Inhalatory stridor, throat pain, difficulty swallowing, chronic coughing, masses in the neck region, and shortness of breath are signs of advanced disease. Depending on the severity and the extent of the cancer, treatment can include chemotherapy, radiation, and surgery. Treatment for malignant laryngeal cancers includes partial or total removal of the larynx. This procedure is usually referred to as a laryngectomy. When the vocal mechanism for generating sound is removed, the trachea (which supplies the lungs with air) is disconnected from the neck and oral cavity. As a result, respiratory functions are routed through a small opening (i.e., stoma) created at the base of the neck (Figure 7.4).

Removal of the larynx has a devastating effect on a person's life. The person is no longer able to phonate by means of vocal fold vibration. The patient and his or her family are usually referred before and after surgery to a speech-language pathologist who is trained in laryngectomee rehabilitation. A temporary means for communicating immediately after surgery is provided to compensate for the loss of voice. Devices that generate sound by means of mechanical vibration include the artificial larynx, pneumatic device, and the electrolarynx. The artificial voice or speech produced by these devices can be perceived as unpleasant, monotonous, or robot-like. The client must be trained by the clinician to use these devices optimally.

The patient also can be taught to speak using his or her esophagus by inhaling air into this muscular tube and generating sound by means of a belch. Although some patients find it difficult to master esophageal speech, the speech-language pathologist can introduce different methods and techniques to facilitate generating vibration or sound. A combination of procedures has also been performed to augment sound production in the laryngectomy patient. These procedures include surgical adjustments to the neck region and implantation of prosthetic devices.

Endocrine Conditions

Hormonal disorders are associated with dysphonia. Hypothyroidism results from a deficit of the hormone thyroxin. Hyperthyroidism results from excessive secretions of thyroxin. Vocal characteristics related to hypothyroidism include hoarseness, excessively low pitch, and dysphonia associated with ataxic dysarthria (in more severe cases with neurologic involvement). In contrast, hyperthyroidism results in breathy vocal quality and reduced loudness believed to be due to weakness of the respiratory and phonatory systems.

Malfunction or lesions of the pituitary gland produce a condition known as *hyperpituitarism*. In this condition, the vocal folds and laryngeal structures, as well as other bony structures, can become enlarged due to oversecretion of the hormone produced in the pituitary gland. Excessively low pitch and hoarseness are characteristics of hyperpituitarism.

In addition, hormonal changes due to normal aging processes, such as menopause, have been related to changes in pitch. Lower pitch levels caused by vocal-fold thickening are characteristic of menopause.

Trauma

Injury to the larynx and vocal folds caused by automobile accidents, stab wounds to the neck, physical and surgical injury to the larynx, and improper vocal techniques (as can occur in professional and amateur singers) produces a variety of voice disorders. The nature of the voice disorder depends on the extent of physical and neurologic damage to the phonatory system. The dysphonia can range from mild hoarseness and breathiness to severe aphonia.

Dysphonia due to injury of the left recurrent laryngeal nerve is common following coronary artery bypass surgery. This nerve is highly susceptible to injury because of its proximity to the aortic artery.

Professional and amateur singers, as well as professional voice users (e.g., business and sales persons, public speakers, clergy, lawyers, and telephone operators) are susceptible to abuse and misuse of their respiratory and phonatory systems. Vocal nodules are common in singers and public speakers.

Neurologic Disorders

Motor speech impairment due to particular neurologic conditions is associated with particular dysphonias. The tenth cranial nerve, which innervates the muscles of phonation, is subject to breakdown caused by neurologic disease or injury to this nerve or its neuronal pathways. A unique dysphonia can result, depending on the location of the lesion or breakdown and the number of processes affected along the central nervous and peripheral nervous systems.

The relationship between the acoustic perceptual qualities of phonation and the location of the lesion to aid in the differential diagnosis of clinical voice disorders and motor speech disorders was established by Darley and colleagues (1969a; 1969b). This landmark study identified and distinguished vocal characteristics and motor speech symptoms that are consistent with particular dysarthrias and dysphonias caused by breakdown in one or several regions within the central nervous and peripheral nervous systems. On the basis of these findings, subjective clinical symptoms, such as hoarseness, breathiness, and strained-strangled phonation, gave new meaning to the study and science of speech-language pathology and neurology.

By applying the procedures and criteria outlined by Darley and colleagues, the speech-language pathologist trained in clinical voice disorders and motor speech disorders can interpret a breathy voice as suggestive of possible vocal fold weakness or paralysis due to neurologic involvement of the vagus nerve, which innervates the muscles of phonation. In the absence of neurologic involvement, a hoarse voice may signify possible vocal fold pathology, such as paralysis, weakness, vocal nodules, and vocal ulcers. Moreover, strained-strangled phonation can indicate musculoskeletal tension of the laryngeal muscles or a voice disorder caused by bilateral upper motor neuron disease, which suggests damage to the central nervous system involving both cerebral hemispheres (Table 7.3).

Anatomic and Structural Problems

Cleft Palate

A cleft is an opening between two bony structures that are normally fused or sealed off. Cleft palate is a congenital condition that can involve one or numerous anatomic structures and physiologic

TABLE 7.3   Dysphonias Associated with Major Types of Dysarthria

Dysarthria Type	Associated Dysphonia	Neuromuscular Implication	Location of Lesion
Spastic	Strained Hoarse Hypernasal	Spasticity	Bilateral upper motor neuron
Flaccid	Varies per lesion Breathy or hoarse Diplophonia Aphonia Hypernasa	Weakness	Lower motor neuron
Hyperkinetic	Voice arrests Strained Hoarse	Involuntary movement	Basal ganglia
Hypokinetic	Breathy Reduced loudness Monopitch	Rigidity Reduced range of movement	Basal ganglia
Organic tremor (essential)	Rhythmic voice tremor (4–7 Hz)	May accompany body and extremity tremor	Basal ganglia
Myoclonus	Rhythmic voice arrests (1–4 Hz)	May accompany similar movements of body and oral structures	Varies in brain stem: dentate nucleus inferior olive superior cerebellar peduncle red nucleus restiform body
Ataxic	Excess loudness Voice tremor	Discoordination	Cerebellum
Mixed	Dependent on location and systems affected	Varies	More than one location

Source: Adapted from JR Duffy. Motor Speech Disorders: Substrates, Differential Diagnosis, and Management. St. Louis: Mosby, 1995;12.

processes. Congenital clefts usually involve the hard palate, the soft palate, the lip, and the bony ridges of the palate. The extent of the cleft can be unilateral, bilateral, complete, or incomplete. Cleft palate is more prevalent in males than females. Cleft palate results in a breakdown in communication, particularly involving articulatory, resonatory, auditory, linguistic, and phonatory systems. Other problems are also associated with cleft palate. Such problems include feeding difficulties, middle ear disease or hearing impairment, and dental problems. Treatment and management of this condition is multidisciplinary, involving specialists in dentistry, orofacial and plastic surgery, audiology, speech-language pathology, and special education.

The major resonatory problems related to cleft palate are due to excessive nasal emission. Hypernasality is a common feature in children with cleft palate that has not been repaired. In addition, varying degrees of hypernasality in children with surgically repaired clefts can exist due to velopharyngeal insufficiency. Disorders of phonation include reduced loudness, hoarseness, harshness, and breathiness caused by excessive tension of the vocal folds and poor vocal fold adduction.

Velopharyngeal Insufficiency

When the velum does not adequately seal off the nasal cavity from the oral cavity for production of non-nasal sounds, velopharyngeal insufficiency results. Causes can include a cleft of the soft palate, a short velum, and neurologic involvement of the pharyngeal branch of the vagus. Hypernasality is the resonatory problem associated with velopharyngeal insufficiency.

Restricted Movement Due to Arthritis

Restricted movements of the arytenoids on the cricoarytenoid joint can result from arthritis of this joint region. Vocal symptoms include hoarseness and stridor. Redness and inflammation around the tissue surrounding the cricoarytenoid joint may be observed by the otolaryngologist.

Inorganic Etiologies

A voice problem or voice disorder due to psychological, behavioral, and emotional factors is referred to as an *inorganic voice disorder*. An inorganic voice disorder exists when there is an absence of structural, neurologic, and physiologic findings and the clinical symptomatology and examination findings support a psychological or behavioral basis. A multidisciplinary approach, involving the speech-language pathologist, otolaryngologist, medical practitioner, specialists in psychiatry and psychology, and the patient's family, is important in the diagnosis and treatment of inorganic voice problems. Voice problems that are psychogenic in origin are similar in that (1) the vocal folds and laryngeal examinations are normal in most cases, (2) the voice disorder frequently is the only overt physical symptom, (3) there is substantial evidence obtained from the patient's psychosocial history to support the development of the voice disorder around personal and emotional issues, and (4) the client's voice improves or returns to normal with removal of the personal conflict with and without counseling (Aronson 1990) (Table 7.4).

Musculoskeletal Tension

The laryngeal musculature is sensitive to emotional stress. Conditions, such as anger, anxiety, and frustration, induce the extrinsic and intrinsic laryngeal muscles to overcontract. Musculoskeletal tension in the neck region produces elevation of the larynx (as a unit) and the hyoid bone. Increased tension of the vocal folds can also be present. Palpation of the neck region on exam usually reveals tightness or phys-

TABLE 7.4   Disorders of Phonation and Resonation Due to Inorganic Etiologies

Etiology	Specific Condition
Emotional stress	Musculoskeletal tension
Behavioral factors with vocal abuse and misuse	Vocal nodules
	Contact ulcers
Psychoneurosis	Conversion reaction
	Dysphonia
	Aphonia

Source: Adapted from AE Aronson. Clinical Voice Disorders (3rd ed). New York: Thieme, 1990.

ical discomfort. Vocal quality associated with musculoskeletal tension includes strained and high-pitched phonation.

Behavioral Problems Associated with Vocal Abuse and Misuse

Vocal nodules and contact ulcers are two conditions in which laryngeal pathology exists at the level of the vocal fold. Although vocal nodules and contact ulcers are actual physical changes that occur on the vocal folds, they are symptoms of the pathophysiology or abnormal systems underlying these conditions. The primary etiology of nodules and ulcers is believed to be behavioral, resulting from abnormal and abusive speaking behaviors perpetuated by emotional and personality factors.

Vocal Nodules

Vocal nodules are small protrusions or nodules that develop on the vocal folds at the junction of the anterior and the middle third section of the fold. At first, vocal nodules are pink; however, they take on a gray color as they become more fibrous. Vocal nodules can be unilateral but are more commonly bilateral. Vocal nodules are caused by constant friction between the two folds. As a result, they increase the mass and reduce the rate of vibration of the vocal fold. Vocal quality is usually low pitch, hoarse, and breathy.

Specific behavioral and personality characteristics have been associated with children who have vocal nodules. Compared to a control group of children with normal voices, children with nodules were found to exhibit acting-out behaviors, distractibility, immaturity, and disturbed peer relationships (Greene 1991). Adults with vocal nodules manifest similar habits and personality traits. Vocal abuse appears to be the primary cause in adults. Associated behavioral characteristics in adults include socially aggressive personality, tension, anxiety, anger, depression, and interpersonal conflict.

Contact Ulcers

In contrast to vocal nodules, contact ulcers result from an erosion of tissue in the middle-to-posterior third portion of the vocal folds due to hyperadduction. Contact ulcers occur unilaterally or bilaterally.

They occur predominantly in men from 40 to 50 years of age. The constellation of symptoms exhibited by persons with contact ulcers include excessively low-pitched voice, hoarseness, limited pitch range, hard glottic attack, and excessive subglottal air pressure with abrupt speech patterns. In addition, a constant need to clear the throat, vocal abuse and misuse, musculoskeletal tension, chronic smoking, and alcohol consumption are common features. Behavioral traits associated with this condition include chronic emotional stress and tension. The vocal folds are believed to hyperadduct due to increased musculoskeletal tension.

Psychoneurosis and Psychogenic Problems

Aphonia and Dysphonia

Voice disorders can result from sensory and motor problems in the absence of neurologic or physical problems. This condition is frequently referred to as *conversion reaction* by neurologists and *hysteria* by psychiatrists. Apparently, the person with a psychogenic aphonia or dysphonia suffers from an interpersonal conflict or emotional condition that is psychological in origin. The conflict remains unresolved and the person is oblivious to the problem and clinical symptoms. As a result, the person may experience voice-related problems ranging from dysphonia to complete loss of voice. The speech-language pathologist must work in conjunction with specialists in otolaryngology, neurology, psychiatry, and psychology to accurately diagnose and treat this condition.

Mutational Falsetto

Puberphonia, or mutational falsetto, is a condition in which the adolescent fails to acquire a lower pitch level or more mature voice consistent with the normal developmental process in teenagers. This voice disorder occurs in both boys and girls. It is most common in teenagers between the ages of 13 and 15 years. In boys, the lower-pitched voice is not developed despite normal laryngeal and vocal fold development. The boy continues to speak with the high-pitched voice associated with adolescents. In girls, a baby-like voice characteristic is maintained. It is important to rule out other conditions that can affect the voice from maturing (e.g., endocrine conditions retarding growth of the larynx, severe hearing loss, general illness, respiratory, and neurologic conditions).

Spasmodic or Spastic Dysphonia

A family of disorders for which there is no definite etiology to date is referred to as *spasmodic* or *spastic dysphonia* (Table 7.5). In fact, researchers of this topic disagree with respect to the name of this condition (i.e., spasmodic versus spastic), the constellation of symptoms, the etiology, and the treatment. This condition includes a variety of vocal symptoms ranging from strained quality, effortful phonation, intermittent voice arrests, breathiness, and hoarseness. The two predominant vocal

TABLE 7.5 Dysphonia Arising from Organic Versus Inorganic Etiology

Voice Disorder	Specific Condition
Indeterminate dysphonia	Spasmodic dysphonia
Neurologic versus psychogenic	Spastic adductor
etiologies	Spastic abductor

characteristics are strained phonation and voice tremor or voice arrests. Similar vocal symptoms have been noted in people with dysphonias due to neurologic conditions (e.g., strained phonation in spastic dysarthria and voice tremor in hyperkinetic dysarthria). Likewise, strained phonation and quavering tremor have been observed in voice disorders due to psychogenic musculoskeletal tension.

Persons with spasmodic or spastic dysphonias may or may not exhibit other signs of neurologic disease. In many cases, the dysphonia is the only symptom. However, signs of tremor or rigidity may be observed in other parts of the body (e.g., the extremities). Traditionally, a neurologic etiology is suspected when the spastic dysphonia coexists with other soft neurologic signs (e.g., body or hand tremor). In the absence of neurologic signs, a psychogenic etiology is contemplated in the presence of emotional and interpersonal issues.

Spastic adductor dysphonia results when hyperadduction of the vocal folds occurs with brief, intermittent voice arrests. In contrast, spastic abductor dysphonia is marked by hyperabduction of the vocal folds with intermittent voice arrests. The etiology of spastic dysphonia is indeterminate. However, research to date supports involvement of the extrapyramidal system and possible cortical involvement (Aronson and Hartmann 1981; Aronson and Lagerlund 1991; Finitzo and Freeman 1989; Finitzo and Freeman 1991). One of the current treatments for spastic dysphonia is a botulinum toxin injection into the vocal fold to eliminate the strained/strangled quality of the voice.

Incidence of Voice Disorders

Several surveys have been conducted on various age groups and sample populations to determine the incidence of voice disorders in children and adults. The studies vary according to age and number of subjects studied, sampling techniques, methodology, criteria used for identification, and cultural environment (Moore and Hicks 1994). Of studies conducted on elementary and school-age children, the incidence of voice disorders ranges from 2% to 23% (Senturia and Wilson 1968; Milisen 1971; Yairi et al. 1974; Silverman and Zimmer 1975). The largest survey study representative of school-age children with voice disorders reported the incidence of voice disorders to be 6% of 32,500 school-age children studied in the St. Louis area (Senturia and Wilson 1968).

The prevalence of voice and resonatory problems among African-American children is estimated to be comparable to that of white children, when the data are controlled for socioeconomic status (Haller and Thompson 1975). However, African-American children of low socioeconomic status (i.e., those falling in the poverty range) were found to have a higher incidence of voice and resonatory problems than the national averages. Of 1,000 African-American children in Harlem, New York, 22% exhibited dysphonia marked by hoarseness due to laryngeal problems (Haller and Thompson 1975).

Most of the voice disorders reported in school-age children are related to vocal abuse and misuse with or without vocal fold nodules and inflammation. More than half of the children who are considered to have deviant voices are diagnosed with vocal nodules (Wilson 1979). Vocal nodules are one of the most common laryngeal pathologies found in school-age children (Allen et al. 1991). Moreover, vocal nodules are seen three times more often in boys than girls and more often in children who are not the first born (Kay 1982; Toohill 1975).

Survey studies on the incidence of voice disorders in adults are limited. Of 428 adults sampled in one study, approximately 7% of men and 5% of women were reported to have voice disorders (Laguaite 1972).

Researchers have also reported the incidence of specific types of voice disorders in certain populations. In 1,406 child and adult patients seen in clinical practice in one study, 37% were reported to have voice disorders related to vocal abuse and misuse, 18% had vocal nodules, 6% had contact ulcers, 4.8% had vocal polyps, 4.5% had polypoid degeneration, 4.2% had voice disorders related to neurologic disease, 3.9% had had a laryngectomy, 3% had spastic or spasmodic dysphonia, and the remainder had miscellaneous diagnoses (Cooper 1973).

The incidence of abnormal voice and laryngeal pathology according to age, sex, and occupation was investigated in 1,262 patients drawn from several otolaryngology medical practices. According to this study, 22% had vocal nodules, 14% had voice disorders related to inflammation (edema), 11.4% had vocal polyps, 9.7% had cancer of the larynx, 8% had paralysis of the vocal folds, and 7.9% had abnormal voices without any evidence of laryngeal pathology (Herrington-Hall et al. 1988). When age was the primary factor of consideration, laryngeal pathologies were most common in older adults: Fifty-seven percent of the patients were older than 45 years of age. Voice disorders due to cancerous lesions occurred with greater frequency in adults between the ages of 45 and 65 years. Vocal fold paralysis was common in adults older than 65 years. Young adults between the ages of 22 and 44 years were found to have vocal nodules and edema. Inorganic voice disorders with psychogenic etiologies were more prevalent in women: Eighty-five percent of the patients diagnosed with psychogenic voice disorders were women (Herrington-Hall et al. 1988).

With respect to occupation, the most common of 73 different occupations surveyed in the study by Herrington-Hall and colleagues were factory workers, unemployed and retired persons, nurses, homemakers, company executives and managers, teachers, students, amateur and professional singers, and secretaries. Thirty-five percent of the psychogenic voice disorders were found in female homemakers. Factory workers frequently exhibited dysphonia due to laryngeal pathology (Herrington-Hall et al. 1988).

Diagnosis of Voice Disorders

Evaluation of voice disorders involves a variety of procedures and assessment protocols. The speech-language pathologist must systematically (1) test the structure and function of the vocal mechanism, (2) interpret and measure acoustic perceptual properties of the dysphonia, (3) correlate abnormal and normal vocal parameters with their respective structures and systems, (4) differentially diagnose the condition given the symptoms and pathophysiology, and (5) refer for proper treatment after the diagnosis. An otolaryngologic examination is a prerequisite. Information regarding the health, integrity, and function of the vocal folds and vocal mechanism is essential in understanding the underlying cause of the voice disorder. Medical and neurologic examinations may be warranted to rule out health- and disease-related conditions. A summary of the diagnostic protocol is outlined in Table 7.6.

Treatment

The management of voice disorders is multifaceted. The treatment protocol depends on the nature of the voice disorder and its etiology, the extent of communication deficit, the number of systems involved, the magnitude of the problem, and the education of the patient and other significant members of the patient's family and medical team. A multidisciplinary approach involving the speech-language pathologist and other specialists may be deemed necessary to manage the voice-disordered client. A medical diagnosis should always precede treatment for voice disorders.

Psychosocial, Cultural, and Technologic Aspects of Voice Disorders

The human voice has many purposes. From a medical perspective, the human voice is an indicator of the state of health and the severity or progression of disease. From an intellectual perspective, the human

TABLE 7.6   Voice Evaluation

History
Referral source
Medical
Otolaryngology
Psychosocial
Neurologic
Environmental
Occupational
Oral peripheral examination
Anatomic structures
Teeth
Hard palate
Soft palate
Pharynx
Larynx
Neurologic motor speech examination
Neuromuscular integrity and function
Lips
Tongue
Velum
Vocal fold function
Voice evaluation
Resonation
Phonation
Respiration

voice is a means for communicating linguistic information. From a cultural standpoint, the human voice signifies the community and society associated with the speaker.

According to Boone (1991), approximately 25% of adults in the United States are displeased with the way they sound to the extent that they believe their careers and social lives have been affected. This phenomenon seems to be independent of the existence of identifiable voice problems. According to Ramig (1994), the degree of the communication impairment resulting from a voice disorder relates to both the severity of the problem and its impact on the voice user. Moreover, Aronson (1990) stated:

> In addition to abnormal voice as an index of health or illness, it is also valued as an instrument of communication. Within this framework, the following questions are pertinent: 1) Is the voice adequate to carry language intelligibly to the listener? 2) Are its acoustic properties aesthetically acceptable? 3) Does it satisfy its owner's occupational and social requirements? Voice, in other words, has personal, social, and economic significance. The higher one ascends the socioeconomic scale the greater the emphasis placed on pleasant effective voices. With few exceptions, the greater the dependence on voice for occupational and

social gratification, the more devastating the effects of a voice disorder on the person.

The role of the human voice differs from person to person, and the concern about one's voice does not necessarily relate to objective performance. Instruments that measure the human voice objectively lack reliability and validity, in that they fail to correlate particular vocal characteristics to their etiology, community, society, and psychosocial aspects. To date, the trained ear remains the best instrument with which to diagnose the human voice in context of medical, cultural, dialect, and psychosocial dimensions. In the future, professionals in speech-language pathology and clinical voice disorders must train practitioners to recognize and measure characteristics of the human voice across all these dimensions, by using objective procedures and instrumentation that are reliable and valid.

References

Allen MS, Pettit JM, Sherblom JC. Management of vocal nodules: a regional survey of otolaryngologists and speech-language pathologists. J Speech Hear Res 1991;34:229–235.

Aronson AE, Hartmann DE. Adductor spastic dysphonia as a sign of essential (voice) tremor. J Speech Hear Res 1981;46:52–58.

Aronson AE, Lagerlund TD. Neuroimaging studies do not prove the existence of brain abnormalities in spastic (spasmodic) dysphonia. J Speech Hear Res 1991;34:801–805.

Aronson AE. Clinical Voice Disorders (3rd ed). New York: Thieme, 1990.

Boone DR. Is Your Voice Telling on You? San Diego: Singular Publishing, 1991.

Cooper M. Modern Techniques of Vocal Rehabilitation. Springfield, IL: Thomas, 1973.

Darley FL, Aronson AE, Brown JR. Clusters of deviant speech dimensions in the dysarthrias. J Speech Hear Res 1969;12:462–496.

Darley FL, Aronson AE, Brown JR. Differential diagnostic patterns of dysarthria. J Speech Hear Res 1969;12:246.

Duffy JR. Motor Speech Disorders: Substrates, Differential Diagnosis, and Management. St. Louis: Mosby, 1995.

Finitzo T, Freeman F. Spasmodic dysphonia, whether and where: results of seven years of research. J Speech Hear Res 1989;32:541–555.

Finitzo T, Freeman F. Whether and wherefore: a response to Aronson and Lagerlund seven years of research. J Speech Hear Res 1991;34:806–811.

Greene G. Psycho-behavioral characteristics of children with vocal nodules: WPBIC ratings. J Speech Hear Res 1991;54:306–312.

Herrington-Hall BL, Lee L, Stemple JC, et al. Description of laryngeal pathologies by age, sex, and treatment seeking sample. J Speech Hear Disord 1988;53:57–64.

Haller RM, Thompson EA. Prevalence of speech, language, and hearing disorders among Harlem children. J Natl Med Assoc 1975;4:299.

Johnson W, Brown SF, Curtis JF, et al. Speech Handicapped School Children. New York: Harper and Brothers, 1965.

Kay N. Vocal nodules in children-etiology and management. J Laryngol Otol 1982;96:731–736.

Laguaite JK. Adult voice screening. J Speech Hear Disord 1972;37:147–151.

Milisen R. The Incidence of Speech Disorders. In LE Travis (ed), Speech-Language Pathology Disorders. New York: Appleton-Century-Crofts, 1971.

Moore GP, Hicks DM. Voice Disorders. In GH Shames, EH Wiig, W Secord (eds), Human Communication Disorders: An Introduction. New York: Merrill, 1994.

Perkins WH. Vocal Function: A Behavioral Analysis. In LE Travis (ed), Handbook of Speech Pathology and Audiology. Englewood Cliffs, NJ: Prentice-Hall, 1971.

Ramig LO. Voice Disorders. In FD Minifie (ed), Introduction to Communication Sciences and Disorders. San Diego: Singular Publishing 1994.

Senturia BH, Wilson FB. Otorhinolaryngic findings in children with voice deviations. Ann Otol Rhinol Laryngol 1968;77:1027–1042.

Silverman EM, Zimmer CH. Incidence of chronic hoarseness among school-age children. J Speech Hear Disord 1975;40:211–215.

Toohill RJ. The psychosomatic aspects of children with vocal nodules. Arch Otolaryngol 1975;101:591–595.

Wilson DK. Voice Problems of Children (2nd ed). Baltimore: Williams & Wilkins, 1979.

Yairi E, Currin LH, Bulian N, Yairi J. Incidence of hoarseness in school children over a 1 year period. J Commun Disord 1974;7:321–328.

Chapter 7   Study Questions

1. What are the social, psychological, and emotional implications of clinical voice disorders? Cite some specific examples to support your answer.
2. Describe the difference between organic and inorganic voice disorders. Cite examples of voice disorders that fall into each category.
3. What are the three branches of the vagus nerve and what structures do they innervate?
4. What is the difference between a dysarthria and a dysphonia? Cite examples of conditions that are both dysarthrias and dysphonias.
5. Describe three voice disorders that are inorganic in origin.
6. What is laryngectomy? Describe postlaryngectomy symptoms, etiology, and treatment to enhance communication.
7. What are the problems associated with cleft palate? Describe the vocal and resonatory characteristics of this craniofacial problem.

8   Stuttering

Carolyn Conrad and Charlena M. Seymour

A single, precise definition of stuttering has always been controversial among persons who have studied the disorder. No one knows for sure what causes stuttering. Also, due to stuttering's complex nature, few agree on what aspects of stuttering should be emphasized in its definition. Perhaps the only one who knows what stuttering is is the stutterer (Van Riper 1973). Most experts agree that the word *stuttering* can be defined in three major ways: (1) to describe what the speaker does, (2) to classify what the listener hears, and (3) to describe the overt and covert behavior and the negative emotions that evolve for some persons who stutter as a result of their attempt to avoid, hide, disguise, or stop the moment of stuttering.

Most speech-language pathologists agree that stuttering is a speech behavior characterized by the audible repetitions of sounds, syllables, and words and the audible prolongations of sounds and syllables in words. Other verbal behaviors, such as interjecting, and nonverbal behaviors, such as hesitating and blocking, are also sometimes considered as the primary symptoms of stuttering. When the speaker stutters, he or she involuntarily produces repetitions, prolongations, or both of sounds and syllables in words. Sometimes the speaker interjects pauses, such as *uh*, *er*, and *um*, between words in phrases. He or she may also appear to be hesitant about saying a particular word or may experience a temporary stoppage or blocking in trying to talk.

The repetitions, prolongations, interjections, hesitations, and blocking are verbal behaviors that are considered to be the primary or core symptoms of stuttering. The person who stutters may produce only one type of these stuttering symptoms or a combination of these symptoms. *Repetitions, prolongations, interjections, hesitations,* and *blocking* are also the terms that the listener uses to describe some of the audible features of stuttering. What differentiates stuttering behavior from normal interruptions in the flow of speech is that stuttering interruptions occur more frequently, last longer, and are produced in a hard, tense manner. Because similar speech interruptions also occur in the speech of persons who do not stutter, the speech-language pathologist should observe the speaker for both auditory and visual clues when identifying stuttering (Seymour et al. 1983). Other behaviors that are related to the stuttering moment are described as secondary symptoms of stuttering. These symptoms are atypical features (e.g., irregular eye blinking, distorted facial grimacing, exaggerated head or body jerking, or excessive clearing of the throat) that are used to avoid, hide, or disguise the moment of stuttering or to prevent the moment of stuttering from occurring.

Underlying feelings that precede, follow, or accompany the moment of stuttering can also be considered secondary symptoms. Often within the stuttering cycle, the person who stutters feels anxious, frustrated, or angry when stuttering occurs. In a larger sense, then, stuttering reflects a person's emotions as well as his or her speech pattern (Murphy 1974). Underlying negative emotions provide insight into how well the person copes with stuttering. Indeed, the negative feelings that accompany stuttering also influence the severity of the stuttering moment and the treatment outcomes. Therefore, when speech-language pathologists treat persons who stutter, they not only have to consider the nature of the speech interruptions but also the influence stuttering has on the person's attitude and self-esteem. People who stutter know what they want to say: They just have difficulty saying some sounds in words in a smooth, effortless way. Because their speech patterns are different and because the listener may have a low tolerance for these differences, the person who stutters feels pressured to be fluent when speaking. The speaker becomes tense and anxious when attempting to speak fluently. The more the speaker tries not to stutter, the more the accompanying tension and anxiety make the stuttering worse. In other words, stuttering is what a speaker does when he or she expects stuttering to occur, dreads it, and becomes tense in anticipation of it and in trying to avoid it (Johnson 1973).

Identification of Stuttering

Identification of stuttering begins with an investigation into the environment that determines the appearance and severity of the stuttering moment (Van Riper 1971). Although some features of stuttering are always present, the frequency, intensity, and duration of the stuttering moment are not the same for everyone who stutters. These variables change according to the conditions under which the person is talking. People who stutter do not stutter all of the time. People tend to stutter more when they are talking to someone who is authoritative, of the opposite sex, older, bigger in size, or nonattentive. Stuttering also tends to increase when people are talking to a group, as opposed to an individual, and when talking on the telephone. When using a telephone, the speaker must convey the message with a procedure that is completely verbal. Stuttering tends to occur less when the speaker sings, whispers, role plays, speaks alone, repeats material in succession, or speaks in the presence of masking noise or with a chorus.

There are some linguistic peculiarities about stuttering. Stuttering has a tendency to occur at the beginning of a sentence, usually on the first word, and on the first syllable or accented syllable of words in the sentence. Longer words tend to be stuttered more than shorter words. However, no single sound or sound classes stand out as more difficult to produce or more frequently stuttered. Emotionally loaded words tend to trigger more stuttering than familiar words. In general, content words, such as nouns, verbs, and adjectives, tend to be stuttered more frequently than articles, conjunctions, and prepositions. Van Riper (1982a) found that grammatical class has only a minor effect in determining the place in which a person is likely to stutter. It is also likely that learned fears of certain sounds and words influence the place in which stuttering occurs.

Development of Stuttering

Stuttering is first noticed in most persons during childhood. It is considered a developmental problem of childhood. Parents (or caretakers) often complain that their child is having difficulty getting the words out. This difficulty is typically noticed when the child is between 2 and 4 years of age, a time when parents are carefully scrutinizing the child's language performance to determine normalcy. Most people who stutter begin stuttering before they reach their fifth birthday. Rarely does stuttering begin in adulthood. When it does, the stuttering appears suddenly (Van Riper 1982a).

It is not clear whether stuttering begins in the mouth of the child or the ear of the parent (Johnson 1942; Johnson et al. 1959; Johnson 1961). Most researchers believe that all children are normally disfluent when learning how to talk and eventually grow out of the disfluent speech pattern. It is not clear why some children do not outgrow the disfluency. According to Wendell Johnson and many of his proponents, children would probably not develop stuttering if it were not for the misperception and subsequent misdiagnosis of normal speech production by overly critical parents or caretakers. Because normal disfluency and mild stages of stuttering sound alike, it is understandable that a listener may misdiagnose normal disfluency for stuttering.

Making a differential diagnosis of mild stuttering from normal disfluent speech behavior in children is a difficult task for even the most experienced clinician. In the early stages of stuttering development, stuttering tends to be episodic, inconsistent, and irregular. The following early warning signals help detect stuttering: multiple repetitions of sounds or syllables (rather than whole words or phrases); exaggerated, prolonged stress on sounds in words; and the appearance of being stuck or blocked on a word. When such warning signals occur too frequently and the child appears to struggle to speak, then professional help should be sought.

Coping with Stuttering

The effect of stuttering on the lifestyle of the person varies. People who stutter are sometimes successful when they try to speak fluently, thus experiencing a feeling of relief and satisfaction. Those who do not experience some level of fluency are left with feelings of doubt, uncertainty, and anxiety. Some people accept their stuttering and make no attempt to change their speech. Others spend their lifetime in therapy trying to change their speech and trying to cope with the effects of stuttering. In countries where great emphasis is placed on how well a person communicates, being a poor communicator has a great effect on how one is perceived and how one socially interacts. It is not surprising, therefore, that many people who stutter have low self-esteem, particularly about speaking situations. Among adults who stutter, many think that their stuttering has influenced their educational, vocational, and social achievement.

What should be remembered when meeting individuals who stutter is that they are much like other people. They are not trying to be funny by stuttering: They are not slow-witted: They are not crazy. However, the media has created a negative image of the person who stutters that has been hard to overcome. Stuttering advocacy groups, such as the National Stuttering Project and the Stuttering Foundation of America, have challenged these negative portrayals, increased the public's awareness of the damage brought about by stereotyping persons who stutter, and enlightened the public to positive role models of persons who stutter.

History contains biographies of famous people who stuttered and were considered successful in spite of their speech disorder, including Winston Churchill (Prime Minister of Great Britain during World War II), Clara Barton (founder of the American Red Cross), Jimmy Stewart (actor), Carly Simon (singer), and John Updike (novelist), just to name a few. There are many more people who stutter who are authors, movie stars, singers, scientists, Olympic athletes, preachers, speech-language pathologists, and audiologists.

Some people who stutter are in high-profile positions that require a lot of talking, and they have prevailed. Others who stutter have deliberately chosen careers in which a great emphasis is not placed on communication skills and have been satisfied with their choice. A third category of persons who stutter is those for whom stuttering has made no difference in their career selection: Persons who have not felt compelled to change their speech to be successful. However, a strong positive attitude like that is rare and may be a form of self-denial. Murphy (1974) explained that denial of self as a stutterer is self-deception. Some find it impossible to look at themselves in a mirror while stuttering or to look into the double-barreled mirrors of their listener's eyes. They may shut their eyes, sometimes as a tension reflex, but sometimes to separate themselves from their painful environment.

Persons Who Stutter

Stuttering is a speech disorder that cuts across gender, race, socioeconomic level, and culture. Although at one time it was believed that persons from complacent, less-aspiring societies were less likely to stutter, stuttering is now considered a worldwide phenomenon that is not endemic. In the United States, stuttering affects an estimated 1% of the population. It is most prevalent among preschool children and is less prevalent in adults. Regardless of age, about seven persons in every thousand stutter nationally. About 80% of children who begin to stutter grow out of it. It appears that more boys than girls stutter, and that girls are less likely to be referred for therapy than boys (Silverman 1986). In today's society, women encounter the same pressures to succeed as men. This may alter the gender ratio in stuttering and, subsequently, the motivation to refer more girls for therapy if identified as having stuttering symptoms.

Stutter Among Minority Groups

A limited amount of research has been conducted regarding stuttering among minority groups in North America. Early investigators, interested in documenting the influence of environment on the development of stuttering, were eager to locate American cultures in which stuttering was absent or low in incidence. These early studies focused on Native American tribes and are indicative of the nature of early research in the field of stuttering among minority cultures in that they lacked quantitative data and relied upon interviews collected with the help of a translator (Snidecor 1947; Stewart 1960).

Studies of the Shoshone and Bannock tribes of the Northwestern United States (Snidecor 1947); the Salish, Kwatkutl, and Nootka tribes of British Columbia and Vancouver (Lemert 1953); and the Ute and Cowichan tribes (Stewart 1960) indicated that the prevalence of stuttering was influenced by the type of child-rearing practices and the attitudes of the tribes toward disabled speech. A later study refuted the findings of these early investigators (Zimmerman et al. 1983). Zimmerman and colleagues were able to obtain more direct information from the Bannock and Shoshone, because one of the researchers spoke the language of these Native Americans and was himself a stutterer. However, because of the conclusions of the earlier research, for many years speech-language clinicians identified strict discipline of young children as one of the factors increasing the likelihood of the development of stuttering.

Stuttering Among African-Americans

Investigation of stuttering among African-Americans is still in the beginning stages, and much more research needs to be conducted before the nature of stuttering in this population can be accurately described. Two studies of the prevalence of stuttering among African-Americans indicated a difference in the gender of stutterers within this group, which matches findings from other groups, and a higher prevalence of stuttering among African-American women than among white women (Goldman 1967; Conrad 1980). Goldman surveyed school children in Tennessee and found that the ratio of stuttering was 2.4 boys to 1.0 girls among African-Americans, compared with a ratio of 4.9 boys to 1.0 girls among whites (Goldman 1967). In a sample of 1,271 African-American adults at an urban community college, Conrad found that, among students who stutter, the man-to-woman ratio was 2 to 1. She also found a prevalence of stuttering in the student sample of 2.7%. The indication that stuttering occurs more frequently among African-American women than among white women could result from the differences of environmental stress on the minority population.

Results of a study by Leith and Mims (1975) suggested that stuttering behavior in adolescent and young-adult African-American male patients differed from that of their white counterparts. The authors compared the performance of the two groups on a behavior-profile rating scale designed to evaluate each stuttering behavior independently. Results indicated that white males who stuttered tended to exhibit overt stuttering behaviors (i.e., prolongations and repetitions), whereas African-American males who stuttered tended to mask core stuttering behaviors and even avoid speech, exhibiting severe speech modifying behaviors, such as eye blinks, head and body movements, and facial contortions, rather than speech stuttering behaviors.

In her dissertation research evaluating the conversations of African-American pairs of mothers and their stuttering and nonstuttering children, Conrad (1985) identified differences in the interactions of mothers and their stuttering children compared with mothers and their nonstuttering children. Mothers of nonstuttering children tended to repeat the utterances of their children, possibly as a cue that they are listening or as a turn-taking signal. Mothers of stuttering children did not repeat their children's utterances as frequently, and their children produced longer utterances and took longer turns. This study did not compare African-Americans to other racial groups. The identified difference in conversational interaction between the subjects and their matching controls may also be true of white mother–stuttering child pairs.

Stuttering Among Other Minority Groups

Research describing stuttering behavior among other minority groups is sparse. A study comparing bilingual people who stutter to monolingual people who stutter found no significant influence of language difference on stuttering. The study also found similar patterns, within both subject groups, of syntactic complexity affecting the stuttering moment (Jayaram 1983). The lack of research in the area of stuttering among minority groups is perhaps related to the limited number of minority speech-language pathologists and researchers. Fewer than 6% of the members of the American Association of Speech-Language Pathology and Audiology are members of minority groups. Further research of stuttering in minority persons would enhance the knowledge base and help to improve treatment of stuttering in minorities.

Intervention Strategies for Stuttering

Stuttering has perhaps the longest history of treatment efforts among all the communication disorders. Treatment approaches, as well as attitudes about the stuttering, have changed over the years. From the time when Demosthenes was told to place pebbles in his mouth to stop stuttering to the variety of technologic biofeedback devices employed today to increase fluency, clinicians have developed a broad range of techniques that are useful in achieving some level of success in the correction of stuttering.

Theoretic Approaches to Stuttering Intervention

Treatment of stuttering before the twentieth century consisted primarily of a number of techniques that trained the stutterer to speak in a novel fashion. Examples of such techniques are speaking in rhythmic or singsong patterns, speaking in time to movements of the finger or the hand, and speaking in a monotone. Other early techniques (i.e., relaxation therapy and shadowing) are still used by some speech-language pathologists. Shadowing is a method that requires the stutterer to mirror another's speech by speaking a few seconds after the first speaker. All of these techniques demonstrated some success during the initial stages of therapy. However, such success was not usually permanent.

In the 1920s and 1930s, researchers interested in stuttering remediation began to approach treatment differently. They proposed theories that attempted to explain either (1) the cause of stuttering (Orton and Travis 1929; Eisensen 1958; Glauber 1958) or (2) the cause of the moment of stuttering (Perkins et al. 1976; Sheehan 1953; Brutten and

Shoemaker 1967). In both cases, it was thought that effective, lasting improvement resulted from treatment based on a logical theory explaining the stuttering behavior. It is, therefore, helpful to review these theories because they shaped treatment approaches during the following six decades.

The plethora of theories that explain either the etiology of stuttering or the source of the stuttered movement have been classified by Bloodstein (1981) as follows:

- Breakdown theories
- Repressed-need theories
- Anticipatory-struggle theories
- Cybernetic (feedback) theories
- Learning theories

Breakdown Theories

The theories that arose in the first half of the twentieth century were breakdown theories. These attributed stuttering behavior to some type of breakdown in the physical makeup of the person who stuttered. Breakdown theories described either the etiology of stuttering, the cause of the stuttered moment, or both. One example of a breakdown theory is the cerebral dominance theory, which attributes stuttering to a lack of clear dominance of one of the hemispheres and cites the practice of forcing left-handed children to write with their right hand as a causative factor (Orton and Travis 1929; Travis and Lindsley 1933). Another breakdown theory is the genetic predisposition theory, which describes stutterers as having an innate weakness that is triggered by stress and manifests itself as stuttering behavior (Eisenson 1958; West 1958).

Later research suggested that early theorists who proposed a physiologic breakdown as the cause of stuttering were on the right track. Investigators later identified subcortical systems that govern motor speech control (Watson et al. 1992; Smith 1990). Investigators have also successfully measured neurophysiologic aspects of listening and speech behaviors of subjects who stutter, thus pinpointing breakdown occurring in these systems (Dietrich et al. 1995).

Repressed-Need Theories

As interest in the etiology of stuttering continued, other researchers attempted to apply principles of psychoanalysis to the problem of stuttering (Froeschels 1943; Glauber 1958). These scholars explained stuttering by describing the behavior as an attempt to satisfy a repressed need. Two examples of repressed-need theories are (1) the description of stuttering behavior as a manifestation of an infantile need for oral gratification (Glauber 1958), and (2) the consideration of stuttering behavior as a covert expression of an emotional response (Barbara 1954).

Anticipatory-Struggle Theories

Anticipatory-struggle theories propose that the speaker is disfluent because he or she thinks of speech as a difficult task and expects failure (Johnson 1933; Johnson and Solomon 1937). Each anticipatory-struggle theory attempts to explain why the young person who stutters has a negative view of speech. As described earlier in *Development of Stuttering*, one such theory attributes this negative viewpoint to the parents' high expectations. Another, the diagnosogenic theory, identifies the parents' diagnosis of the child as a stutterer, which is often based on normal disfluencies exhibited by the child, as a primary cause of the negative expectations of the child who stutters (Johnson 1942).

More recently, researchers have been exploring a theory that is based on findings that the person who stutters experiences difficulty coordinating articulation, phonation, and respiration (Perkins et al. 1976; Peters et al. 1989). This theory, termed the *covert repair hypothesis*, postulates that stuttering is the speaker's covert attempt to repair errors in the phonetic motor plan, before such errors are overtly produced (Louko et al. 1990; Yaruss and Conture 1996).

Cybernetic Theories

Cybernetic etiology theories proposed complex models to explain that the system of monitoring speech is deficient or malfunctioning in the stutterer (Lee 1950; Fairbanks 1955).

Learning Theories

Learning theorists proposed that stuttering was a result of (1) approach-avoidance conflict (Sheehan 1953), (2) classical conditioning (Froeschels 1943), (3) operant conditioning (Flanagan et al. 1959), or (4) some combination of these processes (Brutten and Shoemaker 1967).

The Speak More Fluently versus Stutter More Fluently Debate

The array of theories led to an expansion of treatment approaches and an increase in controversy over selection of treatment techniques. The entrance of learning theories into the mélange of theoretic approaches sparked a division among speech-language pathology researchers that has been described as the *speak more fluently versus stutter more fluently* controversy (Gregory 1979).

To understand this controversy, it is helpful to consider the theories described above and take note of the implications of each. Breakdown theories imply that something is broken or defective and, therefore, cannot be fixed completely. Feedback or cybernetic theories are a complex variation of breakdown theories that describe a malfunctioning of the speech monitoring system. The repressed-need theories imply that a deep-seated neurosis exists in the person who stutters, which is difficult to repair or cure. The anticipatory struggle theories describe an abstract behavior, anticipation, or expectation that is difficult to delineate or change. Learning theories imply that a behavior is acquired through a tangible process that involves manipulation of stimuli. To carry this one step further, learning theories suggest that the behavior can also be extinguished by manipulation of stimuli. Accordingly, the speak more fluently versus stutter more fluently controversy is a debate over whether persons who stutter can successfully achieve complete fluency or whether therapy can only help them to speak better and accept their disability.

Advocates of the speak more fluently school of thought believe that the person who stutters can become completely fluent, particularly if appropriate interventions are undertaken before the age of 10 years (Goldiamond 1965; Perkins 1974; Webster 1974; Ryan and Ryan 1995). Moreover, these speech-language professionals think that the application of operant conditioning to fluency therapy provides a means of reinforcing the fluency that occurs in every patient's speech, motivates the patient, and indirectly improves the negative self-image of the patient.

In contrast, researchers in the stutter more fluently school of thought believe that most persons who stutter demonstrate some level of abnormal disfluency all of their lives, that many persons who stutter have developed a self-image of a stutterer that prevents the achievement of permanent fluency, and that these attitudes and self-image must be addressed directly (Van Riper 1973; Sheehan 1970; Bloodstein 1981). These clinicians advocate treatment approaches that help the person who stutters become a mild stutterer and methods that enable the patient to cope with the stuttering before or during its occurrence. The attainment of this coping strategy, rather than the elimination of stuttering behavior, is the goal of treatment.

An Integrated Approach to Treatment

As clinicians and researchers evaluated these two therapy approaches, a third position developed that draws from the strengths of both sides (Peters and Guitar 1991). As a result, clinicians began to recognize that an integrated approach permits selection from a broad array of techniques and encourages the clinician to take into consideration the patient's social and cultural background, his or her community, his or her role in society, and his or her attitude toward certain behaviors. Although the selection of the appropriate techniques for the patient is sometimes determined on the basis of the clinician's theoretic perspective regarding the cause of stuttering and his or her belief concerning the possibility of complete remediation, many speech-language pathologists base the design of a patient's treatment program on the patient's needs, not on a specific theory.

The modern clinician recognizes that each patient presents a unique profile of behavior. He or she also realizes that the patient must accept the technique and practice it systematically to achieve fluent speech. There are many methods of treating stuttering, but treatment must be determined on a case-by-case basis. Because there are different factors contributing to the cause of each patient's stuttering disorder, no one method is a panacea. There are certain common strategies that can be found in most treatment methods, and the skilled clinician uses the strategy that best meets the needs of the patient. Even when a clinician is an advocate of a certain treatment procedure, sometimes modification of that procedure is necessary to help the patient improve. More important, the patient must be treated by someone with the proper credentials. That person must be a certified speech-language pathologist, preferably someone who specializes in the treatment of stuttering.

One strategy that enhances treatment is allowing people who stutter to speak for themselves. The stuttering behavior only becomes more severe if the speaker feels that someone is going to complete or interrupt his or her statements. The listener should let the person finish the statement, regardless of how long it takes. When the listener interrupts or completes statements, the stutterer becomes dependent on the listener to finish statements. To reduce the fear of stuttering, the person who stutters has to confront stuttering, not avoid it. Most persons who stutter and who have received speech therapy have been able to decrease, control, or eliminate their stuttering behavior.

Evaluation of Social and Cultural Factors in the Treatment of Stuttering

Research has indicated that stuttering behavior fluctuates according to the status of the speaker, the nature of the speaking situation, the type of language used by the speaker, and the role and attitude of each participant in the conversation. Therefore, the speech-language pathologist who wishes to maximize treatment success considers the patient from a cultural-social perspective and evaluates the following factors:

- The phonologic, syntactic, semantic, and prosodic features of the patient's first language or dialect
- The role the patient is expected to play in the family setting
- The roles expected of other family members
- The variety of speaking situations the patient encounters and the nature of the patient's expected speech in these situations
- The family's, community's, and peer group's attitudes toward stuttering

- The family's, community's, and peer group's attitudes toward artificial forms of speech
- The family's, community's, and peer group's attitude toward medical intervention

In addition to evaluation of the above factors, the clinician evaluates the total spectrum of speech-language behavior exhibited by the patient. He or she assesses the patient's language competency, articulation skills, vocal loudness level, pitch and quality, and respiratory pattern.

Techniques for Remediation of Stuttering

Once the speech-language pathologist has a complete profile of the patient's speech-language behavior, including social and cultural features, selection of the appropriate techniques for remediation are made. The clinician may wish to consider the focus of the technique (i.e., the area of speech behavior intended to be changed by its application) and select methods that match the patient's needs within his or her social and cultural framework. Techniques for remediation of stuttering can be divided into five broad areas of focus (Figure 8.1): (1) attitudes and secondary behaviors, (2) language and prosody, (3) overall speech change, (4) physical speech targets, and (5) the stuttered moment (Table 8.1).

Attitudes and Secondary Behaviors

A variety of techniques have been employed to change attitudes and secondary behaviors. Some require the patient to directly confront his or her attitudes: Examples are counseling and cognitive therapy. Such direct confrontation may be viewed by many cultural groups negatively. African-Americans and some Asian cultural groups may find it difficult to discuss personal feelings with persons outside the family or cultural group. In other methods that address attitudes, the patient talks about what he or she is feeling as he or she participates in a staged speaking situation: Examples are role playing and systematic desensitization. However, the clinician may find that patients from some social and cultural backgrounds will not transfer attitudinal change achieved in an artificial situation to real-life speaking. Relaxation therapy has been used to eliminate secondary behaviors. Operant conditioning, counterconditioning, and deconditioning (all methods based on learning theory) also address attitudes and secondary behaviors. The clinician should carefully explain the purpose of these techniques and ensure that the patient is comfortable with the selected approach before initiating therapy.

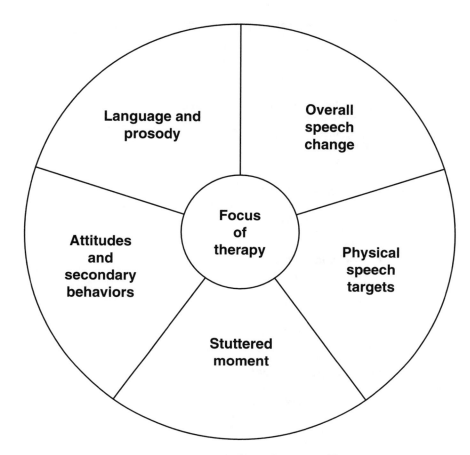

FIGURE 8.1 *Foci of therapy for stuttering. (Reprinted with permission from C Conrad. Teaching Cultural Diversity in Professional Education—Fluency and Fluency Disorders. In L Cole, V Deal [eds], Multicultural Professional Education. Rockville, MD: American Speech-Language-Hearing Association, 1990.)*

Language and Prosody

A standard technique often paired with other methods is one that gradually increases the length and complexity of the utterance that the patient is required to produce fluently (Ryan 1971). This method, designated by the acronym *GILCU* (gradual increase in length and complexity of utterance), encourages success by controlling the difficulty of the task presented to the patient. Ryan and Ryan (1995) found GILCU to be particularly successful in transfer and maintenance activities, assignments that the patient performs outside the therapy setting.

Other methods addressing language or prosody demand an artificial or atypical form of speech and may not be acceptable to some patients

TABLE 8.1   Foci and Types of Therapy Used for Stuttering

Attitudes and secondary behaviors
    Counseling
    Relaxation therapy
    Systematized desensitization
    Counter-conditioning
    Deconditioning
    Cognitive therapy
    Operant conditioning
    Role playing
    Biofeedback

Language and prosody
    GILCU (gradual increase in length and complexity of utterance)
    Exaggerated stress
    Junctured speech
    Rate reduction

Overall speech change
    Prolonged speech
    Rate reduction
    Delayed auditory feedback
    White noise
    Metronome/rhythm
    Choral speech
    Shadowing

Physical speech targets
    Breath flow management
    Easy phonatory onset
    Smooth articulation contacts
    Fluency initiating gestures
    Biofeedback

Stuttered or fluent moment
    Cancellations
    Pullouts
    Motor planning
    Preparatory set
    Punishment
    Negative practice
    Operant conditioning

Source: Reprinted with permission from C Conrad. Teaching Cultural Diversity in Professional Education—Fluency and Fluency Disorders. In L Cole, V Deal (eds), Multicultural Professional Education. Rockville, MD: American Speech-Language-Hearing Association, 1990.

for transfer activities because their cultural group may ridicule use of an artificial speech pattern. Examples of these are rate reduction or slowed speech; exaggerated stress, which is a technique requiring the person who stutters to use an artificial intonation pattern; and junctured speech, in which the patient lengthens the normal pause time at grammatical junctures.

Overall Speech Change

The goal of techniques of overall speech change is to immediately produce fluent speech in patients who stutter. Often the fluent speech is artificial in nature and has the same disadvantages for use with certain cultural groups as those described in the previous section. Prolonged speech and rhythmic speech using a metronome are examples of techniques of overall speech change. Other techniques that effect an overall speech change require the use of some artificial device. *Delayed* auditory feedback is a device that produces prolonged fluent speech in the patient by presenting his or her speech to the patient through earphones at a 1- or 2-second delay. Another technique is to present *white noise*, or masking noise, through earphones to the stutterer while he or she is talking to produce fluency. These techniques demonstrate to the patient his or her fluent capabilities, but they are often not practical for transfer activities. Persons from several cultural groups may resist public use of an artificial device. Choral speech, in which the person who stutters speaks simultaneously with one or more speakers, and shadowing, in which the patient initiates with another speaker with a brief delay, are both methods that produce immediate fluency. These methods can be effective for classroom activities for the school-age patient with the teacher or a fluent classmate serving as a simultaneous speaker or model. However, both techniques should be evaluated carefully for individual acceptability.

Physical Speech Targets

Because a number of research studies have documented abnormal functioning of physical speech processes during stuttering behavior, as well as during fluent speech in persons who stutter (Perkins et al. 1976; Peters et al. 1989; Adams 1974; Zimmerman 1980; Yaruss and Conture 1996), speech-language pathologists often train the patient to control one or more of these physical processes to achieve fluent speech. Breath-flow management, easy phonatory onset, and development of smooth articulatory contacts are examples of techniques that focus on speech targets. The modern speech-language pathologist uses computerized applications of these techniques that are focused on physical speech targets. Using biofeedback, computer software permits the speaker to monitor his or her behavior and use that information to modify the target speech behavior. Developing appropriate and acceptable transfer assignments using these approaches is the challenge clinicians face as they employ techniques to change the patient's ability to control his or her physical speech processes.

Traditional stuttering therapy developed by the Iowa Group at the University of Iowa in the 1930s focused on helping the patient cope with each stuttered moment (Johnson 1933; Bryngelson et al. 1944; Van Riper 1982b). The Iowa Group consisted of three speech pathologists, Bryng Bryngelson, Wendell Johnson, and Charles Van Riper, who were major contributors to the development of the field of speech-language pathology. Van Riper (1982a) described techniques that the person who stutters could use to modify his or her speech so that it would be more acceptable to the listener. These techniques are preparatory set, pullout, and cancellation. Preparatory set is a technique in which the patient changes the tense articulatory position with which he or she typically initiated disfluent speech. The patient begins speech with his or her articulators at a state of rest, initiates the first sound as a movement into the second sound, and initiates voice as he or she begins to say the word. Pullout is a technique the patient uses when he or she begins to stutter a word. Instead of allowing the stuttered movement to continue, the patient prolongs the word to "pull out" of the stuttering pattern. Cancellation is used by the patient when preparatory set and pullout fail. With cancellation, the stutterer repeats the stuttered word to cancel the disfluency. In addition to Van Riper's techniques, Bryngelson and colleagues (1944) developed the negative practice technique to enable the patient to develop motor control by deliberately stuttering on a word, or "bouncing" in a controlled form of stuttering. The goal of all of these techniques is to help the patient cope with stuttering.

Another method that focuses on the stuttered moment is based on learning theory. Punishment is a technique that presents an aversive stimulus (e.g., mild electric shock or the word *no*) with the occurrence of each stuttered moment (see Table 8.1).

Transfer and Maintenance of Fluency

Fluency is often achieved in the clinical therapy setting and fades away in the classroom and at home. Typically, permanent fluency is the gauge that patients and their families use to measure the success of therapy. Transfer describes the ability of the stutterer to be fluent outside of the therapy setting. It is crucial that the speech-language pathologist plan transfer activities that fit the patient's lifestyle, his or her social setting, and his or her cultural milieu. When considered in the evaluation process, social and cultural factors maximize the success of the transfer process and the ability of the patient to maintain the level of fluency attained over a long period of time.

Treatment of the Child Who Stutters

Treatment of the preschool or school-age child who stutters differs from that of the adult who stutters (Ham 1990). For the child, the family and the teacher are included as essential members of the treatment team. This means that the clinician must be especially aware of the social and cultural factors identified in *Evaluation of Social and Cultural Factors in the Treatment of Stuttering.*

Because family members are frequently participants in conversations with the stutterer, they should be considered in the development of the treatment plan. In addition, the parents will most likely decide to implement therapy. Consequently, the parents must feel comfortable with the treatment plan. The successful clinician develops a plan that incorporates transfer activities that address the conversations occurring in the home, in the classroom, and among peers.

References

Adams MR. A physiologic and aerodynamic interpretation of fluent and stuttered speech. J Fluency Disord 1974;1:35–47.

Barbara DA. Stuttering: A Psychodynamic Approach to Its Understanding and Treatment. New York: Julian Press, 1954.

Bloodstein OA. A Handbook on Stuttering (3rd ed). Chicago: National Easter Seal Society, 1981.

Brutten GJ, Shoemaker DJ. The Modification of Stuttering. Englewood Cliffs, NJ: Prentice-Hall, 1967.

Bryngelson B, Chapman M, Hansen O. Know Yourself: A Guide for Those Who Stutter. Minneapolis: Burgess Publishing, 1944.

Conrad C. An incidence study of stuttering among black adults, Ph.D. diss., Northwestern University, Evanston, IL, 1980.

Conrad C. A conversational act analysis of black mother-child dyads including stuttering and non-stuttering children, Ph.D. diss., Northwestern University, Evanston, IL, 1985.

Dietrich S, Barry SJ, Parker D. Middle latency auditory responses in males who stutter. J Speech Hear Res 1995;38:5–17.

Eisenson J. A Perseverative Theory of Stuttering. In J Eisenson (ed), Stuttering: A Symposium. New York: Harper & Row, 1958.

Fairbanks G. Selective vocal effects of delayed auditory feedback. J Speech Hear Disord 1955;20:333–346.

Flanagan B, Goldiamond I, Azrin N. Instatement of stuttering in normally fluent individuals through operant procedures. Science 1959;130:979–981.

Froeschels E. Pathology and therapy of stuttering. Nerv Child 1943;2:148–161.

Goldiamond I. Stuttering and Fluency as Manipulatable Operant Response Classes. In L Krasner, LP Ullmann (eds), Research in Behavior Modification. New York: Holt, Rinehart & Winston, 1965.

Glauber IP. The Psychoanalysis of Stuttering. In J Eisenson (ed), Stuttering: A Symposium. New York: Harper & Row, 1958.

Goldman R. Cultural influences in the sex ratio in the incidence of stuttering. American Anthropologist 1967;69:78.

Gregory HH. Controversies About Stuttering Therapy. Baltimore: University Park Press, 1979.

Ham RE. Therapy of Stuttering Preschool Through Adolescence. Englewood Cliffs, NJ: Prentice-Hall, 1990.

Jayaram M. Phonetic influences on stuttering in monolingual and bilingual stutterers. J Commun Disord 1983;16:287–297.

Johnson W. An Interpretation of Stuttering. Q J Speech 1933;19:70–76.

Johnson W. A study of the onset and development of stuttering. J Speech Disord 1942;7:251–257.

Johnson W. The Onset of Stuttering. Minneapolis: University of Minnesota Press, 1959.

Johnson W. Stuttering and What You Can Do about It. Minneapolis: University of Minnesota Press, 1961.

Johnson W. What is Stuttering? Stuttering Words (3rd ed). Memphis, TN: Speech Foundation of America, 1973.

Johnson W, Solomon A. Studies in the psychology of stuttering: IV. A quantitative study of expectation of stuttering as a process involving a low degree of consciousness. J Speech Disord 1937;2:95–97.

Lee BS. Effects of delayed speech feedback. J Acoustical Soc Am 1950;22:639–640.

Leith W, Mims H. Cultural influences in the development and treatment of stuttering: a preliminary report on the black stutterer. J Speech Hear Disord 1975;40:459–466.

Lemert E. Some Indians who stutter. J Speech Hear Disord 1953;18:168–174.

Louko LJ, Wolk L, Edwards ML, Conture EG. Phonological characteristics of young stutterers and their normally fluent peers. Preliminary observations. J Fluency Disord 1990;15:191–210.

Murphy A. Feelings and Attitudes. Therapy for Stutterers. Memphis, TN: Speech Foundation of America, 1974.

Orton S, Travis LE. Studies in stuttering: IV. Studies of action currents in stutterers. Arch Neurol Psychiatry 1929;21:61–68.

Perkins W. Replacement of stuttering with normal speech. III. Clinical effectiveness. J Speech Hear Disord 1974;39:416–428.

Perkins W, Rudas J, Johnson L, Bell J. Discoordination of articulation with phonation and respiration. J Speech Hear Res 1976;19:509–522.

Peters HFM, Hulstijn W, Starkweather CW. Acoustic and physiological reaction times of stutterers and non stutterers. J Speech Hear Res 1989;32:668–680.

Peters TJ, Guitar B. Stuttering: An Integrated Approach to Its Nature and Treatment. Baltimore: Williams & Wilkins, 1991.

Ryan BP, Ryan BV. Programmed stuttering treatment for children: comparison of two establishment programs through transfer, maintenance, and follow-up. J Speech Hear Res 1995;38:61–75.

Ryan B. Operant procedures applied to stuttering therapy for children. J Speech Hear Disord 1971;36:264–280.

Seymour CM, Ruggiero A, McEaneaney J. The identification of stuttering: can you look and tell? J Fluency Disord 1983;8:3.

Sheehan JG. Theory and treatment of stuttering as an approach-avoidance conflict. J Psychol 1953;36:51–63.

Sheehan JG. Stuttering: Research and Therapy. New York: Harper & Row, 1970.

Silverman EM. The Female Stutterer. In KO St. Louis (ed), The Atypical Stutterer. Orlando, FL: Academic, 1986;35–63.

Smith A. Factors in the Etiology of Stuttering. In JA Cooper (ed), Research Needs in Stuttering: Roadblocks and Future Directions [ASHA Reports 18, 39–47]. Rockville, MD: American Speech-Language-Hearing Association, 1990.

Snidecor JC. Why the Indian does not stutter. Q J Speech 1947;33:493.

Stewart JL. The problem of stuttering in certain North American Indian societies [monograph]. J Speech Hear Disord 1960;6:1.

Travis LE, Lindsley DB. An action current study of handedness in relation to stuttering. J Exp Psychol 1933;16:258.

Van Riper C. What is Stuttering? Stuttering Words (3rd ed). Memphis, TN: Speech Foundation of America, 1973.

Van Riper C. The Nature of Stuttering (1st ed). Englewood Cliffs, NJ: Prentice-Hall, 1971.

Van Riper C. The Treatment of Stuttering. Englewood Cliffs, NJ: Prentice-Hall, 1982a.

Van Riper C. The Nature of Stuttering (2nd ed). Englewood Cliffs, NJ: Prentice-Hall, 1982b.

Watson BC, Pool KD, Devous MD, et al. Brain blood flow related to acoustic laryngeal reaction time in adult developmental stutterers. J Speech Hear Res 1992;35:555–561.

Webster RL. A Behavioral Analysis of Stuttering: Treatment and Theory. In KS Calhoun, HE Adams, KH Mitchell (eds), Innovative Treatment Methods in Psychopathology. New York: Wiley, 1974.

West R. An Agnostic's Speculations About Stuttering. In J Eisenson (ed), Stuttering: A Symposium. New York: Harper & Row, 1958.

Yaruss JS, Conture EG. Stuttering and phonological disorders in children: examination of the covert repair hypothesis. J Speech Hear Res 1996;39:349–364.

Zimmerman G, Liljeblad S, Frank A, Cleeland C. The Indians have many terms for it: stuttering among the Bannock-Shoshone. J Speech Hear Res 1983;26:315–318.

Zimmermann GN. Articulatory dynamics of fluent utterances of stutterers and nonstutterers. J Speech Hear Res 1980;23:95–107.

Chapter 8   Study Questions

1. Why is understanding social and cultural features of the patient critical?
2. What are two of the theories that have been proposed to explain the etiology of stuttering?
3. What portion of therapy is critical to the patient achieving permanent fluency outside of the therapy setting?

4. Describe the two sides of the major controversy about stuttering therapy that developed in the 1970s.
5. What is a technique used to change the attitudes of the person who stutters?
6. What is a technique that can be useful to help a student who reads aloud in the classroom avoid stuttering?
7. How will the clinician's knowledge of the patient's culture affect transfer and maintenance of fluency, especially in the young child who stutters?

9 Adult Cognitive, Linguistic, and Speech Disorders

Judy Perkins Walker

Talking is one of the fine arts. … and its fluent harmonies may be spoiled by the intrusion of a single harsh note.

—Oliver Wendell Holmes

The human brain is capable of executing multiple cognitive computations, enabling humans to perform complex acts and communicate thousands of thoughts and ideas. When brain damage disrupts cognitive abilities, it has dire consequences for a person's capabilities to function within his or her society. Brain damage has many different etiologies, including stroke, head injury, and progressive diseases. It is not selective, but it affects people from different economic, cultural, and religious backgrounds. This chapter addresses the sequelae of aberrant behaviors that result from brain damage in adults. An overview of the anatomy of the brain is followed by sections that outline behaviors resulting from damage to different brain regions.

Organization of the Cerebral Cortex

To understand language and cognitive impairments resulting from neurologic damage, one must consider the relationship between brain and behavior. The human brain is divided into two halves—a left cerebral hemisphere and a right cerebral hemisphere. The two hemispheres are connected by fibers called the *corpus callosum*. The cells in each hemisphere depend on blood, which provides oxygen and metabolic agents that enable them to survive. Permanent damage to the brain tissue occurs if the blood supply is disrupted for more than 2–3 minutes. Cells within the brain communicate with one another via axons and dendrites, which are extensions of the cell. Thousands of interconnections

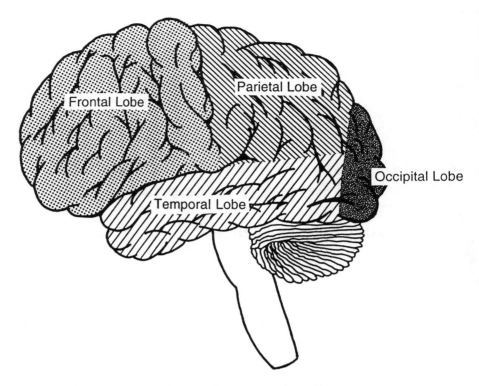

FIGURE 9.1 *Four lobes within each hemisphere of the brain.*

between cells form vast arrays of neural networks, which provide a rapid means for many cells to exchange information.

Each hemisphere is divided into four lobes: the temporal lobe, the occipital lobe, the parietal lobe, and the frontal lobe (Figure 9.1). Processing of sensory information from the environment occurs through the posterior portion of both cerebral hemispheres. The temporal lobe specializes in processing auditory stimuli. The occipital lobe processes visual stimuli. The parietal lobe processes stimuli related to the senses of touch, pain, and body temperature. The olfactory system and taste buds located on the surface of the tongue are responsible for the senses of smell and taste, respectively, but are not discussed in this chapter. The frontal lobes, located anteriorly within each hemisphere, specialize in planning and execution of motor responses to the environment.

Each lobe is further divided into primary, secondary, and tertiary areas. The primary sensory cortex is the first "place" that sensory information in its raw form is received in the cortex. This information is then sent to secondary and tertiary areas via neural networks for analysis of more complex characteristics of the stimulus. Once the information is processed, the frontal lobes are engaged to formulate and execute a response. For example, the primary visual area in the occipital lobe may receive visual sensory input of a basic line configuration.

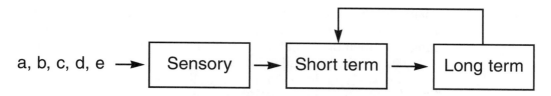

FIGURE 9.2 *Schematic of sensory, short-term (working), and long-term memory. A representation of a stimulus (i.e., alphabet) enters into sensory memory and is transferred to short-term memory for temporary storage. If the stimulus is to be retained, it is transferred to long-term memory, where it can be recalled and transferred into working memory at a later time.*

The secondary and tertiary areas may further analyze the line configuration by shape, color, and texture and visually recognize a bell. Additional sensory information, such as "ringing sound" and "cold and smooth to touch," may be added from the temporal and parietal lobes, respectively. This combined information may then be sent to the frontal lobe and a motor response of "ringing the bell" may be initiated.

Attention and Memory

Humans are not conscious of all stimuli that are detected by sensory organs. Attention refers to the ability to selectively attend to certain stimuli over others within the environment. These chosen stimuli are ultimately entered into memory. Attention cannot be separated from memory, because only the stimuli that are attended to can be learned and remembered. Selective attention can be controlled by certain properties of the stimulus (e.g., its intensity) or by task demands. For example, a loud clap of thunder immediately draws attention to that sound, and taking a written test draws attention to the words on the page.

After a person attends to information, it must be retained in memory for further processing. There are three forms of memory (Figure 9.2). Sensory memory is the form of memory in which the stimulus lasts for only a brief period of time. Sensory memory accurately represents the stimulus in its original form. Visual or iconic sensory memory contains a brief visual image of an object that was just seen, and auditory or echoic sensory memory contains a fleeting echo of the sound that was just heard. This brief stimulus is then transferred to short-term, or working, memory, which refers to the temporary storage of information that has just been perceived. Working memory has limited capacity (e.g., up to seven digits plus or minus two) and duration. For example, after dialing directory assistance for a phone number, a person rehearses the seven-digit number in working memory while hanging up the phone and preparing to dial. If there is no future use for the phone number, it is erased from working memory. However, if there is a need to permanently retain the phone number, it is transferred from working memory to long-term memory for storage and retrieval at a later time.

Long-term memory has an unlimited capacity and duration as indicated by the ability to recall childhood memories. Both attention and memory are susceptible to brain damage that interferes with the ability of each cerebral hemisphere to process and access the kind of information specialized within that hemisphere.

Lateralization of Function: Damage to the Left Hemisphere

In most people, the left hemisphere is specialized for analytical processing (i.e., analyzing individual parts that comprise the whole). Because of this, the left hemisphere has a dominant role in the processing and production of language and in sequential organization and deductive reasoning abilities (i.e., inferring specific instances from general rules). The left hemisphere also controls motor movements on the right side of the body that are necessary for speaking, swallowing, and arm and leg movement.

Aphasia

Damage to the left hemisphere often results in aphasia. Aphasia is an acquired disruption in the processes involved in understanding and producing language. The most common cause of aphasia is a cerebrovascular accident, or stroke, which disrupts the blood supply to the left cerebral hemisphere, causing the brain cells to die. Each year, strokes occur in approximately 550,000 people in the United States (Agency for Health Care Policy and Research 1995). These strokes are primarily attributed to hypertension and heart disease. The incidence of strokes is higher in men than in women. Strokes tend to affect African-Americans more than any other cultural group, as this group has a greater susceptibility to heart disease (Agency for Health Care Policy and Research 1995). Stroke etiologies can be classified as embolic, thrombotic, or hemorrhagic in nature.* Once the brain tissue is deprived of oxygen and metabolic agents provided by the blood supply, it cannot be rejuvenated. Other neurologic insults to the left hemisphere, such as a head injury and progressive diseases, can also result in aphasia.

---

*A thrombus is an obstruction that forms in an artery partially blocking the blood supply to the brain. An embolism is a clot that travels from another part of the body, becomes lodged within a cerebral artery, and blocks the blood supply. A hemorrhage results from a weakening of an arterial wall.

People with aphasia have deficits in language comprehension and production that are believed to stem from difficulty in accessing and/or retrieving linguistic information from long-term memory. Consequently, deficits can manifest in one or more stages of language comprehension and production. They can manifest in the retrieval of words (i.e., lexical access) and morphologic markers (i.e., bound morphemes, such as those showing verb tense, and free-standing morphemes, such as the function words *the* and *a*) and in the organization of grammar (i.e., syntax), all essential language components that form sentences that make some sort of semantic sense. Although there is considerable debate as to whether deficits can be localized to specific regions in the brain, distinct variations of deficient language patterns have been found to emerge from damage to certain areas of the left hemisphere. These patterns of aphasic deficits have been described according to the Boston Classification System (Goodglass and Kaplan 1983). This system makes an initial, broad distinction between types of aphasia according to fluent and nonfluent speech production.

Patients with fluent aphasia can be described as having little difficulty in speech production, but the content of the sentences may or may not make sense. They also have problems with auditory comprehension and repetition of words and sentences. Conversely, patients with nonfluent aphasia can be described as having effortful speech production and varying degrees of auditory comprehension deficits. The Boston Classification System also further subdivides fluent and nonfluent types of aphasia. Table 9.1 provides a brief summary of different classifications of aphasia.

Types of Aphasia

Wernicke's Aphasia
Wernicke's aphasia is an example of a fluent aphasia (see Table 9.1). It is caused by damage to Wernicke's area in the left temporal lobe resulting in both comprehension and production deficits (Figure 9.3). Auditory comprehension is often severely impaired at the lexical, syntactic, and semantic stages of sentence processing. Verbal production, which is typically severely impaired, can be described as fluent, well-articulated, language of confusion. Sentences are usually devoid of meaning, containing semantic paraphasias (e.g., "spoon" for *fork*, "coffee pot" for *cup*, "rubber" for *eraser*) and neologisms (i.e., nonsense words). Although grammatical structures appear to be intact, sentences often do not make sense. These patients tend to be compelled to talk without stopping and have a lack of awareness of their deficits (i.e., anosognosia).

Consider the following patient. SZ is a 55-year-old, right-handed woman who had a hemorrhagic stroke causing damage to the left temporal lobe that resulted in Wernicke's aphasia. SZ was asked to

TABLE 9.1   Types of Aphasia According to the Boston Classification System

Aphasia Type	Classifications of Aphasia		
	Auditory Comprehension	Repetition	Verbal Expression
Fluent			
Wernicke's	Poor	Poor	Poor; grammatical structure intact but presence of semantic paraphasias and neologisms make verbal expression resemble jargon
Transcortical/sensory	Poor	Good	Poor; similar to Wernicke's aphasia
Conduction	Good	Poor	Good; occasional paraphasias and grammatical errors
Anomic	Good	Good	Good; word finding difficulties in the presence of grammatically well-formed sentences
Nonfluent			
Broca's	Good	Poor	Poor; effortful; agrammatic sentences with content words but few function words; literal paraphasias
Transcortical/motor	Good	Good	Poor; incomplete sentences; paraphasias; naming better than spontaneous speech
Global	Poor	Poor	Poor; effortful; spontaneous speech characterized by limited recurring utterances

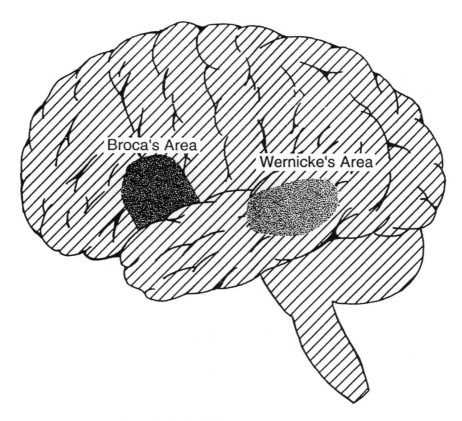

FIGURE 9.3 *Broca's and Wernicke's areas.*

describe the picnic scene from the *Western Aphasia Battery* (Figure 9.4):

Examiner: Tell me what you see. Try to talk in complete sentences.
SZ: Wayne now is a things. They're continuing on the things. Brown considers the things now. I don't know for sure. It might have a continued look, I don't know. A complete message. Ah, there a badder brought home a thing. Well, there is a failure that I couldn't understand. Well, I could understand the future of the fly, but got confused when I couldn't.

As can be seen in this example, SZ's spontaneous speech is fluent, but the message is meaningless. There is a prevalence of empty content words (e.g., thing) used as fillers. However, the sentences have relatively intact grammatical structures. SZ clearly had difficulty conveying her thoughts about this picture but did not demonstrate an awareness of the problem.

Broca's Aphasia

Broca's aphasia is an example of a nonfluent aphasia. It is caused by damage to Broca's area within the left frontal lobe (see Figure 9.3).

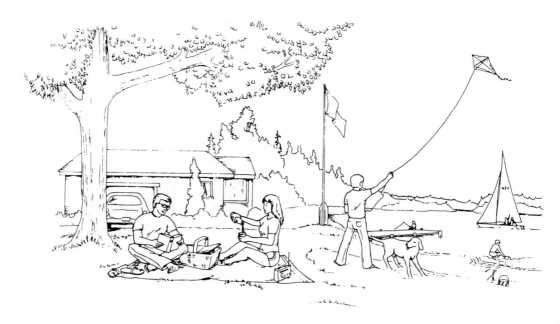

FIGURE 9.4 *Picnic scene from the Western Aphasia Battery. (Reprinted with permission from A Kertesz. Western Aphasia Battery. New York: Grune & Stratton, 1982.)*

Verbal production is described as nonfluent. Patients have trouble with the processes involved in accessing and retrieving the appropriate words, morphology, and syntax to produce semantically coherent sentences. In general, the sentences of patients with Broca's aphasia reflect word-finding difficulties in that they contain many content words (i.e., nouns and verbs) but few function words (i.e., articles). In addition, many of the content words are literal paraphasias, in which incorrect sound substitutions render the words meaningless (e.g., "knipe" for *knife*, "sopey pin" for *safety pin*, "bubber bad" for *rubber band*, "poom" for *spoon*). Bound morphemes also tend to be absent. Sentences often are agrammatical, containing incomplete or incorrect syntactic constructions. Although there may be auditory comprehension deficits, they tend to be disproportionately mild when compared to the severe production deficits. Consequently, these patients may understand or express the gist of a message but miss relevant linguistic details necessary to convey a complete thought. They tend to be acutely aware of their deficits and often try to self-correct mistakes, which interferes with the forward flow of speech.

Consider the following patient. BK is a 59-year-old, right-handed woman who sustained damage to the left frontal lobe from a hemorrhagic stroke that resulted in Broca's aphasia. When asked what had happened to her, BK responded with the following:

Examiner: Tell me what happened to you.

BK: It was ... um, fifty, forty. I didn't ... talk three years ... and I talking and ... um , I went doctor ... um, I went teacher ... was very good and ... um, want to test ... test something in brain. I did, dit, didn't try ... and talking.

As can be seen, BK had a great degree of difficulty retrieving the correct words. The ellipses indicate pauses where she was searching for the appropriate words. She was able to produce content words but had more difficulty with function words. Sentences were incomplete and lacked the appropriate syntactic structures. Although she clearly had difficulty speaking, BK's answer was sufficient to convey the gist of her problem.

Other Types of Aphasia

Other types of fluent and nonfluent aphasias have also been described by the Boston Classification System. As seen in Table 9.1, the distinguishing characteristics of transcortical sensory aphasia include the relative ability of patients to repeat words and sentences in spite of poor auditory comprehension and verbal expression abilities. In contrast, patients with conduction aphasia have poor repetition abilities with intact auditory comprehension and verbal expression abilities. Anomic aphasia is characterized primarily by subtle word-finding difficulties in spontaneous speech. Of the remaining nonfluent aphasias, transcortical motor aphasia is characterized by relatively good auditory comprehension and repetition abilities but impaired spontaneous speech. This is different from Broca's aphasia in that patients with transcortical motor aphasia tend to have good repetition abilities in spite of having poor naming abilities and difficulty initiating spontaneous speech. Global aphasia results from massive damage to the left hemisphere and usually severely impairs all modalities. Patients with global aphasia are often unable to comprehend simple one- and two-word combinations, and their production is limited to continuous repetition of the same utterance.

Aphasia in Bilingual Populations

The discussion of aphasia thus far has focused on monolinguals (i.e., people who speak only one language). However, in a multicultural society there are many people who speak two or more languages. Because bilingual people have the ability to mix the languages at the lexical, syntactic, and semantic stages of sentence processing and production, it is interesting to determine the impact of brain damage on each of their languages.

Although there are many bodies of research on aphasia in bilingual populations, a central question to all of this research is whether cerebral representation of the languages of a bilingual speaker is the same as that of a monolingual speaker. One view suggests that there are different anatomic regions for different languages (Rapport et al. 1983). However, there is sufficient evidence to support an opposing view that all languages are represented in the same anatomic regions, those regions being the classical language areas as brain damage in one area can impact multiple languages (Paradis 1987). For example, Paradis and colleagues (1982) reported on patients who lost selective linguistic abilities in all of their languages after brain damage and also lost their ability to translate in either direction. But the impact is not necessarily equivalent across languages, as bilingual speakers with aphasia do not always lose language capabilities proportional to the degree of mastery of the languages before the brain injury. There are reports of differential recovery in which the skill in one language recovers better than that in another (Rapport et al. 1983; April and Han 1980). There are also reports of the recovery of one language before another (Rapport et al. 1983). In other cases, the patient's recovery results in systematic mixing of languages inextricably (Perecman 1984). These findings present challenges to the practicing clinician in diagnosing and treating aphasia in the bilingual or multilingual speaker, because several factors must be considered when addressing aphasia in this population.

Deficits That Accompany Aphasia

Reading and Writing Deficits

In addition to deficits in auditory comprehension and verbal production of language, patients with damage to the left hemisphere of the brain may also exhibit complications with reading and writing. A literate person may experience a sudden onset of reading difficulties, which is referred to as *acquired dyslexia*. Acquired dyslexia can affect the ability to recognize whole words, as well as the ability to sound out words letter by letter, which results in difficulty reading individual words and sentences. Writing deficits, referred to as *dysgraphia*, can also be experienced by patients with left-hemisphere damage. If motor deficits do not affect the dominant hand, patients can write words and sentences that reflect word-finding and grammatical deficits that exist in their spontaneous speech. The words may contain numerous spelling errors. For example, it can be seen in Figure 9.5 that the patient has relatively intact, but simplistic, syntactic constructions. The patient also has word-finding difficulties.

Motor Deficits

Damage to the left hemisphere can result in motor deficits that cause difficulty with speaking, swallowing, and arm and leg control. Cortical damage to the precentral motor strip above Broca's area in the frontal lobe can cause apraxia (i.e., difficulty in voluntarily executing learned motor sequences not caused by muscle weakness). Apraxia is divided into three general categories: oral apraxia, apraxia

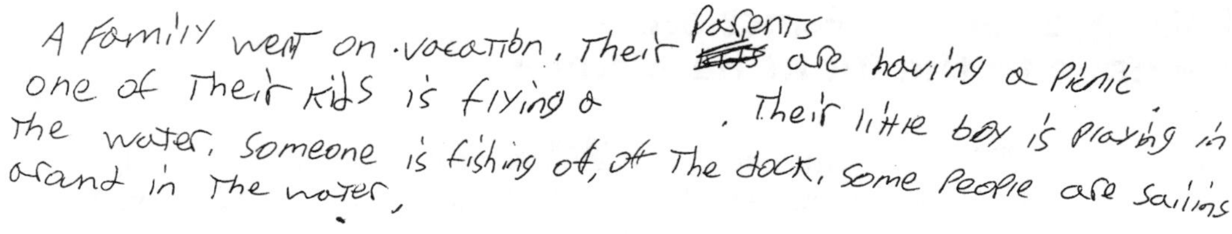

A Family went on vacation, Their parents ~~kids~~ are having a Picnic
one of Their kids is flying a . Their little boy is playing in
The water. Someone is fishing of, off The dock, some people are sailing
around in The water,

FIGURE 9.5   *Writing deficits associated with left-hemisphere damage to the brain. Description of the picnic scene from the Western Aphasia Battery (see Figure 9.4). (Reprinted with permission from A Kertesz. Western Aphasia Battery. New York: Grune & Stratton, 1982.)*

of speech, and limb apraxia. Oral apraxia affects the ability to execute nonverbal oral motor sequences, such as blowing and sticking out the tongue. Apraxia of speech affects the ability to execute motor sequences for speaking. Patients with apraxia of speech may know what they want to say but are unable to properly program their articulators to say it. Speech production is often effortful and nonfluent, consisting of numerous articulatory errors. Limb apraxia affects the ability to execute motor sequences related to arm and hand movement, such as using a screwdriver or saluting.

Dysarthria is described as a slurring of speech resulting from muscle weakness. Patients often know what they want to say, but their utterances are often slurred and unintelligible.

Patients who have difficulty speaking as a result of apraxia or dysarthria may also have dysphagia (i.e., impairment in swallowing), as many of the same motor sequences and muscle groups are involved in both speaking and swallowing. Patients who have difficulty swallowing liquids and foods by mouth may require feeding tubes to prevent aspiration pneumonia caused by liquids or foods entering the lungs.

Patients with left-hemisphere damage may experience gross motor deficits in the form of weakness (i.e., hemiparesis) or paralysis (i.e., hemiplegia) of the right side of the body. As a result, patients often have trouble using their right extremities for activities such as writing, eating, dressing, and walking.

Sequential Organization and Deductive-Reasoning Deficits

Left-hemisphere damage can also cause deficits in the analysis of crucial steps in a sequence that lead to the organization and correct resolution of tasks. Patients with left-hemisphere damage know what they want to accomplish but often leave out steps while performing a task. For example, when baking cookies, the patient may forget to add sugar. Furthermore, analytical abilities are also necessary for deductive reasoning. For example, the aforementioned patient may also have difficulty deducing that sugar makes food sweet. Hence, the patient may be unable to correct the problem.

Lateralization of Function:
Damage to the Right Hemisphere

As with left-hemisphere damage, the most common cause of right-hemisphere damage to the brain is stroke. However, patients with right-hemisphere damage present a number of behavioral sequelae that are different from those of patients with left-hemisphere damage. Unlike the left hemisphere, the right hemisphere is dominant in holistic processing, which organizes and integrates individual parts into the whole. These processes are essential to pragmatic interactions, visuo-perceptual and spatial abilities, and the overall organization of information required to complete tasks. Furthermore, the right hemisphere appears to be dominant for inductive reasoning (i.e., inferring general rules from specific instances).

Deficits in Pragmatics

Right-hemisphere damage often results in deficits in pragmatics or social interactions. According to Davis and Wilcox (1985), three contexts must be considered for successful pragmatic interactions: linguistic context, paralinguistic contexts, and extralinguistic contexts. Linguistic context is the understanding of and production of complex linguistic units beyond sentence level, such as in conversations and stories. Paralinguistic contexts provide information that is expressed through implicit information (e.g., inflectional changes that convey emotion and sarcasm). Extralinguistic contexts refer to the understanding of implicit social conventions for successful pragmatic exchanges determined by the shared knowledge of participants and situational cues.

Linguistic Contexts

Although the left hemisphere of the brain in most people is dominant in language, deficits can stem from right-hemisphere damage, which can affect the ability to exchange the complex linguistic information required for conversing and telling coherent stories. Aphasia that is associated with left-hemisphere damage affects the ability to use the correct sounds, words, and syntax to understand and produce semantically correct sentences. Conversely, right-hemisphere damage disrupts the organizational and inferencing abilities necessary to comprehend and produce lengthy linguistic units comprised of several sentences.

When engaged in conversation or when telling a story, patients with right-hemisphere damage often fail to use the appropriate microstructure, which consists of cohesive devices that tie one sentence to another. These cohesive devices can take several linguistic forms, such as pronominal references (e.g., *Bob* bought a car. *He* drove the car home) and determiners (e.g., Bob bought a *car*. *The* car was red.). Cohesion can also occur by making the appropriate inferences regarding information that is missing between sentences. Causal inferences are often used as implicit cohesive devices to tie sentences together. For example, when hearing the two sentences, "The lamp was on the table. Now it's in a million pieces," a listener could infer that the cause of the lamp being in a million pieces is that it fell off the table. Causal inference ties these two sentences together, but the cause is not explicitly stated.

Consider the following description of the picnic scene from the *Western Aphasia Battery* told by AJ, a 76-year-old man who sustained a right frontoparietal embolic stroke following heart surgery (see Figure 9.4):

Examiner: Tell me a story about this picture. Try to talk in complete sentences.

AJ: Must be a camp on Western Ontario lake. It is a family affair, dog little fella, sailors, dog and the family. People been up in that area before, like the area. Lunch basket is open. So they must have traveled somewhere; Canada. To there, could be carrying things to that part of Canada, I don't know. Evidently it is a happy family, even the dog. I don't see a cat. It is probably a winter camp. They make them up there sometime for ice skating. It is probably a young professor. And they are spending the summer up there. It was back in 1980 too.

It is evident that AJ had difficulty telling a story about the picture. Because of the appropriate word selection and sentence structure, it can be determined that this difficulty is not attributed to aphasia. Instead, AJ had difficulty producing a cohesive story about this picture. He frequently used incorrect cohesive devices (i.e., the underlined words), which had no clear referents in preceding sentences. He also demonstrated a lack of causal cohesion (e.g., "Lunch basket is open. So they must have traveled somewhere").

Right-hemisphere damage to the brain also disrupts the ability to use the appropriate macrostructure, which is required to follow the proper overall organization necessary for engaging in conversation or telling stories. Most conversations and stories have a setting and opening event, in which all of the characters involved are identified (e.g., "Once upon a time, there was a queen that lived in a big castle in England. One day, she was kidnapped from the castle by an evil knight …"). The story then follows a series of episodes that ultimately lead to some kind of closure (e.g., "The king killed the evil knight, rescued the queen, and they lived happily ever after"). Typically, it would be surprising and confusing to hear the conclusion or closing event of a story at the beginning. However, patients with right-hemisphere damage often wander from the point, providing strings of unrelated details that cause a conversation partner to miss the gist of a story or conversation.

As seen in AJ's story, coherence is lacking, because there is no clear structure to the story. Although AJ provides an initial setting (i.e., camp on Western Ontario lake) and attempts to identify characters (e.g., dog, little fella, sailors, family), he fails to provide an initiating event, episodes, or closure to the story. He wanders from the point by giving tangential information related to Canada and imposing irrelevant details.

Paralinguistic Contexts

In addition to linguistic contexts, there is implicit pragmatic information (e.g., changes in prosody, facial expression, and situational cues) exchanged during a conversation that allows the participants to abstract more information than is contained in the words. This implicit information is referred to as the *paralinguistic context*.

Prosody refers to the stress, rhythm, and intonation that provides additional information about a message, such as a speaker's gender, emotional status, sarcasm, and humor. For example, sarcasm can be conveyed by increasing stress on one word in a sentence: "Oh yea, Joan is *really* fat," meaning that Joan is thin. Right-hemisphere damage to the brain disrupts the holistic processing necessary to analyze and produce prosodic patterns that convey implicit information. Consequently, patients tend to interpret sentences, such as the one above, literally and form a concrete interpretation (e.g., Joan *is* fat).

Furthermore, right-hemisphere damage can disrupt inferential abilities necessary to understand or express metaphors, idiomatic expressions, and indirect requests, all of which often require situational cues for correct interpretation. As with prosody, patients with right-hemisphere damage tend to focus on the concrete information explicitly stated in words, resulting in a literal interpretation of metaphors, idiomatic expressions, and indirect requests. For example, a right hemisphere–damaged patient may interpret the expression, "It takes two to tango," concretely and believe that the speaker is saying that you need two people to dance.

Extralinguistic Contexts

The participants in a conversation recognize certain conventions, termed the *extralinguistic contexts*, that must be considered to carry out appropriate pragmatic interactions. These conventions include making inferences about the purpose and setting of a conversation, and about the participants, including their roles, shared knowledge, emotional state, physical orientation, and body position. Because right hemisphere–damaged patients have trouble recognizing the whole scene and focus instead on individual parts, they often make the wrong inferences regarding the rules they must follow to interact appropriately. Patients with right-hemisphere damage often make the wrong judgment about the context and roles of the participants and make the wrong adjustments. For example, in a formal situation (e.g., talking to his or her boss) a patient with right-hemisphere damage might speak as if he or she were in an informal situation (e.g., talking

to a friend). Furthermore, because they have trouble making inferences, right hemisphere–damaged patients often do not recognize their
inappropriate behavior (i.e., anosognosia).

Visuoperceptual, Visuospatial, and Visuoconstructional Deficits

Right parietal lobe damage has a pronounced impact on visual processing abilities, which results in a variety of visuoperceptual, visuospatial, and visuoconstructional deficits. These deficits do not stem
from a visual acuity problem but rather from a higher-level impairment
in the ability to integrate parts into a meaningful whole in spite of
receiving sufficient sensory information.

Visuoperceptual Deficits

Patients with visuoperceptual deficits experience difficulty in visual
discrimination. An example of such a difficulty is a patient's inability to
visually recognize an object when it is placed in front of him or her
(i.e., visual object agnosia), although the patient can often name the
object if allowed to process other features through different sensory
modalities (e.g., sound or touch). These patients may also have pro-
posagnosia, which is the inability to recognize faces. Family members
often report walking into hospital rooms and not being recognized by
the patient until they speak, when the patient recognizes the voice.

Some patients who recognize individual objects lack visual analysis
and synthesis capabilities and may not understand the interrelationships among an array of complex stimuli. These patients may have
trouble separating figure from ground or recognizing incomplete figures because of difficulty synthesizing the disparate parts into a complete form. Consider the performance of MC, who sustained a closed
head injury with significant right-hemisphere damage, when asked to
name incomplete pictures from *The Hooper Visual Organization Test*
(Figure 9.6). When presented with Figure 9.6A, he responded, "I can't
really make it out. I think it might be a cup because I can see a handle." He was unable to put together the pieces of Figure 9.6B to formulate a correct response and ultimately responded, "I just don't know
what it is."

Visuospatial Deficits

Visuospatial deficits involve the visual processing of interrelationships
of items within a spatial domain. Patients with right-hemisphere damage often have difficulty making directional judgments and locating
points in space necessary for depth perception and judgment of
width, length, and distance. For example, a patient who worked as a
bartender remarked that he had trouble judging how far or near an
object was and frequently grabbed air when reaching to take a glass
off a shelf.

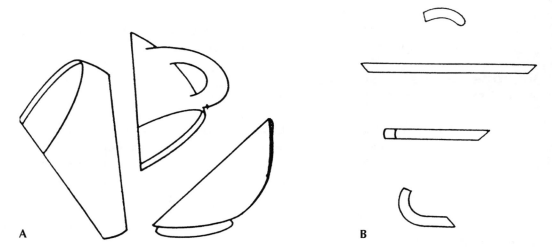

FIGURE 9.6 *Test items from The Hooper Visual Organization Test. (A) is a cup, and (B) is a cane. (Reprinted with permission from HE Hooper. The Hooper Visual Organization Test. Los Angeles: Western Psychological Services, 1957.)*

Right-hemisphere damage can also cause poor topographical orientation and the inability to create a visuospatial representation of a place within working or long-term memory. Patients with this deficit often get lost even in familiar surroundings. One patient commented that he could not remember the layout of a store he had worked in for several years after the lights were turned off. This indicated that he had no mental representation of the spatial layout of the store in memory. Another patient was unable to draw a map of her small town, although she had lived there for 20 years.

One of the most interesting visuospatial deficits is unilateral spatial agnosia, or unilateral visual neglect. Right hemisphere–damaged patients with this problem do not attend to visual stimuli that is left of the midline of their bodies. The left neglect can also extend to auditory and tactile information. Unilateral visual neglect is rarely seen in patients with left-hemisphere damage. Clinical observations of these patients have revealed interesting behaviors. For example, patients with left neglect may not attend to people or objects on their left side. They may bump into doorways and walls on the left side and never make left turns. They may even forget to eat food on the left side of their plate. One interesting way to test for left neglect is to have patients draw figures (e.g., a clock face or a person) and look for completeness and symmetry or have them dissect a horizontal line into two equal halves.

Consider the drawings of a clock face in Figure 9.7. Figure 9.7A was drawn by a patient, RS, who had sustained a right frontoparietal lesion from a cerebral vascular accident. Figures 9.7B and 9.7C were drawn by a patient, BG, who sustained damage in the same area

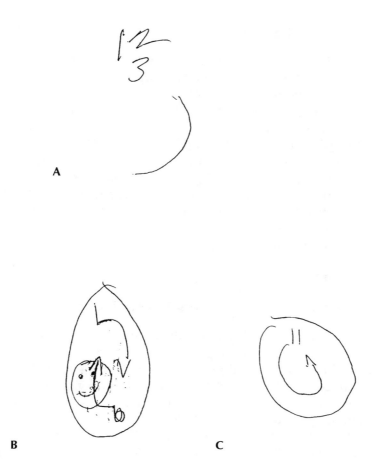

FIGURE 9.7 *Drawings of a clock face. (A) reveals both left neglect and visual analysis and synthesis deficits. (B) (drawn without a model) reveals both visual analysis and synthesis and direction deficits, as well as a literal interpretation of the task. (C) (drawn by the same patient as B when given a model to copy) is by a patient who continues to demonstrate analysis, synthesis, and direction deficits.*

from a head injury that occurred in a snowboarding accident. As seen in Figure 9.7A, RS demonstrated both visual analysis and synthesis deficits, as indicated by the incomplete drawing. Furthermore, the drawing reveals unilateral left visual neglect, because he only identified pieces of the clock located on the right side. In Figure 9.7B, BG has drawn a clock face that clearly reveals analysis and synthesis deficits, because the drawing is incomplete. The figure also shows difficulty in determining whether the arrow should go clockwise or counter-clockwise. Furthermore, he demonstrated a literal interpretation of the instructions and drew a face on the clock. Figure 9.7C is another attempt at drawing the clock face after being given a visual model. However, he continued to demonstrate the same analysis, synthesis, and directional deficits as seen in the previous figure.

Visuoconstructional Deficits

Patients with visuoconstructional deficits have difficulty perceiving the spatial relations between parts to organize or construct them into a two- or three-dimensional object. Two-dimensional deficits can be detected by requesting that patients copy complex figures or draw to verbal command. Three-dimensional deficits are often seen when asking a patient to assemble objects (e.g., block construction) along both horizontal and vertical planes. Visuoconstructional deficits can have a devastating impact on people who require these skills to earn a living. An experienced carpenter, who had sustained a right frontoparietal lesion from a head injury, told a story of trying to build three stairs leading to a doorway. He was unable to complete the project because he had no idea how the pieces should go together.

Additional Impairments

General Organization and Inductive Reasoning

Right-hemisphere damage to the brain can also cause deficits in the holistic processing of steps in a sequence that lead to the general organization and completion of tasks. Unlike patients with left hemisphere damage who are able to complete tasks but often do so incorrectly because they have left out details, right hemisphere–damaged patients tend to get caught up in details and fail to see tasks through to completion. A typical story that illustrates the disorganization experienced by right hemisphere–damaged patients was told by MC, a patient with a right frontoparietal lesion stemming from a head injury he sustained after being hit in the head.

MC: I am never able to finish any housework and my wife always gets mad at me and tells me I'm lazy. The other day, she left a list of things for me to do around the house. One of the things she wanted me to do was to vacuum both the upstairs and downstairs. So, I started to vacuum my daughter's room and saw clothes on the floor. I picked up some clothes and went to put them away and found that the closet door was loose. So, I went down to the basement to get my tool box and saw a birdhouse I had started to build. I decided to work on the bird house for awhile and the phone rang. I went upstairs to answer the phone and talked about 10 minutes. It was my wife. When I got off the phone, I saw the laundry basket full of clothes and began to do the laundry.

Needless to say, MC never completed any of the tasks on his wife's list. He lacked the organizational skills to execute one task through completion, instead he focused on details that led him from the task.

In addition, right hemisphere damage can cause deficits in inductive reasoning, which is the ability to infer general rules or principles from specific instances. These general rules are concepts that are formed from experience, so that when similar experiences occur a prototype in long-term memory guides the correct response. For example, when a person is lost in a strange place, a typical response is to go to the next gas station or stop a person on the street to ask directions or consult a map. A response typically given by right hemisphere–damaged patients is that they would go to the police station for help. They generalize the wrong concept to the specific instance—that is, they reason that "When I need help, I go to the police station," as opposed to "When I am lost, I ask the next person I see for directions." They also fail to see the logic of not being able to find the police station in a strange place. Because of deficits in inductive reasoning skills, these patients have the tendency to use poor judgment, which often makes them unsafe for independent living.

Motor Deficits

Damage to the right hemisphere can result in motor deficits to the left side of the body that interfere with speaking, swallowing, and arm and leg control. Like left hemisphere–damaged patients, these patients may have dysarthria, which impairs their speech intelligibility, and dysphagia. They may also have a left hemiparesis or hemiplegia.

Conclusion

Brain damage is not selective and can occur in any cultural or socioeconomic group. The impact the damage can have in disrupting a person's life is largely contingent on the society the person lives in. A person with aphasia would be at a tremendous disadvantage living in a culture that relies heavily on verbal communication (e.g., many technologically advanced countries). Likewise, a person with right-hemisphere damage would have difficulty surviving in a culture that requires excellent spatial and navigational skills (e.g., nomadic tribes). The interaction between socioeconomic status and cognitive deficits must always be considered when designing a diagnostic program or a therapy program that accurately targets a patient's abilities.

References

Agency for Health Care Policy and Research. Post-Stroke Rehabilitation. Rockville, MD: U.S. Department of Health and Human Services, 1995.

April R, Han M. Crossed aphasia in a right-handed bilingual Chinese man. Arch Neurol 1980;37:342–345.

Davis GA, Wilcox MJ. Adult Aphasia Rehabilitation: Applied Pragmatics. San Diego: College Hill Press, 1985.

Goodglass H, Kaplan E. The Assessment of Aphasia and Related Disorders. Philadelphia: Lea & Febiger, 1983.

Paradis M. The Assessment of Bilingual Aphasia. Hillsdale, NJ: Lawrence Erlbaum, 1987.

Paradis M, Goldblum MC, Abidi R. Alternate antagonism with paradoxical translation behavior in two bilingual aphasic patients. Brain Lang 1982;15:55–69.

Perecman E. Spontaneous translation and language mixing in a polyglot aphasic. Brain Lang 1984;23:43–63.

Rapport RL, Tan CT, Whitaker HA. Language function and dysfunction among Chinese and English-speaking polyglots: cortical stimulation, Wada testing, and clinical studies. Brain Lang 1983;18:342–366.

Chapter 9   Study Questions

1. Describe the organization of the human brain. What are neural networks? What are general functions of different areas of the cerebral hemispheres?
2. How do humans learn new information?
3. What is aphasia?
4. Describe deficits associated with Wernicke's aphasia and Broca's aphasia.
5. What are two different views regarding location of languages in a bilingual speaker?
6. What motor deficits are associated with left-hemisphere damage to the brain?
7. What three contexts must be considered when analyzing pragmatic deficits associated with right hemisphere damage to the brain?
8. What is the difference between the macrostructure and microstructure of narratives?
9. What are three different types of visual processing abilities associated with the right parietal lobe? Provide an example of deficits in each area that can result from damage to the right parietal lobe.
10. Brain damage affects people in all cultures and socioeconomic groups. Give an example of how a specific left-hemisphere deficit may impact a person in a specific culture. Give an example of how a specific right-hemisphere deficit may impact a person within a specific culture.

10 Augmentative and Alternative Communication for Persons with Severe Speech Impairments and Severe Speech and Physical Impairments

Myrna P. Cronen and Patricia A. Mercaitis

This chapter discusses augmentative and alternative communication (AAC) as it pertains to persons with severe speech impairment (SSI) and severe speech and physical impairment (SSPI) throughout the life span and across different cultures. The American Speech-Language-Hearing Association (ASHA) defines *AAC* as an area of clinical practice that attempts to compensate (either temporarily or permanently) for the impairment and disability patterns of persons with severe expressive communication disorders (i.e., the severe speech-language and writing impaired) (American Speech-Language-Hearing Association 1989).

This chapter focuses on several topics that help to develop a perspective on persons with SSI or SSPI. Beginning with the social complications of SSI and SSPI and their implications, the following are examined: (1) issues of self-esteem and self-worth, (2) the impact of the impairment on the family, (3) cultural attitudes toward disability, and (4) a partnership philosophy of intervention. Intervention strategies and suggestions for interactions are also discussed. Some important educational issues include early intervention for infants, toddlers, and their families; inclusion; assistive technology in the classroom; social interaction in the classroom; literacy development; and the transition from high school to higher education. This chapter also discusses the effect of SSI and SSPI on obtaining and keeping a job and on independent living and long-term adult relationships. Future trends in AAC are also identified.

Terminology

The terms *SSI* and *SSPI* are derived from the World Health Organization model of disorder, which defines the consequences of chronic injury, disease, or syndromes; organizes them into a conceptual model; and divides them into three areas of disorder: impairment, disability, and handicap. According to this model, the term *impairment* refers to "any loss or abnormality of psychological, physiological, or anatomical structure or function" (Wood 1980). The term *disability* refers to "any restriction or lack (resulting from an impairment) of ability to perform an activity in the manner or within the range considered normal for a human being. Disabilities reflect the consequences of impairment in terms of functional performance and activity, thus indicating that the illness experience is objectified." The term *handicap* refers to "a disadvantage for an individual, resulting from an impairment or a disability, that limits or prevents the fulfillment of a role that is normal … for that individual. Handicaps … represent socialization of an illness experience."

Other key words include *symbol, aid, strategy, technique, scanning, message encoding, communication board,* and *communication system.* People with SSPI and SSI may need to use symbols other than speech to represent concepts. ASHA defines *symbols* as "visual, auditory, and/or tactile representations of conventional concepts (e.g., gestures, photographs, manual sign sets/systems, picto-ideographs, printed words, objects, spoken words, Braille)" (American Speech-Language-Hearing Association 1991). The symbols can be used with an aid to communicate. The term *aid* refers to "a physical object or device used to transmit or receive messages (e.g., a communication book, board, chart, mechanical or electronic device, or computer)" (American Speech-Language-Hearing Association 1991). The term *strategy* refers to a "specific way of using [AAC] aids, symbols, and/or techniques more effectively for enhanced communication. A strategy, whether taught to an individual or self-discovered, is a plan that can facilitate one's performance." The term *technique* refers to "a method of transmitting messages (e.g., … scanning, encoding)" (American Speech-Language-Hearing Association 1991). The term *scanning* refers to a type of item-selection process used by persons whose motor control does not allow for pointing or selecting items in an array (Beukelman and Mirenda 1992). *Message encoding* refers to "any technique where the individual gives multiple signals which, taken together, specify the desired item from the individual's selection vocabulary" (Vanderheiden and Lloyd 1986). *Communication board* refers to a type of aided, augmentative communication approach that can be constructed of paper, cardboard, wood, plastic, or other durable material. It displays letters, pictures, words, or symbols from which an individual selects to send a message.

A *communication system* for most persons without SSPI consists of many different components that vary depending on the rate of communication, the environmental constraints, the communication partner, and the goal of the communication task. These issues are also important when considering a communication system for someone with SSPI. In addition, the "communication system for an individual [with SSPI] should include a collection of symbols, aids, strategies, and techniques that the individual can use interchangeably" (Vanderheiden and Lloyd 1986).

Causes of and Extent of Disability Involved with Severe Speech Impairment and Severe Speech and Physical Impairment

It is estimated that there are approximately 2 million people, or 0.8% of the population, in the United States with an SSPI or SSI (American Speech-Language-Hearing Association 1991). This group includes people of all ages, from different ethnic and racial groups, and from all socioeconomic levels. SSPI or SSI can be caused by a variety of congenital or acquired problems that can be progressive or temporary in their course. Congenital impairments include mental retardation, cerebral palsy, developmental apraxia of speech, autism, severe hearing impairment, and dual sensory impairment (Vanderheiden and Yoder 1986). Some of the most commonly acquired conditions include head injury, spinal cord injury, stroke, and cancer of the larynx that results in laryngectomy. Progressive, degenerative diseases include multiple sclerosis, muscular dystrophy, Parkinson's disease, Huntington's disease, acquired immunodeficiency syndrome, and amyotrophic lateral sclerosis, or Lou Gehrig disease. Temporary conditions include shock and surgery.

SSI results in a significant loss or abnormal functioning in a person's ability to speak. For example, a child with a severe speech disorder may be understood when saying single-syllable words but may be severely unintelligible when saying longer words or sentences. A person with SSPI has significantly reduced abilities in both speaking and motor movements. For example, an adolescent with cerebral palsy may have severely impaired ambulation and speech.

SSI and SSPI are used to describe the type and extent of a person's impairment, without assuming that the presence of a severe impairment means that the person has a severe disability. In addition to the severity of the impairment, the extent of a person's disability depends on such factors as the person's communication "lifestyle and the extent of the individual's compensation for the impairment through self-learning, specialized instruction, or prosthetic intervention, such as glasses, hearing aids, arm rests, and communication aids" (Beukelman 1986).

In many individuals, the degree of impairment does not change during a lifetime, but the level of disability can be influenced by changes in the person's lifestyle. Some examples of influencing factors include beginning school, beginning specialized communication training, changing the employment situation, and retirement from employment.

Historical Perspective

Since the 1960s, there have been numerous advances in several aspects of United States society that have impacted the lives of persons with SSI or SSPI. Legislative, social, technologic, cultural, and economic developments are among those that have contributed dramatically to the changing picture for persons with SSI or SSPI.

The Americans with Disabilities Act, which was signed into law in 1990, prohibits discrimination on the basis of disability in the areas of transportation, employment, public accommodation, communication, and activities of the state and local government. The passage of this legislation has had a profound impact on American society. Societal attitudes toward persons with disabilities are changing gradually as a result of its passage. Many aspects of the Americans with Disabilities Act are currently in effect: Additional requirements will become effective in 2010 (see Chapter 1).

The explosive advancements in technology have resulted in major advancements in dedicated communication devices, adaptive software, hardware, interface (switch) mechanisms, and environment-control systems. Access to such technology has also improved, as service providers and families have learned to work as partners to obtain appropriate communication technology for the person with SSPI and SSI.

Since the early 1970s, there has been a dramatic improvement in the quality, type, and availability of communication services for persons who cannot use speech to communicate. The improvement has been witnessed with enthusiasm and a sense of impatience, owing to the pace at which changes occur in our society. The improvement in communication service delivery has been fueled by changes in attitudes, legislation, technology, and disability rights movements.

The most recent, remarkable changes have resulted from the growing awareness by parents, teachers, advocates, and other professionals of the communication needs of persons with SSI or SSPI. The impetus for change has been the passage of federal and state legislation that guarantees a free, appropriate, public education for all persons regardless of disability. In addition, technologic advances in the telecommunications field have expanded the variety of dedicated communication devices and environmental-access devices available to those whose speech or mobility is impaired. Finally, communication professionals have begun to emphasize the need to focus on functional communication skills.

Severe Speech Impairment and Severe Speech and Physical Impairment: Social Complications and Implications

The inability to speak—to make one's wants and needs known, to be able to tell about one's day, to express emotion—strikes at the very essence of what it is to be human. In her autobiographical book *I Raise My Eyes to Say Yes*, Ruth Sienkewicz-Mercer (Sienkewicz-Mercer and Kaplan 1989), a former client of ours who has had SSPI since infancy, states to her coauthor through the use of her communication boards

> *Without a doubt, my inability to speak has been the single most devastating aspect of my handicap. If I were granted one wish and one wish only, I would not hesitate for an instant to request that I be able to talk, if only for one day, or even one hour.*

When a person does not speak, those around tend to ignore him or her, underestimate the person's understanding or intellectual level, and, in some cases, treat them as objects to be acted on rather than persons with whom to interact.

Self-Esteem

There is the danger among persons with SSI or SSPI of experiencing *learned helplessness* (Seligman 1975). Learned helplessness is learned dependent and passive behavior. It is easily developed when speech, cognitive, motor, visual, or hearing limitations make persons dependent on caregivers for most or all of their daily needs. It is frequently fostered by well-meaning caregivers and can handicap people well beyond their level of impairment. However, it need not develop.

People define who they are and what they will become as a result of social contacts, which begin in early childhood, with parents, teachers, therapists, and peers (Blackstone 1993a). Parents, teachers, and other service providers can be instrumental in fostering self-esteem by encouraging and praising children's abilities, fostering their aspirations, and listening to their ideas and concerns. Social skills should be developed early, and opportunities should be provided for friendships to emerge. Young children with SSI should have a balance of opportunities to interact with others with and without disabilities. Older children need to have role models among the disabled community. Efforts should be made to extend the world experiences of children with SSI and provide them with opportunities to develop interests beyond home and school (Blackstone 1993b).

For persons with acquired disabilities, sense of meaning and self-worth can diminish as they experience the loss of their ability to contribute to society and maintain control of their lives. Adults with acquired SSI or SSPI can experience social isolation when members of their former social network limit or even end their interactions because of the difficulty of maintaining conversations.

In recent years, changes in societal attitudes and laws, the disability rights movement, the availability of assistive technology, and integration experiences have had a positive effect on persons with SSI and SSPI. They have become self-advocates, and peers have begun to regard them as friends, classmates, and coworkers.

Family

Communication constitutes meaningful relationships and the establishment of social networks (Blackstone 1994). When a family member has an SSI or SSPI, the stress on the family is dramatically increased. Before the 1970s, physicians typically advised families of children with severe disabilities to institutionalize the child. This was because physicians believed that the child had limited potential, and the stress of caring for the child at home would be too much for the family. However, due to changes in attitudes and in public law and policy, even the most severely physically and cognitively impaired are currently raised at home.

When there is a person with an SSI in the family, everyone is affected. Caring for a person with a disability can put severe stress on the family emotionally, physically, and economically. Persons with severe disabilities require extensive and time-consuming care. Family members may decrease their out-of-home work and social commitments to devote more time to the care of the person with a disability. Frequently, one person's life (typically the mother's) revolves around the care of the disabled person. Unresolved feelings of guilt can cause a marriage to deteriorate. Siblings of a disabled child may be slighted or given heavy responsibilities when one or both parent's energy and concern is directed toward the disabled child.

When professionals intervene in families with disabled members, services should enable entire families to have a lifestyle that encourages personal development, growth, and autonomy (Gartner et al. 1991). Professionals should focus on the capacity, not the dysfunction, of the family (Blackstone 1994).

Some families have successfully found ways of involving the disabled member in family activities, and others make participation in AAC activities a family affair. We know of a father and son who participate every year in the Boston Marathon. The father runs the race pushing his son's wheelchair. Parents and siblings of young AAC users can learn about AAC in overnight recreational settings. AAC camps give youngsters and parents opportunities to meet other families who use AAC (Trace 1993a). Local support groups also provide opportunities for parents and siblings to share their concerns and benefit from the experiences of others.

When the disabling condition occurs in an adult after role relationships have been established, difficulty can result from changing roles. When changed roles are in direct conflict with cultural norms, additional tensions arise. For example, in cultures in which the husband speaks for the family, it can be difficult for the husband, wife, and community to accept the wife's new role as the family spokesperson.

Family Attitudes Toward Disability, Intervention, and Technology

How a family responds to the presence of a severely disabled member is influenced by a number of factors. These factors include the family's cohesiveness and strength; education level; socioeconomic status; religion; racial, ethnic, and cultural beliefs; prior experience with disability; and the family's assimilation into the mainstream culture. One cannot make assumptions about a family's response to disability or intervention on the basis of their cultural, religious, linguistic, or geographic background. Practitioners need to be aware, however, that family attitudes are influenced by a combination of factors. Practitioners should also attempt to understand an individual family's beliefs and view of the world.

While Western health practice looks to biomedical reasons to explain disability, traditional non-Western beliefs about health and disorders share a basic belief in the connection between disability and an external force. They may believe the disability is a result of disharmony with nature. This belief can result from a specific cultural orientation toward guilt, shame, or fatalism. Others may accept the family member as fate, their "cross to bear," or a gift from God. Some cultures have a wide range of tolerance for differences and easily accommodate the disabled person, while others may attempt to hide a disabled family member because of the stigma attached to disability (Trace 1992; Brecker 1992; Matsuda 1989).

Not all families have access to, actively seek, or enthusiastically embrace intervention from mainstream service providers. They may prefer to seek treatment from healers or practitioners of folk medicine. They may mistrust technology. Mainstream professionals must be aware of their own values and attitudes toward disability and intervention. They must also recognize the way in which these beliefs influence what they see and how they interpret it. They must also be aware of how their interpersonal communication style may conflict with that of a different cultural group. They must avoid a collision of mainstream professional beliefs and goals with those of a family from another cultural background. Professionals can be more effective if they adapt their approach to work with the family's belief system and its interpersonal style (Matsuda 1989; Cohen 1986).

Some families object to the use of AAC. They may not trust technology, or they may be uncomfortable using it. They may believe AAC prevents a child from acquiring natural speech. They may fear that it calls adverse attention to a person with SSI. They may react to the added burden of being responsible for maintaining the technology. Additionally, they may object to altered family interaction patterns (Blackstone 1994).

There are many cases of abandoned technology. This usually occurs (1) when the technology is not appropriate for the user's needs and abilities, (2) the user and communication partners receive inadequate training and education, (3) there are frequent breakdowns in the technology, or (4) the user and communication partners are not truly committed to using AAC for communication purposes.

Families determine the success of persons with SSI or SSPI who become AAC users (Blackstone 1994). Efforts should be made to create a family-professional partnership. The family should be empowered to act as an advocate for the disabled family member. In most cases, professionals come and go, while the family remains the constant in the life of a person with SSI or SSPI. Among some cultural groups, deference to authority can inhibit the family's willingness to accept this advocacy role (Matsuda 1989).

Intervention: A Partnership Between the Family and Professionals

Persons with SSI and SSPI require the services of many specially trained professionals. In most cases, the role of assembling and coordinating the team's activities is assumed by a speech-language pathologist. The interdisciplinary AAC team can include any or all of the following: speech-language pathologist, AAC consultant, physician, physical therapist, occupational therapist, special education teacher, literacy specialist, psychologist, vision specialist, hearing specialist, computer technologist, rehabilitation engineer, social worker, and vocational specialist. Family members and the disabled person (if older than 14 years of age) complete the team membership.

Because lifelong planning is necessary for those with SSI or SSPI, teams assemble at key times throughout the person's lifetime. Key times include early intervention, the transition to elementary school, the transition from school to work, and the transition to independent living. Critical decision-making points occur when communication needs are unmet, have changed, or will change substantially in the near future (Cohen 1986; Yorkston and Karlan 1986).

Because so many people provide services, every attempt must be made to build consensus and provide integrated services and systems. Without consensus building, members may disagree or fail to understand the goals or process. These members could later sabotage the intervention either consciously or unconsciously (Beukelman and Mirenda 1992).

When working on a team, it is also important to understand the interpersonal style of a family. Cultural differences, for example, could contribute to an Asian patient's difficulty saying "no," because direct disagreement is considered confrontational and a threat to the harmony of the group (Matsuda 1989).

Family input and cooperation are essential when planning assessment and intervention. It is important to know what languages are used by family members and for what purposes. Language or languages of interviewing, assessment, and intervention need to be considered. The use of translators and interpreters can be required. A cultural informant, who can report on normal communicative behaviors within a culture and who can compare the individual with SSI or SSPI to other members of the family or community, may be needed (Mattes and Omark 1991; American Speech-Language-Hearing Association 1985).

Professionals should determine how the family perceives the goals, perceptions, expectations, and aspirations of the person with SSI and SSPI (Blackstone 1993b). Frequently, families regard the disabled member as more communicatively competent than do professionals. Family members can be aware of subtleties of expression, such as facial or body movements, or the meaning of seemingly unintelligible sounds.

It is also important to understand that while AAC can remove some of the frustration of being unable to communicate, it is not for everyone, nor is it appropriate for use in every situation. Many persons with SSI use a combination of communication methods throughout their lifetime (e.g., natural speech or sounds, gestures, facial expressions with familiar partners, and AAC with less familiar partners). Frequently, AAC is introduced along with treatment directed toward speech development.

Education

Critical educational issues for persons with SSI include early intervention for infants, toddlers, and their families; inclusion in the mainstream classroom; assistive technology in the classroom; development of social interaction skills; literacy development; and the transition from high school to higher education.

Early Intervention

Ideally, intervention begins early in the home with primary caregivers. In the United States, Public Law (PL) 99-457 mandates services for handicapped infants and toddlers ages birth to 2 years who experience developmental delays in one or more of the following areas: cognitive development, physical development, language and speech development, psychosocial development, or self-help skills.

The primary goal of early intervention in the area of communication is to develop interactional and social strategies, so that children learn the power of communication in affecting their environment (Beukelman and Mirenda 1992). Interventionists should take into consideration that cultural groups differ from one another in the extent to which particular language functions are emphasized, how children are expected to behave during communicative interactions, how children are acculturated, who is responsible for raising the child, and the role of parents as teachers (Mattes and Omark 1991; Anderson and Battle 1993).

Numerous communication opportunities occur in the context of daily routines of eating, diaper changing, dressing, bathing, and play. Caregivers are taught to facilitate opportunities for communication by establishing predictable routines. Caregivers are also taught to identify and respond to children's signaling behaviors. When caregivers respond to what are initially random behaviors, young children learn to initiate these behaviors intentionally to signal attention seeking, acceptance, and rejection (Beukelman and Mirenda 1992).

As children grow older, they can be given opportunities to make choices about the foods to eat, toys to play with, people to sit with, and clothes to wear. Communication boards that use symbols (e.g., line drawings of objects and actions) that occur in daily activities can be used to teach receptive and expressive language and to teach children to associate the line drawings with the object or action in naturally occurring situations (Beukelman and Mirenda 1992). Culturally sensitive and relevant symbols should be used. For example, symbols to represent family members of an African-American child should be African-American, food items for Hispanic children should include tortillas, and winter holiday symbols for Jewish children should include a Chanukah menorah. Communication devices with speech output can be used to give the child a voice and provide auditory feedback to the child. Some devices can be programmed with age-, gender-, and dialect-appropriate voices.

A second goal of early intervention is to foster the social, linguistic, and operational competencies children need to participate in the school environment. The Education for All Handicapped Children's Act of 1975 (PL 94-142) and the Individuals with Disabilities Education Act Amendments of 1991 (PL 102-119) mandate that all children receive a publicly funded education in the least-restrictive environment. These public policies make all children with SSI and SSPI eligible for public education. They also require that some children with SSI and SSPI be placed in traditional classrooms with nondisabled peers for at least part of each day (Beukelman and Mirenda 1992).

Inclusion

The concept of inclusion or inclusive education emerged in the 1980s. This concept differs from other forms of integration, because it allows greater fusion of special education within the framework and process of general education. According to this concept, the student with disabilities has full general education class membership. Both special education and general education teachers have "ownership" of and responsibility to the student with disabilities and participate as a team in designing the curriculum and providing educational services and support to the student. The curriculum is designed to meet the needs of the student. Providing support to students so their inclusion can be socially and academically meaningful is the challenge to school personnel in an inclusive school program. The inclusion program differs from the special education class model, in which the child is mainstreamed for a portion of the day for activities selected by the teacher (Sailor et al. 1993).

There has been significant resistance to this model from both special educators and general educators. Special educators fear that children may lose some of their entitlement to specialized instruction and services and the protections of due process. General educators see special education students as one more responsibility in an already overburdened system of large class sizes, shrinking budgets, and difficult students (Sailor et al. 1993).

Studies have documented enhanced educational outcomes associated with integrated placements when compared with the outcomes of their segregated counterparts. There is evidence that when children with disabilities are included in regular classrooms, their independence, skill acquisition, friendships, and social integration increase as a direct function of increased school and community interactive contacts with nondisabled, similar-aged peers (Sailor et al. 1993).

Mainstream preschool classes provide a challenging and developmentally appropriate, socially communicative environment, in which disabled youngsters can participate. Opportunities need to be created that allow children to participate as fully as possible. SSI and SSPI children can use AAC devices to announce a change in activities, they can hit a switch that turns on an audiotaped song, or they can deliver a snack to other children with a battery-operated toy truck. They need access to the vocabulary appropriate to the preschool situation. Some vocabulary can be programmed into a child's personal communication device and some can be made available throughout the preschool environment. Play areas can have miniature communication boards with symbols denoting materials and activities. A child in the sandbox corner can have available symbols denoting sand, shovel, pail, dump, and so on to use in "talking" about the play activities. Teachers and nondisabled peers can point to these symbols to narrate the child's actions.

Assistive Technology in the Classroom

Assistive technology is necessary for children to benefit from education—that is, to communicate, achieve independent mobility, and be active and competitive in classroom settings. AAC systems that are age- and context-appropriate are critical tools for school success. Children with SSI and SSPI should learn to use communication systems for interaction, writing, drawing, and reading that permit them to participate in the regular classroom (Beukelman and Mirenda 1992).

Assistive technology is not a curriculum (Blackstone 1990). Assistive technology is a tool that supports the student's active participation in a curriculum that should include reading, writing, and math. Software programs and switch-activated technology are available to teach language and preliteracy skills to young children. Simple software programs are also available to encourage early drawing skills and to teach letter and number recognition, preliteracy concepts (e.g., matching), and basic keyboarding skills.

The Technology-Related Assistance for Individuals with Disabilities Act of 1989 (PL 100-407) provides financial incentives in the form of grants that enable states to make assistive technology service equitably available. Ideally, assistive technology should move with the student, so that he or she can participate in school and classroom activities where they occur in the classroom or building. This is preferable to confining the student to a workstation in a corner of the room. Battery-operated laptop computers and portable communication aids that can be attached to a wheelchair or lap tray are suited to this need.

For the student to be successful using technology, all persons involved with the student (e.g., teacher, speech-language pathologist, instructional aide, and family) must be trained in the use of the technology. In addition, students need people to support them (e.g., instructional aides) throughout the day, so they can actively and independently participate in the classroom activities. Assistive technology also increases functional and social independence. Persons with SSPI can activate switches to control lights, appliances, televisions, video cassette recording equipment, and tape recorders. Communicating via the Internet puts persons with disabilities in touch with peers (with and without disabilities), which facilitates social interaction, access to information, empowerment, and equal opportunities (Blackstone 1991a).

Social Interaction in the Classroom

Providing technology and mainstreaming children does not guarantee social integration and peer interactions. Observations of children with SSI and SSPI often reveal that they have few social interactions with their peers and most of their interactions are with adults. A critical factor in accomplishing integration is the promotion of positive social interaction through systematic integration.

How do children make friends when they cannot speak? One innovative method, termed the *Circle of Friends Intervention*, brings together a small group of classmates who volunteer to learn about the disabled child and to arrange opportunities for them to spend time together (O'Brien et al. 1989). In other programs, peers are trained to teach social skills and to work as tutors.

Most able-bodied children are intrigued by AAC devices and eager to see them used, particularly when they contain age-appropriate communications. Knock-knock jokes and silly riddles help make SSI and SSPI youngsters part of the crowd. Preteens and teens respond enthusiastically to "cool" bids for interaction (e.g., "Hey guys, how's it going?") using up-to-date slang expressions. These communications should match the gender, socioeconomic, and ethnic characteristics of the user.

Literacy Development

Literacy is the key to social, academic, and vocational success. Literacy provides access to unrestricted vocabulary and allows for self-expression. It also allows the person with SSI to use a range of adaptive technology options both in school and in the workplace.

However, most persons with SSI and SSPI experience severe literacy-learning difficulties. While some learn to read at the same time as their able-bodied peers, most children with SSI or SSPI learn to read and write slowly, if at all. In some cases, the problems can be traced to general cognitive abilities. However, there are many children with SSI and SSPI who, despite average or above-average intelligence, enter adulthood without developing fluency in reading (Blackstone 1989).

Understanding of the reasons for literacy-learning difficulties among persons with SSI and SSPI is just beginning. Literacy programs and curricula need to be developed that take into account the special needs of persons with SSI and SSPI. One method is to use the symbols from a communication display to make a storybook, thus using the symbol system as a bridge to literacy (Blackstone 1989).

Strategies used by adult AAC users with congenital disabilities who learned to read as children have been identified by Koppenhaver et al. (1991). They consistently cited the high expectations and encouragement of family members and teachers, as well as the person's persistence and talents, as having a major role in literacy-learning success. In addition, they noted the following as contributing to success in learning to read: (1) being raised in a literate environment in which print materials are widely accessible and others read, (2) being read to for both pleasure and academic tasks, (3) following the text with the eyes, and (4) being engaged in interaction about the text (Koppenhaver et al. 1991).

Because reading and other literacy activities are not promoted among some cultural groups, professionals may need to educate families as to the importance of reading in the home and strategies for involving the child in literacy activities. The language of the material is not as important as the exposure to literacy activities.

Writing activities must also be encouraged. For writing and note taking, a predictive word-processing system can increase the quantity and quality of written work of users with both physical impairments and spelling difficulties. Message prediction is a process in which logical word choices are offered based on the portion of the message already formulated, using spelling and grammatical rules.

Transition from High School to Higher Education

Few high school graduates with SSI or SSPI enroll in postsecondary courses in the years immediately following graduation from high school. For those who do enroll in postsecondary courses, the challenges are formidable.

To be successful in college, persons with SSI and SSPI must be provided with adequate academic preparation and have access to a range of support services provided by a coordinated interdisciplinary effort. A reduced course load is usually taken. The Disabilities Resource Office should be involved in coordinating overall services. These services can include class note takers, writing tutors, AAC assessment, interventionists, and staff trained in educational and vocational applications of adaptive technology. Students with SSPI who live away from home need personal care assistants (PCAs) to assist with bathing, dressing, and grooming. Because neither physical proximity nor tolerance ensure acceptance, social integration needs to be addressed before the student arrives, so that roommates or suitemates can be identified as interested in rooming with peers with SSI or SSPI.

Effect on Vocation

Finding a Job

Only a small fraction of persons with SSI or SSPI in the United States are fully employed. Thousands of people who depend on AAC are being trained and educated in schools but cannot find work. For those who do work, the most frequent work sites are sheltered workshops (segregated facilities where disabled individuals perform subcontracted work for low wages with assistance) or supported work environments (Blackstone 1993b; Trace 1993b) Societal attitudes, the generally slow rate at which workers with SSI or SSPI communicate and work, low aspirations of many persons with SSI or SSPI, poor literacy skills, and lack of prior job experience have diminished the ability of many of these persons to compete in the workplace. To combat the current situation, these persons need to be encouraged to dream. They should also be exposed to successful role models with SSI or SSPI. They need to develop skills, talents, and interests as they are growing up that lend themselves to future employment (Blackstone 1993b). Participation in clubs, teams, and work forces in the community enables students to realize their individual capabilities (Blackstone 1990).

For a successful transition from school to work, persons with SSI or SSPI need a team effort. The team should determine if adaptive technology currently in use is applicable or should be changed to accommodate and be integrated into the new work environment (Cohen 1986). Successful transitions to a new or first job frequently involve a job coach. Job coaches train the person in the skills needed in the work environment and accompany the person to the work environment for generalization of these skills to on-the-job training. Job coaches can be hired by rehabilitation agencies or employers and are helpful in providing on-the-job support for AAC users. Job coaches also demonstrate to the employer and coworkers the way the AAC user communicates and the accommodations needed in the workplace (Trace 1993b).

Keeping a Job: Adults with Acquired Severe Speech Impairment and Severe Speech and Physical Impairment

Adults who acquire motor or severe speech impairments that interfere with their ability to carry out their work responsibilities can continue their vocation if they can benefit from the use of adaptive technology. Employers are likely to recognize their wisdom and experience and make accommodations in the workplace. For example, a college professor with amyotrophic lateral sclerosis (a degenerative, neurologic condition) that affects his or her ability to speak can continue to lecture and write through the use of a computer with a speech synthesizer. An accountant with a degenerative, neurologic disease affecting his or her ability to speak and write can use a computer with appropriate software and adaptive-switch technology to maintain accountancy records and communicate with clients.

A survey of the employment of persons who use AAC was conducted in 1993 (Blackstone 1993b). Jobs held by the 727 respondents, listed from most frequently held to least frequently held, were data entry, assembly work in sheltered workshops, custodial, laborer, clerical, AAC-related jobs (e.g., consultant, rehabilitation counselor, and aide in speech department), service jobs (e.g., in a supermarket or in food preparation), and professional jobs (e.g., lawyer, physicist, professor, engineer, architect, librarian, or policy analyst). Those who work confront multiple barriers. Barriers include problems with communication, technology, transportation, architecture, and attitudes (Blackstone 1993b).

The Americans with Disabilities Act prohibits employment discrimination against persons with disabilities. As long as a person has the physical and mental capacities to do the job, he or she should have equal access to employment opportunities. Some state offices of vocational rehabilitation are training AAC users and securing jobs for them, but many vocational rehabilitation counselors are not fully aware of the potential of AAC users. There is no universally accepted or supported infrastructure that allows the AAC user to develop appropriate work skills. Choice of work is limited. However, each person with SSI or SSPI has a unique set of skills and interests to offer (Trace 1993b).

Effects on Independent Living and Long-Term Adult Relationships

Goals of most young adults are to live independently in the community, to develop long-term adult relationships, and to marry. Most young adults with SSI or SSPI have a prolonged and delayed adolescence. During this period, they must resolve problems of separation, independence, body image, and sexual identity (Blackstone 1993a). While some persons with SSI or SSPI are encouraged by families to live independently, others have overprotective parents who are reluctant to let their adult children live on their own. Learned helplessness can prevent a young adult from making the transition from family to independent living arrangements. At this time, few persons who have grown up with SSI or SSPI live independently, are involved in long-term adult relationships, or have married (Blackstone 1993a).

Researchers have examined gender differences among persons with disabilities who marry (Whyte and Ingstad 1995). They found that women with disabilities are less likely to marry than men with disabilities. They also found that when women with disabilities marry after the onset of impairment, they are more likely than men with disabilities who marry to have a spouse with a disability.

Some strategies for preparing young adults with disabilities to marry or live in the community include (1) organizing support and discussion groups for parents and the young adult; (2) providing sex education and encouraging the development of sexual identity and healthy sexual attitudes; (3) introducing successful role models; (4) offering more opportunities for young adults to assume increased responsibility for their own care, food shopping, and finances; and (5) providing instruction on how to hire and manage PCAs (Blackstone 1993a).

In most communities, there are two living options for adults with SSI or SSPI. Some persons with SSI or SSPI live in group homes with professional staff. Others are able to live in handicapped-accessible apartments with the assistance of PCAs. In either case, adults with SSI or SSPI need communication devices that are appropriately programmed with messages and used effectively with PCAs, van drivers, store clerks, waitpersons, friends, lovers, and so on.

Projected Trends for Persons with SSI and SSPI and for AAC Professionals

Advances in technology, declining financial resources, improved services for culturally diverse populations with SSI or SSPI, and specialty recognition in AAC will all have an effect on the future of persons with SSI or SSPI.

Advances in Technology

The number of persons with SSI or SSPI in the population will increase in the future. Improved medical care and technology are saving the lives of persons who in the past may not have survived infancy, illness, or trauma. Advances in medicine and technology are also prolonging the lives of the aging population. As mainstream technology expands, available AAC technology will continue to improve. Each year, communication aid manufacturers introduce new and enhanced devices. Telecommunication technologies will provide increased opportunities for persons with SSI or SSPI to communicate in non–face-to-face environments.

Declining Financial Resources

The population of persons with SSI or SSPI is increasing, laws are creating a greater demand for services, and equipment and technologic options are increasing. However, at the same time, government resources are dwindling, and health care and education systems are limiting financial support for services. Belt-tightening and rationing of health care will require the establishment of priorities. In this climate, AAC professionals will need to address issues, including (1) taking a proactive role in determining for whom technology is appropriate by conducting outcome studies, (2) looking at alternative delivery systems, (3) conducting cost-benefit analyses for assessment, (4) training for delivery of technology, and (5) establishing best-practice patterns given a multitude of settings (Blackstone 1991b).

Augmentative and Alternative Communication Specialists

As the body of knowledge associated with AAC and the need to stay current with the rapid advances in technology increase, professionals from a variety of fields will choose to specialize in this professional area. The Rehabilitation Engineering Society of North America (RESNA) is an organization composed of individuals from a variety of professions involved in AAC, including speech-language pathologists, computer engineers, and occupational therapists. In 1997, RESNA adopted a voluntary examination and will issue AAC specialty certification to those professionals who meet the criteria. For speech-language pathologists specializing in AAC, ASHA has a special interest division. Specialty recognition may be offered by ASHA in the future, although there are no definitive plans at the time of this writing. Other AAC specialists include occupational therapists, physical therapists, special educators, reading teachers, computer software developers, and computer engineers. Many of these professionals will work together in regional centers across the country in universities, hospitals, and regional school districts. Local speech-language pathologists will look to these specialists for recommendations on equipment, training strategies, and educational materials.

Improved Services for Culturally Diverse Populations with Severe Speech Impairments and Severe Speech and Physical Impairments

Efforts are underway by ASHA and many graduate programs to offer more courses in AAC. Graduate programs and ASHA are also attempting to recruit persons who are bilingual, bicultural, or fluent in languages other than English. In addition, there is an increased emphasis on providing graduate clinicians with education on multicultural issues that will increase the number of culturally sensitive and knowledgeable service providers. Services are now being provided to people who, because of disability or distance, have been unable to travel to a center where AAC services are available. Typically, vans travel to remote areas where services are limited, such as Native American reservations (Trace 1994). These trends should result in improved services to all persons with SSI and SSPI.

References

American Speech-Language-Hearing Association. Clinical management of communicatively handicapped minority language populations. ASHA 1985;27:29–32.

American Speech-Language-Hearing Association. Competencies for speech-language pathologists. Providing services in augmentative communication. ASHA 1989;31:107–110.

American Speech-Language-Hearing Association. Report: augmentative and alternative communication. ASHA 1991;33:9–12.

Anderson NB, Battle DE. Cultural Diversity in the Development of Language. In DE Battle (ed), Communication Disorders in Multicultural Populations. Boston: Butterworth–Heinemann, 1993;158–185.

Beukelman DR. Evaluating the Effectiveness of Intervention Programs. In S Blackstone (ed), Augmentative Communication: An Introduction. Rockville, MD: American Speech-Language-Hearing Association, 1986.

Beukelman DR, Mirenda P. Augmentative and Alternative Communication: Management of Severe Communication Disorders in Children and Adults. Baltimore: Paul H. Brookes, 1992;62–227.

Blackstone S. The three R's: reading, writing, and reasoning. Augmentative Communication News 1989;1:1–3.

Blackstone S. Assistive technology in the classroom. Augmentative Communication News 1990;3:1–6.

Blackstone S. Access to communication: building a power base for AAC in the 1990's. Augmentative Communication News 1991a;4:1–2.

Blackstone S. Being proactive: health-care rationing and assistive technology. Augmentative Communication News 1991b;4:5.

Blackstone S. Adolescence: reflections of AAC users. Augmentative Communication News 1993a;6:1–5.

Blackstone S. What do you want to be when you grow up? Augmentative Communication News 1993b;6:1–8.

Blackstone S. Being family-centered in AAC. Augmentative Communication News 1994;7:4–7.

Brecker L. A meaning-centered model of cultural influences. Adv Speech-Lang Pathol Audiol 1992;2:14.

Cohen C. Total Habilitation and Lifelong Management. In S Blackstone (ed), Augmentative Communication: An Introduction. Rockville, MD: American Speech-Language-Hearing Association, 1986;447–469.

Gartner A, Lipsky DK, Turnbill AP. Supporting Families with a Child with a Disability: An International Outlook. Baltimore: Paul H. Brookes, 1991.

Koppenhaver D, Evans D, Yoder D. Childhood reading and writing experiences of literate adults with severe speech and motor impairments. Augmentative and Alternative Communication 1991;7:20–33.

Matsuda M. Working with Asian parents: some communication strategies. Top Lang Disord 1989;9:45–53.

Mattes LJ, Omark DR. Speech and Language Assessment for the Bilingual Handicapped (2nd ed). Oceanside, CA: Academic Communication Associates, 1991.

O'Brien J, Forest M, Snow J, Hasbury D. Action for Inclusion: How to Improve Schools by Welcoming Children with Special Needs into Regular Classrooms. Toronto: Frontier College Press, 1989.

Sailor W, Gee K, Karasoff P. Full Inclusion and School Restructuring. In ME Snell (ed), Instruction of Students with Severe Disabilities (4th ed). New York: Macmillan 1993;1–30.

Seligman M. Helplessness. San Francisco: W.H. Freeman, 1975.

Sienkewicz-Mercer R, Kaplan S. I Raise My Eyes to Say Yes. Boston: Houghton-Mifflin, 1989;12–13.

Trace R. Changes in cultural demographics warrant shift in approaches to diagnosis and treatment. Adv Speech-Lang Pathol Audiol 1992;2:5.

Trace R. AAC camps augment learning. Adv Speech-Lang Pathol Audiol 1993a;3:12–13.

Trace R. Vocational specialists working to help AAC users overcome obstacles to employment. Adv Speech-Lang Pathol Audiol 1993b;3:8.

Trace R. Mobile unit provides AAC services in rural areas. Adv Speech-Lang
Pathol Audiol 1994;4:14.

Vanderheiden GC, Lloyd L. Communication Systems and Their Components.
In S Blackstone (ed), Augmentative Communication: An Introduction.
Rockville, MD: American Speech-Language-Hearing Association,
1986;49–161.

Vanderheiden GC, Yoder DE. Overview. In S Blackstone (ed), Augmentative
Communication: An Introduction. Rockville, MD: American Speech-
Language-Hearing Association, 1986;7.

Whyte SR, Ingstad B. Disability and Culture: An Overview. In B Ingstad, SR
Whyte (eds), Disability and Culture. Berkeley: University of California
Press, 1995;3–32.

Wood P. Appreciating the consequences of disease: the WHO classification of
impairments, disabilities, and handicaps. WHO Chronicle
1980;34:376–380.

Yorkston K, Karlan G. Assessment Procedures. In S Blackstone (ed)
Augmentative Communication: An Introduction. Rockville, MD:
American Speech-Language and Hearing Association, 1986;163–196.

Chapter 10   Study Questions

1. What is augmentative and alternative communication?
2. What kinds of persons benefit from the use of augmentative and alternative communication?
3. What are some recent developments that have had a positive affect on the lives of persons with SSI or SSPI?
4. Why is the family's involvement considered essential to the success of the person with SSI or SSPI? How could a well-meaning, concerned family be detrimental to the success of this person?
5. What are some critical educational issues that must be addressed if the person with SSI or SSPI is to succeed in the mainstream educational and vocational environment?
6. What kinds of cultural issues does the service provider need to consider and address when working with severely impaired persons and families from a cultural background different from his or her own?

IV Audiology in Children and Adults

11   Hearing Disorders

E. Harris Nober

A hearing disorder is an anomaly that occurs in the auditory system and usually causes a loss of hearing. Hearing loss is a common anomaly, particularly in older populations. The prevalence of hearing loss is estimated at slightly more than 9% in the overall United States population; however, this statistic varies markedly depending on the method used to analyze data (Adams and Benson 1992; Shewan 1994). In the early stages of some hearing disorders, there is not a demonstrable loss of hearing sensitivity. In other instances, there can be a congenital deafness. The most obvious effect of a hearing loss in an infant or toddler is the disruption of the oral-aural (i.e., speaking-hearing) communicative process that links the speaker and listener. This disruption in communication development varies widely, depending on factors such as (1) the type and degree of the hearing disorder, (2) the age of onset, (3) initial language development, (4) intelligence, (5) associated anomalies, (6) family support, and (7) medical and remedial efforts. In the child without full language development, it is likely that a mild hearing loss will deter communication. On the other hand, a mild hearing loss in an adult with full language development may interfere only minimally with communication (Diefendorf 1996; Downs 1996; Schow and Nerbonne 1996).

Many different specialists are involved with the identification, assessment, effects, and treatment of hearing disorders. An otologist is a physician who specializes in the medical, surgical, and preventative treatment of hearing (and labyrinthine) disorders. The clinical audiologist conducts hearing measurement assessment tests and provides and manages hearing rehabilitation (also called aural or auditory rehabilitation), which includes assistive listening devices, and may work with cochlear implants. Research audiologists study and conduct research on normal and abnormal auditory processes. Research in the 1990s began to focus on the ethnic, cultural, and socioeconomic attributes of hearing disorders (American Speech-Language-Hearing Association 1996).

This chapter reviews the types, loci, and degrees of hearing defects. It also discusses their etiology, symptoms, effects, treatment, and audiogram configurations. Linguistic, ethnic, cultural, and socioeconomic parameters are also addressed.

Normal Hearing Sensitivity Range

The ability to detect sound at a minimal level of intensity is referred to as *auditory threshold detection sensitivity*. This sensitivity is diminished by a hearing disorder. An auditory threshold is the level at which the sound is detected in 50% of the test trials. Thresholds for pure-tone stimuli are expressed as decibel (dB) levels above established norms for a range of sound frequencies (i.e., 125, 250, 500, 1,000, 1,500, 2,000, 4,000, 6,000, and 8,000 Hz). These pure-tone frequencies comprise the functional speech range for daily hearing; however, this range is not the full extent of good human hearing (i.e., 20–20,000 Hz). The critical speech range for auditory discrimination is 500–2,000 Hz (Kaplan et al. 1992).

In hearing measurement, the test stimuli are pure tones presented by air and bone conduction using an audiometer. An audiometer is calibrated on a normal young-adult population. The threshold values for each frequency are 125–8,000 Hz. Because normal ear sensitivity varies at each sound frequency, the intensity of sound at each frequency on an audiometer is calibrated independently to obtain a zero-threshold reference level. Hence, a zero-threshold level on an audiogram indicates that the person's hearing threshold at that frequency is comparable to the norm. A 20-dB threshold indicates that the hearing threshold is 20 dB poorer at that frequency. Normal auditory sensitivity, like vision, tactile, and olfaction sensitivity, follows a U-shaped curve, which demonstrates better mid-range sensitivity and poorer sensitivity at the extremes of the spectral range.

Pure tones are not the only stimuli used for the measurement of hearing thresholds. Speech stimuli are also used for clinical testing to obtain a speech recognition threshold (SRT). SRT words are bisyllabic (e.g., mailman and hotdog) and are referred to as *spondee words*.

There is also a suprathreshold word test that is used to ascertain the auditory discrimination score. With this test, 50 monosyllabic words per list are presented via the audiometer through earphones or a loudspeaker at a comfortable listening level, which is usually 30–40 dB above the speech reception threshold. The word lists are designed to be phonetically balanced, thus the word phonemes are distributed in relative proportion to conversational English. Each phonetically balanced word is weighted as two percentage points. A perfect score of 100% occurs when all the words in the list are identified correctly.

The upper threshold limit for normal hearing at 500, 1,000, and 2,000 Hz (the "critical speech range") in an adult is a 25-dB pure-tone threshold average (PTA). For children, the upper normal limit is 15 dB PTA. An adult with full language development and a 25-dB PTA encounters minimal communication inconvenience (Schow and Nerbonne 1996). On the other hand, a child with a 15-dB PTA and incomplete language development could have communication difficulties, particularly in school settings (Downs 1996). Hence, the term *normal hearing* is relative depending on age of onset and communication demands. It is also relative depending on language development, type of auditory disorder, and site of lesion (Nober 1976).

Parameters Used to Classify Hearing Impairments

Degree of Hearing Impairment

Mild hearing impairment indicates hearing threshold levels from 26 to 40 dB. Moderate hearing impairment indicates levels from 41 to 55 dB, moderately severe is 56–70 dB. Severe hearing impairment indicates levels from 71 to 90 dB. Profound or total deafness occurs at levels 90 dB and above.

Some audiograms, referred to as *corner audiograms*, show ostensible thresholds at 125, 250, and 500 Hz. I first reported that these thresholds do not represent true or valid hearing, rather they represent vibrotactile (exteroception) sensations. Hence, low-frequency sound stimuli presented at high-intensity levels can be felt, not heard, and are, therefore, devoid of any functional residual hearing (Nober 1967b; Nober 1970).

Another system that designates the degree of the hearing deficiency employs the descriptive terms *hard-of-hearing* and *deaf*. Hard-of-hearing implies there is enough residual hearing to enable some aural communication. Deaf depicts a total or nonfunctional hearing reserve. An adult is considered deaf when the PTA average is 90 dB or greater. On the other hand, a child can be considered deaf with a PTA of 70 dB or even less, if there is evidence of language and other related problems (Roeser and Downs 1995).

Age of Onset

Hearing impairments are also classified by the age of onset. Hearing impairments can be either congenital (i.e., present at birth) or adventitious (i.e., delayed). An early-onset hearing impairment, which occurs at or before 2 years of age, is often referred to as a *prelinguistic hearing loss*. A prelinguistic hearing loss imposes a deleterious aftermath. Children with a postlinguistic hearing loss benefit significantly from

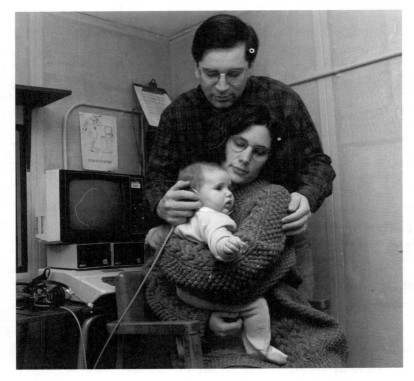

FIGURE 11.1 *A 4-month-old child being screened for a hearing deficit.*

their earlier language acquisition. Figure 11.1 shows a 4-month-old child being screened for a hearing deficit.

Origin or Cause

A hearing impairment can be present at birth or acquired at a later age. Hearing impairments can also be genetic or nongenetic in origin. A genetic hearing loss can be either present at birth or have a delayed onset. An acquired hearing disorder can be caused by perinatal birth complications (e.g., oxygen deprivation [anoxia]) or by postnatal causes, such as bacterial or viral infections, rubella, ototoxic drugs, and fetal alcohol ingestion (Roeser and Downs 1995). Details about origin and etiology of hearing impairments are discussed further in this chapter.

Type of Impairment

The type of hearing impairment relates to the anatomic site of the pathology. The site can be either peripheral or central. A peripheral site occurs in the outer, middle, or inner ear components, the eighth cranial nerve, or some ascending auditory pathways. A central site occurs in the brain, combinations of singular or multiple sites, or some ascending auditory pathways. Depending on the site of lesion, the hearing impairment can be classified as conductive, sensorineural, central, or any combination. Components of the anatomy and physiology of the hearing mechanism are detailed in *Anatomy of the Ear.*

Anatomy of the Ear

Outer Ear

The outer ear consists of the pinna (i.e., auricle) and the external auditory canal or external auditory meatus (Figure 11.2). The pinna is a cartilaginous structure covered by skin with muscular attachments. Major pinna parts include the helix, antihelix, tragus, and antitragus. The external auditory canal is narrow, 1-inch long, and has hairs that catch foreign matter and cerumen (i.e., wax) that is toxic to small insects. Collectively, the pinna and external auditory canal direct sound to the eardrum, protect against foreign bodies, warm and filter the air, selectively resonate some sounds (e.g., 3,000 Hz), and aid in lateralization or localization of the sound source. Disorders of the pinna or ear canal can result in a conductive hearing loss (Gelfand 1997; Northern 1996; Pickles 1988).

Middle Ear

The middle ear connects the outer ear to the inner ear (see Figure 11.2). It is the major component of the peripheral conductive mechanism. The middle ear consists of the eardrum (i.e., tympanic membrane); ossicular chain (i.e., malleus, incus, and stapes); the oval and round windows, which connect to the cochlea; the middle ear cavity (i.e., tympanum); two middle ear muscles (i.e., stapedius and tensor tympani); and other components (Gelfand 1997). The superior end of the eustachian tube terminates in the floor of the middle-ear cavity. Overall, the middle ear amplifies the sound signal, directs the sound to the cochlea, equalizes the middle ear and external air atmospheric pressures during each swallow, and protects the cochlea.

The pearl-white eardrum (i.e., the tympanic membrane) divides the outer ear from the middle ear, and the oval and round windows separate the middle ear from the inner ear. This structural arrangement forms the middle ear cavity (i.e., tympanum), which is bounded by six walls and is normally filled with air supplied from the nasopharynx via the eustachian tube. The middle ear conducts sound to the inner ear and amplifies the sound by about 20–30 dB, depending on the frequency. Amplification is needed to oscillate the cochlea fluids of the inner ear. An impairment to any part of the eardrum or the ossicular chain can result in loss of conductive transmission efficiency and a subsequent conductive hearing loss.

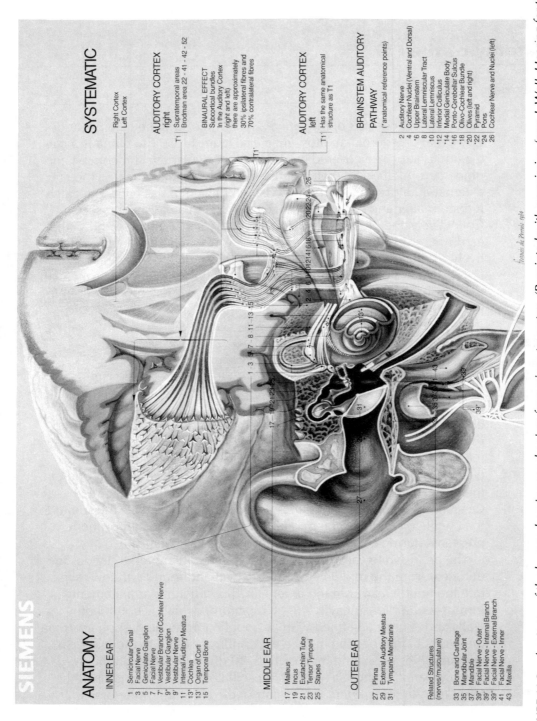

SIEMENS

ANATOMY

INNER EAR

1 Semicircular Canal
3 Facial Nerve
5 Geniculate Ganglion
7 Facial Nerve
7' Vestibular Branch of Cochlear Nerve
9 Vestibular Ganglion
9' Vestibular Nerve
11 Internal Auditory Meatus
13' Cochlea
13' Organ of Corti
15 Temporal Bone

MIDDLE EAR

17 Malleus
19 Incus
21 Eustachian Tube
23 Tensor Tympani
25 Stapes

OUTER EAR

27 Pinna
29 External Auditory Meatus
31 Tympanic Membrane

Related Structures
(nerves/musculature)

33 Bone and Cartilage
35 Mandibular Joint
37 Mandible
39' Facial Nerve – Outer
39' Facial Nerve – Internal Branch
39' Facial Nerve – External Branch
41 Facial Nerve – Inner
43 Maxilla

SYSTEMATIC

Right Cortex
Left Cortex

AUDITORY CORTEX
right

T1 Supratemporal areas
Brodman area 22 · 41 · 42 · 52

BINAURAL EFFECT
Subcortical bundles
In the Auditory Cortex
(right and left)
there are approximately
30% ipsilateral fibres and
70% contralateral fibres

AUDITORY CORTEX
left

T1' Has the same anatomical
structure as T1

BRAINSTEM AUDITORY
PATHWAY

(* anatomical reference points)

2 Auditory Nerve
4 Cochlear Nuclei (Ventral and Dorsal)
*6 Upper Brainstem
8 Lateral Lemniscular Tract
10 Lateral Lemniscus
*12 Inferior Colliculus
*14 Medial Geniculate Body
*16 Porto-Cerebellar Sulcus
*18 Olivo-Cochlear Bundle
*20 Olives (left and right)
*22 Pyramid
*24 Pons
26 Cochlear Nerve and Nuclei (left)

Ivanus de Pernis 1974

FIGURE 11.2 *Anatomy of the human hearing mechanism from pinna to cortex. (Reprinted with permission from L Wall. Hearing for the Speech-Language Pathologist and Health Care Professional. Boston: Butterworth–Heinemann, 1995;2.)*

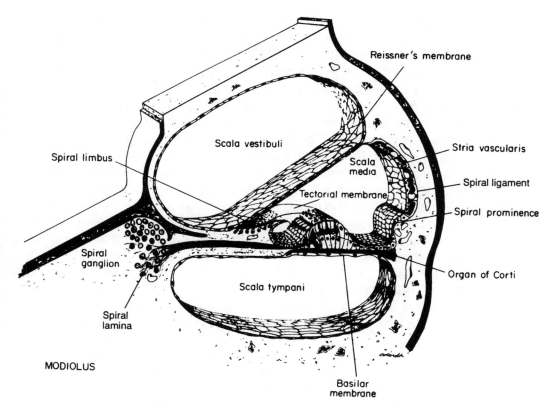

FIGURE 11.3 *Cross section of the cochlear duct shows the organ of Corti situated in the scala media in the basilar membrane. (Reprinted with permission from L Wall. Hearing for the Speech-Language Pathologist and Health Care Professional. Boston: Butterworth–Heinemann, 1995;10.)*

Inner Ear

The inner ear consists of the cochlea, the vestibule system (including the sacculi), and three semicircular canals (see Figure 11.2). It is situated deep in the temporal bone of the skull and is comprised of sacs that are collectively called the *labyrinth*. It consists of a bony (i.e., osseous) labyrinth and a membranous labyrinth with a series of sacs and ducts. Fluid runs through the three parts of the osseous labyrinth, the cochlea, the vestibule, and the semicircular canals.

The cochlea receives sound vibrations transmitted through the middle ear and converts them into electrical impulses for spectral analysis. It then transmits the sound to the neurons of the auditory nerve, which in turn convert the information into neuronal impulses. The snail-shaped cochlea (Figure 11.3) has 2.5 turns (uncoiled, it is about 2 inches long) and a bony axis that is called the *modiolus*. A thin layer of bone, the osseous spiral lamina, projects from the modiolus and, with the basilar membrane attached contiguously to it, extends to the outer wall to form an upper chamber called the *scala vestibuli* and a lower chamber called the *scala tympani.* Both chambers contain a fluid called *perilymph.* The basal end of the scala vestibuli leads to the oval window of the middle ear, and the scala tympani leads to the round window. A third, triangular-shaped duct, the scala media, or cochlea duct, runs the length of the cochlea and contains a fluid called *endolymph.* The base of this delicate but flexible structure is the basilar membrane. The hypotenuse of the triangular-shaped cochlea is Reissner's membrane. The third leg is the spiral ligament.

The cochlea is the end organ of hearing. The vestibule and semicircular canals are the end organ of balance and crude vibration. The sensory component of a sensorineural impairment occurs in the cochlea. The neural component of sensorineural impairment occurs in the eighth cranial nerve of the peripheral nervous system and its retrocochlear pathways to the auditory radiations area in the temporal cortex of the brain.

The basilar membrane holds the structurally complex organ of Corti. This organ has a single row with about 3,500 inner hair cells and three to four rows with 20,000 outer hair cells (Figure 11.4). Inferiorly, the inner and outer hair cells articulate with the reticular lamina. They articulate superiorly with a tectorial membrane. The endolymphatic and perilymphatic fluids that nourish the delicate structures also remove catabolic materials, regulate pressure, aid in vibration, and enable electrolytic energy transformations. Electrolytic energy transformations occur when the hair cells are set into vibration. This vibration is caused when the sound creates a sheering movement against the tectorial membrane. The resultant bioelectric discharge from the hair cells is called the *cochlear microphonic.* The cochlear microphonic maintains the relative intensity and frequency characteristics of the original external acoustic signal. The cochlear microphonic is subsequently transmitted to the eighth cranial nerve (i.e., the acoustic nerve), where it is converted to neuronal discharges for transmission to the brain.

The bilateral ascending auditory pathways to the brain are complex and have a number of synaptic relay stations along the route. In these relay stations, information is modified and recoded for the brain's auditory cortex to encode. Ipsilateral and contralateral pathways transmit and provide protective information redundancy against auditory impairment. The major auditory relay synapse stations of the brain include the medulla, the inferior colliculus, the superior colliculus, and the medial geniculate. The pathways terminate in the auditory cortex in the temporal lobe as an orderly topographical-, spatial-, and frequency-displayed arrangement. Damage along auditory pathway routes produces a sequelae of symptoms for the given area. These symptoms help to identify the locus of any related pathology.

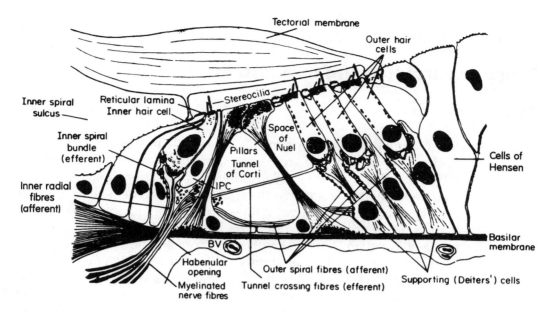

FIGURE 11.4 *Cross section of the organ of Corti. (Reprinted with permission from L Wall. Hearing for the Speech-Language Pathologist and Health Care Professional. Boston: Butterworth–Heinemann, 1995;17.)*

Conductive Hearing Impairment

With conductive hearing loss, word discrimination scores are usually normal (i.e., greater than 90%). In most instances, people with a conductive hearing impairment benefit from compensatory amplification because the defect is structural (or mechanical), meaning that the cochlea hair cells and the neural auditory tracts are intact. An air conductive audiogram is relatively flat or has a greater hearing loss in the lower frequencies (i.e., 125, 250, and 500 Hz). The SRT scores are consistent with PTA levels for 500, 1,000, and 2,000 Hz. Medical intervention, surgical intervention, or both are usually successful and can totally eliminate the conductive hearing loss (Roland 1995). See Chapter 13 for detailed hearing rehabilitation strategies.

When pure-tone thresholds are obtained with a bone oscillator placed on the mastoid bone, the tone stimuli bypass the outer and middle ear and are transmitted directly to the cochlea. Because the cochlea is normal in a conductive impairment, the bone conduction thresholds, which reflect cochlea sensitivity, are also normal with a conductive impairment. With conductive hearing loss, there is excellent tolerance for loud sounds. Patients with conductive hearing loss often hear themselves louder than others, because their normal bone conduction transmission to the cochlea receives less environmental masking interference. Consequently, people with conductive loss tend to speak more softly.

Sensorineural Hearing Impairment

Cochlea Impairment

Sensorineural hearing impairments are usually irreversible. With cochlea impairment, the greater the structural damage to the cochlea, the greater the hearing loss. Sensorineural pure-tone audiograms assume many configurations. These configurations depend on the site and magnitude of the lesion. With sensorineural hearing impairment, there is no air conduction–bone conduction auditory threshold gap on the audiogram. A typical audiogram configuration depicts a progressive increase in hearing thresholds from low to high frequencies. Cochlea impairments can be accompanied by auditory and nonauditory symptoms. These symptoms can yield valuable information about the etiology and prognosis for effective communication. Speech articulation scores, intelligibility, and vocal deficits depend on the extent of the hearing loss, age of onset, type of hearing loss, frequencies involved, native linguistic ability, and family support.

Retrocochlear Impairment

The neural component of sensorineural hearing impairments is formally described as retrocochlear. The eighth cranial nerve and other ascending auditory pathways are described as peripheral in some instances and part of the central auditory processing mechanism in other instances. This neural auditory system provides bilateral innervation that has ipsilateral (i.e., same side) and contralateral (i.e., opposite side) transmission to the auditory radiations of the brain. Damage to the auditory nerve can cause total deafness and is often accompanied by other neurologic symptoms. Elderly people with impairment in the neural component of the auditory processing mechanism can be diagnosed as having presbycusis (Kricos 1995).

Central Auditory Processing Disorder

A central auditory processing disorder (CAPD) involves the central auditory nervous system (CANS). CANS is a large area that includes multiple pathways of the cerebellum, midbrain, and the cerebral cortex. The CANS has its origin at the juncture of the hair cells of the cochlea and the eighth cranial nerve. It terminates in both cerebral hemispheres at Heschl's gyrus (Hood and Berlin 1996; Keith and Jerger 1991). A CAPD can present varying linguistic and educational developmental limitations in a child without full language development and in an adult with full language development. Age of onset, relative to prelinguistic and postlinguistic language acquisition, is a major determinant of future management.

CAPD can manifest in uneven language acquisition and arrested development. Both of these result from abnormal transmission, storage, and integration of language information in the central auditory areas of the brain. The result can be a reduced ability to discriminate, recognize, or analyze speech. Children with CAPD sometimes have other anomalies such as auditory agnosia, aphasia, or a learning disability (see Chapter 12). Learning disabilities vary but can include reading deficit (i.e., dyslexia), minimal brain damage, attention deficit disorder, attention deficit hyperactivity disorder, or an auditory perceptual disorder (Adams and Benson 1992; Christensen and Delgato 1993). Research has shown a correlation between the above deficits and CAPD (Baran and Musiek 1995).

Generally, CAPD occurs more often in males (Roeser and Downs 1995). A broad spectrum of etiologic agents include fevers, anoxia, viral and bacterial infections, meningitis and encephalitis, head trauma, poor nutrition, malnourishment, family impoverishment, and genetic influences. CAPD in adults is associated with brain damage, aging, or a degenerative neurologic disease (Keith and Jerger 1991). There is a greater prevalence of CAPD associated with stroke in blacks. There is also an over representation of CAPD in special education classes (Buchanan et al. 1993; National Institute on Deafness and Other Communicative Disorders 1992).

The audiologic profile of CAPD does not show peripheral hearing loss; therefore, PTA and speech discrimination scores are basically normal. CAPD causes subtle limitations when the listening tasks require precise bilateral auditory integration and sequencing rapid and simultaneous speech. In principle, the CAPD test battery strains the auditory processing system by reducing language redundancy. It also tests the tolerance limits of bilateral transmission to the higher auditory centers.

Symptoms, Syndromes, and Signs Linked to Hearing Impairments

A hearing loss is a symptom or the consequence of a hearing disorder, which is due to an anatomic or physiologic abnormality in the auditory system. Frequently, the basic etiologic agent of the hearing loss causes other nonauditory anomalies and symptoms. If the symptoms are mild, the disorder can go undetected. A syndrome is a composite of related symptoms or signs. A sign is an objective condition of specific diagnostic significance, which is often not apparent to the patient. In contrast, a symptom is apparent to the patient and the diagnostician.

Common signs of pathology include the Babinski's, Bárány's, and Romberg's signs. Common syndromes associated with hearing loss include Down syndrome, Hurler's syndrome, Usher's syndrome, Alport's syndrome, Klippel-Feil syndrome, Noonan's syndrome, Waardenburg's syndrome, Pendred's syndrome, and Treacher Collins syndrome (Northern 1996).

Speech and Language Disorders in Children

Normal connections between audible speech sounds and associated movements are incorporated early into the infant's speech (Boothroyd 1982). Abnormal speech (i.e., phonetic) development and language (i.e., semantic and syntactic) development are often the first symptoms of a peripheral hearing loss or a CAPD (Kretschmer and Kretschmer 1978). Deficient hearing in young children interrupts the learning of linguistic rules that govern the development of sounds, words, and sentences. Ultimately, the interference with language development disrupts meaning and thought acquisition (Bernstein and Tiegerman 1993). Depending on the degree of hearing loss, speech defects of articulation, voice, and pitch can occur. Severe hearing loss causes additional phonetic, rhythmic, inflection, and breath control deficits. The extent of the speech deficit depends on the type of the hearing loss, etiology, age of onset and intervention, family background and bonding, native language ability, and external support (Dagenais and Critz-Crosby 1992; Nober 1967a).

Recruitment

Recruitment is an above-threshold, abnormal, or disproportionate increase in the growth of loudness perception of sound presented with linear increases in intensity. Intensity is the physical dimension of sound, while loudness is the psychological perception of the sound intensity. When the person's perceptual growth of loudness exceeds the linear increment increases in intensity, recruitment is present. Recruitment is a symptom of sensorineural hearing impairment and is not present in conductive hearing impairment. As recruitment causes hypersensitivity to intense sounds, it reduces the effective functional hearing range from the threshold of detection to the threshold of discomfort. Thus, a sound detected at 45 dB can be uncomfortably loud at 75 dB, leaving an operating range of 30 dB (compared to the normal operating range of 100 dB). Recruitment also impacts auditory discrimination and often complicates hearing-aid fitting.

Auditory Discrimination Loss

In sensorineural hearing impairment, there is a reduction in auditory discrimination. Auditory discrimination is measured as the ability to identify monosyllabic words or running speech. Generally, auditory discrimination scores decrease as hearing loss increases; however, auditory discrimination loss can be marked in some instances of mild-to-moderate hearing loss. Auditory discrimination is reduced even further in the presence of competing background noise interference.

Tinnitus

In common speech, tinnitus refers to ear or head noises that occur in the absence of an acoustic stimulus. The person perceives a sound in one ear, both ears, or the center of the head. Tinnitus occurs intermittently in normal-hearing people as a ringing or buzzing in one or both ears. Although it is usually a subjective symptom, in rare instances tinnitus can be detected by the examiner using a special probe microphone. Tinnitus is a symptom of many conditions and diseases, including middle ear and eustachian tube disease, Meniere's disease, cerumen (wax) against the eardrum, acoustic nerve tumors, otosclerosis, presbycusis, cardiovascular disease, acoustic trauma, and ototoxic damage.

Tinnitus can pulsate in rhythm to the heartbeat or can be continuous. It is often heard as ringing, buzzing, hissing, roaring, whistling, or jingling. Tinnitus is debilitating and difficult to treat with any long-range success. It can suddenly appear and disappear. It can last for brief periods or for years, or it may never subside. The etiology is not always apparent and is often never confirmed (Shulman 1991).

Paracusis of Willis

Paracusis of Willis is a condition in which persons with a conductive hearing loss ostensibly hear better in noise. This occurs because the speaker talks louder with excessive background noise, thereby increasing the signal-to-noise ratio. With conductive hearing loss, louder speech against the background noise provides a perceptual advantage that can enhance speech recognition (Nober 1966).

Diplacusis

Diplacusis, which literally means double hearing, occurs with middle ear and inner ear pathologies, either monaurally or binaurally. In monaural diplacusis, a single tone is perceived as more than one tone. In binaural diplacusis, each ear yields the same tone at a different pitch, which causes an echo effect or unclear listening. The causes of diplacusis can be mechanical or due to hair-cell damage in the cochlea.

Nystagmus

Nystagmus is a rhythmic, involuntary oscillation of the eyes in various directions (i.e., rotary, vertical, horizontal, or any combination of these). The movements can be slow, rapid, or both (e.g., slow in one direction and fast in the return direction). Direction and speed are diagnostically significant, particularly if accompanied with other symptoms such as hearing loss, tinnitus, and vertigo. Nystagmus is symptomatic for diseases of the central or peripheral nervous systems, the labyrinth, the inner ear, and the vascular system.

Vertigo

Vertigo is often described as dizziness (i.e., syncope). It is either a subjective sense of rotation (i.e., subjective vertigo) or of the environment in rotation (i.e., objective vertigo). Vertigo is associated with disorders of the semicircular canals and their adjacent structures of the inner ear.

Disorders and Diseases of the Auditory System

Aberrations to the auditory system can occur during the prenatal, perinatal, or postnatal period. The causes can be genetic, viral, bacterial, or traumatic.

Prenatal

Genetic Disorders

A genetic disorder is a congenital, prenatal condition related to a gene aberration. A gene is comprised of coded DNA. Any variation of the gene code is called an *allele*. If a pair of alleles is localized to a specific locus on the chromosome, it can produce a genotype for an auditory disorder. Humans inherit 23 pairs of chromosomes from their parents. One chromosome of each pair is assorted and selected at random as the independent recombination for the offspring. When DNA segments are proximally close on the same chromosome, they may be linked and inherited together with diminished recombination to the offspring (Smith 1995).

Smith provided a detailed summary of genetic syndromes associated with the various types and progressions of hearing impairment. Her classification of genetic disorders accounts for approximately 50% of the deaf population. Genetic types are single-gene mutations that are either autosomal dominant, autosomal recessive, or sex-linked (Jacobson 1995). Overall, one in 750 babies born are deaf (Jacobson 1995). Autosomal-recessive genes account for 90% of genetic hearing loss. The remaining 10% of hearing loss is caused by autosomal-dominant genes. Because of the reduced penetrance (i.e., trait occurring less than 100% of the time) for hearing loss, all carriers of a defective gene do not develop the hearing loss (Smith 1995; Gerber 1990).

Genetic or hereditary deafness can inflict specific outer, middle, or inner ear anomalies in isolation or as part of an expanded syndrome. The hearing loss configurations assume various audiometric patterns and are usually a severe, profound, or total sensorineural hearing loss. One genetic disease, sickle-cell anemia, almost exclusively affects black people. Sickle-cell anemia inflicts damage to the hair cells of the cochlea (Scott 1986). Other genetic disorders that affect the auditory mechanism include Down syndrome, Hurler's syndrome, Usher's syndrome, Alport's syndrome, Klippel-Feil syndrome, Noonan's syndrome, Waardenburg's syndrome, Pendred's syndrome, Treacher Collins syndrome, and Crouzon's disease (Northern 1996). About one-third of the deviant genetic disorder syndromes cause congenital hearing impairments. Some hearing impairments are delayed until periods of physical stress (e.g., puberty or pregnancy) or, in some instances, emotional distress (Smith 1995).

During prenatal ontogenic development, anomalies to any part of the developing ear mechanism can cause disruption of its normal growth and development. Poor fetal position or inadequate uterine space during the critical developmental period can cause deformation and morphologic defects of the ear structures (Mencher et al. 1997). Specifically, deformations that cause partial or even total growth and function disruption are called *aural atresia, microtia,* or *anotia* (depending on the specific magnitude and type). Craniofacial growth disruptions can occur as sequelae to other congenital structural disorders, such as Treacher Collins syndrome and Crouzon's disease.

Diseases

A series of diseases can occur during the prenatal stage of development and damage components of the auditory mechanism. For diagnostic convenience, the acronym *STORCH* has been developed to identify these diseases: *S* for *s*yphilis, *T* for *t*oxoplasmosis, *O* for *o*ther, *R* for *r*ubella, *C* for *c*ytomegalovirus, and *H* for *h*erpes simplex.

Rubella

Rubella, or German measles, is a viral disease that can occur during pregnancy. If rubella occurs during the first trimester or before the full formation of fetal structures, it can have serious multiple consequences, such as (1) severe sensorineural hearing loss, (2) CAPD, (3) learning disabilities, (4) mental retardation, (5) visual anomalies, (6) heart defects, and (7) neurologic deficits. Rubella can also cause hearing loss during the second and third trimesters. The hearing loss at this stage is less frequent and less severe, because the fetal structures are more fully developed. Accordingly, it is rare for hearing loss to occur if the rubella occurs after the sixteenth week of pregnancy (Hanshaw and Dridgeon 1978). The damage risk diminishes from 50% during the first month of pregnancy to 15% by the sixteenth week (Strasnick and Jacobson 1995). Hearing loss, which is the most common consequence of rubella, occurs in one-half of the affected infants.

Cytomegalovirus

Cytomegalovirus (CMV) is an endemic, or transmittable, disease related to a group of herpes viruses (Gerber 1990). It is constantly present in the population. It often lingers a lifetime as dormant or asymptomatic and then suddenly reactivates. There are three ways for the infant to contract CMV: (1) direct contact or contamination during birth, (2) transplacental invasion, and (3) infections in the membranes of the birth canal. CMV is currently the most common cause of viral infection. It is responsible for more than 4,000 sensorineural hearing loss cases annually in the United States (Reynolds et al. 1974). While only 1–2% of newborns have CMV, other consequences include CAPD, mental retardation, learning disorders, sensory and motor dysfunctions, and paralysis. Some symptoms are present at birth, while other symptoms appear later in life (Strasnick and Jacobson 1995). CMV can result from a primary disease in pregnancy or from maternal reactivation: The latter usually has more severe symptoms.

Other Viruses

The word *virus* is derived from the same root as virulent, which denotes a destructive force. Microscopic and resistant to antibiotics, viruses penetrate the cytoplasm of a cell, shed the cell's protective layer, mature there, and then leave the cell. The human fetus is highly vulnerable to any viral or teratogenic infection (i.e., an agent that causes a birth defect or abnormal development) and is protected by the mother's antibodies until 6 months of gestation (Bess 1977). A wide subset of viral agents (e.g., measles, mumps, polio, encephalitis, and meningitis) can cause peripheral hearing loss or central auditory processing disorders.

Fetal Alcohol Syndrome

Fetal alcohol syndrome (FAS) is a preventable, sex-linked, congenital anomaly of children born to mothers who use excessive ethyl alcohol during pregnancy. Approximately one of 30 pregnant women are alcohol abusive, and 6% of their babies manifest FAS (Enloe 1980). Prevalence for FAS is high among African-American and Native-American populations (Shewan 1994; National Institute on Alcohol, Drug Abuse, and Mental Health Administration 1990). The incidence of FAS (i.e., one of 500 to one of 1,000 births) is comparable to that of Down syndrome (Sherman 1994). The symptoms can be congenital or delayed. FAS causes mental retardation; perceptual and motor disorders; speech, language, and hearing problems; behavioral deviance; growth abnormalities; and facial and skull deformities. Sensorineural hearing loss is also prevalent. Conductive hearing disorders occur because of a greater incidence of serous otitis media in this group (Church and Gerkin 1988).

The chemistry of FAS is as follows: The alcohol penetrates the placenta barrier into the fetal bloodstream, where it absorbs fetal water with resulting cellular damage. The alcohol can deprive fetal brain tissue of oxygen and impair the central nervous system. Because the fetus has roughly one-half the mother's ability to eliminate alcohol from its system, the alcohol remains in the fetal bloodstream twice as long as it does in the mother's bloodstream (Gearhart et al. 1991). The effect of alcohol on the fetus is related to the quantity of intake. Inherently, alcohol affects women more than men, because women have a higher body fat to body water ratio (Gearhart et al. 1991). Alcoholism is the third leading cause of death among women (Church and Gerkin 1988).

Perinatal Disorders: Erythroblastosis

Erythroblastosis is usually classified as a perinatal disorder. It is the destruction of red blood cells in the fetus and occurs when the mother's Rh-negative blood produces anti-Rh agglutinin in response to a previous Rh-positive baby. Erythroblastosis occurs in the second and subsequent Rh-positive offspring of an Rh-negative mother. Hyperdevelopment of erythropoietic tissue occurs in infants with erythroblastosis. Immunization techniques have nearly eliminated this problem in the United States.

Kernicterus is a related congenital hemolytic disease caused mainly by erythroblastosis. It produces jaundice, a yellow-bile staining in the basal ganglia. Erythroblastosis is also the major cause of athetosis, a type of cerebral palsy. Athetosis usually involves a severe sensorineural deafness, hence the term *deaf-athetoid* (Nober 1966).

Postnatal Disorders

Otitis Media

Otitis media, a bacterial infection, is an inflammation of the middle-ear mechanism. It is caused by an inadequate or obstructed eustachian tube that prevents normal intratympanic pressure and ventilation in the middle ear cavity (Bluestone 1982). The disease affects the nasopharyngeal structures (i.e., tonsil and adenoid lining) and spreads to the middle ear. It is the most common cause of conductive hearing loss in children and the most common disease of childhood. By the age of 12 years, 90% of all children have one or more bouts of otitis media, but its prevalence declines after puberty. It reoccurs in about 50% of the children. Eighty percent of the children affected are younger than 5 years of age (Martin 1987). Otitis media is two to four times less prevalent in black children than in white children in the United States and

African nations (Buchanan et al. 1993). It is more prevalent in Native, Inuit, and Hawaiian Americans.

It is noteworthy that infants often develop an otitis when milk enters their eustachian tube during feeding and is subsequently trapped in the middle ear cavity, where it becomes contaminated by bacteria. This scenario occurs because the eustachian tube is initially positioned horizontally in infants. (Its position changes to vertical as the child grows.) In such cases, otitis media starts as an infection that reduces the middle ear cavity pressure relative to the external atmospheric pressure. As the middle ear cavity vacuum forms, it draws fluids from the surrounding tissues.

Symptoms of otitis media include pain, reduced hearing, an inflamed and reddened tympanic membrane, eventual fluid buildup, and often an effusion of excessive fluid through a puncture in the eardrum. The pure-tone air conduction threshold audiogram is relatively flat or shows greater low-frequency loss. Because the hearing loss is conductive, the pure-tone bone-conduction thresholds remain normal. Acute otitis media lasts from 10 days to 3 weeks as an isolated incident. When otitis media is prolonged or recurrent, the infection is chronic otitis media. If fluid does not develop, the condition is nonserous otitis media. If the condition is noninfected, it is serous otitis media. If the condition is characterized by infected fluid, it is called *suppurative* or *purulent otitis media.*

Antibiotic treatment is used to eradicate the bacteria that cause otitis media, but the strains are becoming more resistant to the drugs in the process. A surgical treatment is myringotomy, which involves lancing the eardrum to relieve fluid pressure buildup. To maintain aeration and ventilation for middle ear and atmospheric pressure equalization, pressure equalization tubes are inserted into the incision in the eardrum and, on occasion, can facilitate drainage (Clark and Jaindl 1996).

Otitis media has variable effects on the communicative process. A recurrent acute or chronic bilateral middle ear serous otitis media impedes speech and language development and arrests educational progress in children. The standard 25-dB hearing level screening may not identify half of the children affected by serous otitis media. The term *educationally handicapping hearing loss* is used for an otitis media conductive hearing loss in children. Children with mild to moderate conductive hearing loss often do not hear the weaker unvoiced consonants or the weaker vowel sounds, which are essential in preschool and first grade. Reduced auditory discrimination during the first 3 years of life can be confused with a CAPD, an auditory perceptual problem, or a language-learning deficit. It is noteworthy that otitis media can cause excessive absence from school and subsequent loss of classroom continuity, which confounds language and learning development (Maxon and Brackett 1992; Mencher et al. 1997).

Measles

Fewer than 10% of the people who contract measles have subsequent hearing loss. If a loss occurs, it usually appears as a moderate-to-severe, sloping, sensorineural audiogram. Occasionally, otitis media occurs and presents a conductive overlay to the sensorineural hearing loss. Measles is rare in the United States because of the universal immunization policy. However, when a pregnant mother contracts measles, the consequences to her fetus are usually serious (see under *Rubella*).

Mumps

Mumps is the most common cause of a sudden but permanent unilateral sensorineural hearing loss that occurs as a result of damage to the cochlea. Hearing loss occurs in about 5% of those afflicted. Mumps swells the parotid gland and can invade the central nervous system as an encephalitis or meningitis. If such an invasion occurs, the sensorineural disorder is complicated with other aberrations, including mental retardation and motor paralysis.

Meningitis and Encephalitis

Meningitis is an inflammation of one or all three of the meninges (i.e., dura mater, arachnoid, and pia mater), which are the thin tissues that cover the brain. The impairment to the auditory processing mechanism varies with the magnitude of the disease. Other symptoms of brain damage (e.g., mental retardation, sensory and motor deficits, physical aberrations, and emotional distress) can occur. Encephalitis is an inflammation of the brain (i.e., encephalon). The broad array of symptoms and effects are similar to those of meningitis with sensory, motor, mental, and psychological attributes. It is often the sustained high fever that causes damage to the hearing mechanism.

Otosclerosis

Although otosclerosis has a genetic origin, hearing loss does not show until the teenage years or later. It is, therefore, often classified as a postnatal disease. Otosclerosis is a disease of the temporal bone that causes repeated resorption and redeposition of bone tissue. It occurs most frequently in the otic capsule anterior to the oval and round window membranes; however, the primary site is the oval window, including the annular ligament. As otosclerosis progresses, it causes a fixation (i.e., ankylosis) of the stapes that eventually impedes movement of the entire ossicular chain, causing a marked conductive hearing loss. In the advanced stage, inner ear atrophy can occur, adding a sensorineural hearing loss to the conductive loss (Guild 1944; Schuknecht 1974; Derlacki 1996).

Otosclerosis occurs only in humans. It occurs primarily in whites but is also seen in other races. The condition has been identified as microscopic cellular changes seen in the temporal bones of young children and is therefore designated as histologic otosclerosis. When the clinical symptoms of hearing loss and tinnitus appear during the teenage years, the condition is called *clinical otosclerosis* (in contrast to *histologic otosclerosis*). Although the hearing loss is conductive with a relatively flat audiogram, some persons develop a mechanical sensorineural type audiogram configuration, which is caused by obstruction of the round window. Otosclerosis is treated with a surgical reconstruction technique of the middle ear called *stapedectomy*, which can bring excellent restoration of hearing. However, many people with otosclerosis elect to wear hearing aids instead.

Ototoxic Agents

A drug is called *ototoxic* when it passes through the bloodstream to the inner ear, where it damages cochlea structures. Ototoxic damage causes a sensorineural hearing loss that is more severe in the high frequencies. The damage is variable among people. It may not affect certain people. In addition to hearing loss, high-frequency tinnitus and vertigo are accompanying symptoms of ototoxic damage (Fausti et al. 1996). The number of ototoxic drugs currently exceeds 200. Some of the major drug groups are (1) aminoglycosides (e.g., streptomycin, neomycin, gentamicin, kanamycin, and dihydrostreptomycin), (2) diuretics, (3) analgesics, and (4) antipyretics (e.g., salicylates, erythromycin, quinine, and practolol). If the drug is ototoxic to a person, tinnitus and hearing loss often appear within a few days after ingestion. It is noteworthy that aspirin causes tinnitus and hearing loss in some people, when the aspirin intake is high. However, hearing loss due to excessive aspirin intake is usually temporary (Cass 1991).

A high-frequency tinnitus usually precedes the onset of the sensorineural hearing loss caused by ototoxic drugs. The tinnitus is severe and interferes with normal communication. Vertigo results from damage to the vestibular system and causes unsteady posture and gait. The degree of hearing loss, severity of the tinnitus, and the amount of vertigo are related to renal function and the amount of drug intake. Symptoms often abate when drug intake is reduced or withdrawn. Hence, the symptoms can be variable, temporary, or permanent and are usually bilateral (Popelka 1994).

Meniere's Disease

In 1861, Prosper Meniere described a disease, to be named *Meniere's disease*, of excessive endolymph fluid in the cochlear duct. The medical name of the disease is endolymphatic hydrops. Meniere first reported a triad of symptoms (i.e., deafness, episodic vertigo, and tinnitus); however, other symptoms can occur, such as vomiting, nausea, dizziness, and diplacusis. Symptoms of Meniere's disease rarely appear before 20 years of age. As many as 2.5 million people in the United States have Meniere's disease, and 20–30% of this group have bilateral Meniere's disease (Nager 1993).

A Meniere's episode is preceded by a strange sensation of fullness called the *aura*: It is much like the epileptic aura that precedes an epileptic seizure. The Meniere's aura can last from a few hours to days.

In severe cases, the vertigo can confine the patient to bed. The pathology is a reduced reabsorption of fluid in the endolymphatic sac: It is not a defect of the production site (i.e., the stria vascularis) as once postulated (Pulec 1996).

A formidable treatment for severe Meniere's disease is surgical intervention, in which a subarachnoid or endolymphatic shunt is created to redirect the excessive fluid. Less effective, noninvasive treatments include the use of diuretics, modified diet, and antibiotics, all of which have limited benefits. Allergies, blood disorders, and endocrine disorders often complicate the disease (Nager 1993).

The hearing loss from Meniere's disease is sensorineural due to cochlear damage. As the disease progresses, permanent damage exacerbates from the excessive endolymphatic pressure in the cochlea duct. At the outset, the audiogram is often worse in the low frequencies, because the excessive fluid loading increases the mechanical stiffness of the basilar membrane. However, the audiogram begins to slope downward as the disease progresses and more hair cells are destroyed. Loudness recruitment and auditory discrimination are present and often severe, depending on the extent of the damage to the cochlea. The tinnitus, which can be continuous or intermittent, fluctuates in intensity and often keeps the patient awake at night. During Meniere's periods of remission and exacerbation, the symptoms fluctuate accordingly in severity (Nager 1993).

Vestibular Schwannoma

Vestibular schwannoma (i.e., acoustic neuroma) is a tumor of the acoustic nerve. When located in the cerebellopontine angle of the brain, the tumor is called a *cerebellopontine angle tumor*. Although the tumor is usually benign, the secondary symptoms can be fatal if respiration is impeded or if the tumor compresses the cerebellum or pons (Hart 1996). The hearing loss is sensorineural but without loudness recruitment. Distressing tinnitus and a marked speech discrimination loss also occur. If the benign tumor is discovered early, it can be surgically excised (Schuknecht 1974).

Acoustic Trauma

Acoustic trauma is caused by sudden exposure to intense noise (e.g., a gunshot or a sudden explosion) that causes middle-ear damage, cochlear damage, or both. In extreme cases, the eardrum is punctured and the ossicular chain is dislodged. The hearing loss and its effects depend on the type, site, and the extent of the damage. Not infrequently, tinnitus appears.

Contusions to the head have also been known to cause temporal bone fractures, with a resultant loss of hearing, depending on the degree of the physical insult. Contusions to the head differ from noise-impact injuries. Temporal bone fractures can impose a total hearing loss in one or both ears.

Noise-Induced Hearing Loss

Noise-induced hearing loss is a preventable, environmental problem that can be considered a special case of acoustic trauma. It can cause temporary or even permanent hearing threshold shifts. For the most part, hearing loss does not occur if the noise intensity is less than 90 decibels A-scale (dBA), the minimal level for damage risk to the cochlea (Royster 1996). In the early stage, the audiogram shows a temporary threshold shift; however, as the condition progresses, the audiogram depicts a permanent threshold shift. The 4,000-Hz frequency is affected first, and the loss spreads to the other frequencies. Black people have less of a permanent threshold shift than white people. There is a greater permanent threshold shift from exposure to firearms in Inuit-Eskimo people of Northwest Greenland (Counter and Klareskov 1990).

Neoplasms

A neoplasm is a tumor mass of abnormal tissue that is benign or malignant and is caused by rapid cellular growth. A benign tumor form of keratinizing squamous epithelium and cholesterol in the middle ear is called a *cholesteatoma*. A cholesteatoma often occurs from chronic otitis media. In an advanced stage, the cholesteatoma can invade the external auditory meatus or the pinna and add to a conductive loss of hearing. Cholesteatomas are more common in Native Americans and Inuit Americans as a sequela to recurrent otitis media (Buchanan 1993). Other neoplasms include exostoses, osteomas (i.e., bony growths), and malignant tumors.

Fungal Infections

Fungal skin diseases (i.e., otomycosis) of the external auditory meatus are common, because the external auditory canal is dark, moist, and warm, perfect conditions for a fungal infection. The infection often spreads to the pinna in the advanced stage. Accordingly, a nonfungal otitis externa can cause pain, inflammation, redness, and a conductive loss of hearing.

Other acquired disorders of the conductive mechanism include an occlusion from a collapsed ear canal (which can cause a 50-dB hearing loss), impacted wax (cerumen), physical trauma, allergies, eczema, blood clot (hematoma), frost bite, and herpes. Some of the etiologic agents cited above are bacterial and others viral (Becker et al. 1994).

Presbycusis

Presbycusis is a hearing disorder caused by the aging process. The hearing loss is progressive, and, like other aging conditions, the problems tend to increase as time passes. On average, hearing thresholds normally diminish 1 dB per year after the age of 30 years. Presbycusis is the most prevalent hearing disorder in older adults. Its incidence increases as the population ages (Jerger et al. 1994). Presbycusis is sensorineural, involving the sensory and the neural auditory system from the cochlea to the brain. Because there are epithelial and neural anomalies, the terms *epithelial presbycusis* and *neural presbycusis* are used (Kricos 1995). In some instances, the central auditory cortex is involved.

Some people with presbycusis have a mild-to-moderate conductive loss overlay (superimposed) that confounds auditory communication. There is typically a disproportionate reduction of speech discrimination relative to the audiogram, which is called *phonemic regression*. Phonemic regression is caused by poor transmission efficiency due to fewer neurons in the auditory cortex. As a result, presbycusic people often claim that speech is loud enough but unclear. Reducing the speed of the speech delivery is often of considerable assistance (Schuknecht 1955).

Summary

This chapter reviewed an array of disorders of the auditory processing mechanism, as well as their symptoms, etiologies, and pathologies. There are notably different effects for adults and young children, so the educational, medical, and surgical treatments will differ. With the improvement in health care, medical and surgical intervention, and technology, the future is most promising for progress in audiologic techniques, early intervention, and rehabilitative strategies.

References

Adams PF, Benson V. Current Estimates from the National Health Interview Survey. Vital and Health Statistics [Series 10 (176)]. National Center for Health Statistics, Public Health Service. Washington, DC: U.S. Government Printing Office, 1992.

American Speech-Language-Hearing Association. Scope of practice in audiology. ASHA 1996;38:1–4.

Baran JA, Musiek FE. Central Auditory Processing Disorders in Children and Adults. In L Wall (ed), Hearing for the Speech-Language Pathologist and Health Care Professional. Boston: Butterworth–Heinemann, 1995;415–440.

Becker W, Naumann HH, Pfaltz C. In RA Buckingham (ed), Ear, Nose and Throat Diseases (2nd ed). New York: Thieme, 1994.

Bernstein D, Tiegerman E. Language and Communication Disorders in Children. New York: Merrill, 1993.

Bess FH. Childhood Deafness: Causation, Assessment & Management. New York: Grune & Stratton, 1977.

Bluestone CD. Otitis media in children: to treat or not to treat? N Engl J Med 1982;308:1399–1404.

Boothroyd A. Hearing Impairment in Young Children. Englewood Cliffs, NJ: Prentice-Hall, 1982.

Buchanan H, Moore E, Counter A. Hearing Disorders and Auditory Assessment. In D Battle (ed), Communication Disorders in Multicultural Populations. Boston: Andover, 1993;256–286.

Cass SP. Role of medication in otological vertigo and balance disorders. Semin Hear 1991;12:257–269.

Christensen KM, Delgato KM. Multicultural Issues in Deafness. New York: Logman Publishing, 1993.

Church MW, Gerkin KP. Hearing disorders in children with fetal alcohol syndrome: findings from case reports. Pediatrics 1988;82:147–154.

Clark JG, Jaindl. Conductive Hearing Loss in Children: Etiology and Pathology. In FN Marten, JG Clark (eds), Hearing Care for Children. Boston: Allyn & Bacon, 1996;45–72.

Counter A, Klareskov B. Hypoacusis among the polar Eskimos of Northwest Greenland. Scand Audiol 1990;19:149–160.

Dagenais A, Critz-Crosby PC. Comparing tongue positioning by normal hearing and hearing-impaired children during vowel production. J Speech Hear Res 1992;35:35–44.

Derlacki EL. Otosclerosis. In J Northern (ed), Hearing Disorders (3rd ed). Boston: Allyn & Bacon, 1996;139–148.

Diefendorf AO. Hearing Loss and Its Effects. In FN Martin, JG Clark (eds), Hearing Care for Children. Boston: Allyn & Bacon, 1996;3–19.

Downs MP. Contributions of Mild Hearing Loss to Auditory Language Learning Problems. In FN Martin, JG Clark (eds), Hearing Care for Children. Boston: Allyn & Bacon, 1996;188–200.

Enloe CE. How alcohol affects the developing fetus. Nutr Today 1980;15:12–15.

Fausti SA, Henry JA, Frey RH. Ototoxicity. In J Northern (ed), Hearing Disorders (3rd ed). Boston: Allyn & Bacon, 1996;149–164.

Gearhart JG, Beebe DK, Milhorn HT, Meeks GR. Alcoholism in women. Am Fam Physician 1991;44:907–913.

Gelfand S. Essentials of Audiology. New York: Thieme, 1997.

Gerber SE. Prevention: The Etiology of Communication Disorders in Children. Englewood Cliffs, NJ: Prentice-Hall, 1990.

Guild SR. Histologic otosclerosis. Ann Otol Rhinol Laryngol 1944;53:246.

Hanshaw J, Dridgeon JA. Viral Diseases of the Fetus and Newborn. Philadelphia: Saunders, 1978.

Hart MJ. The Acoustic Tumor. In J Northern (ed), Hearing Disorders (3rd ed). Boston: Allyn & Bacon, 1996;213–226.

Hood LJ, Berlin CI. Central Auditory Function and Disorders. In J Northern (ed), Hearing Disorders (3rd ed). Boston: Allyn & Bacon, 1996;227–244.

Jacobson J. Nosology of deafness. J Am Acad Audiol 1995;6:15–27.

Jerger J, Chmiel R, Allen J, Wilson A. Effects of age and gender on dichotic sentence identification. Ear Hear 1994;15:274–286.

Kaplan H, Gladstone VS, Lloyd LL. Audioelectric Interpretation: A Manual of Basic Audiometry. Boston: Allyn & Bacon, 1992.

Keith RW, Jerger S. Central Auditory Disorders. In JT Jacobson, JL Northern (eds), Diagnostic Audiology. Austin, TX: PRO-ED, 1991;235–248.

Kretschmer RR, Kretschmer LW. Language Development and Intervention with the Hearing-Impaired. Baltimore: University Park Press, 1978.

Kricos PB. Characteristics of the Aged Population. In PB Kricos, SA Lesner (eds), Hearing Care for the Older Adult. Boston: Butterworth–Heinemann, 1995.

Martin F. Pediatric Audiology Hearing Disorders in Children. Austin, TX: PRO-ED, 1987.

Maxon A, Brackett D. The Hearing-Impaired Child: Infancy Through High School Years. Boston: Andover, 1992.

Mencher G, Gerber S, McCombe A. Auditory and Auditory Dysfunction. Boston: Allyn & Bacon, 1997.

Nager GT. Pathology of the Ear and Temporal Bone. Baltimore: Williams & Wilkins, 1993.

National Institute on Alcohol, Drug Abuse, and Mental Health Administration. Seventh Annual Report to the U.S. Congress on Alcohol and Health. From the Secretary of Health and Human Services. Washington, DC: Public Health Service, U.S. Department of Health and Human Services, 1990.

National Institute on Deafness and Other Communicative Disorders. Working Group Minutes. Research and Research Training Needs of Minority Persons and Minority Health Issues. Washington, DC: National Institutes of Health, April, 1992.

Nober EH. Articulation of the deaf. Exceptional Children 1967a;611–621.

Nober EH. Cutile air and bone conduction thresholds of the deaf. Exceptional Children 1970;571–579.

Nober EH. The Auditory Processing Mechanism and Cerebral Palsy. In W Cruickshank, G Raus (eds), Cerebral Palsy: Its Individual and Community Problems (2nd ed). Syracuse, NY: Syracuse University Press, 1996;36–180.

Nober EH. Vibrotactile sensitivity of deaf children. Laryngoscope 1967b;12:2128–2146.

Northern J. Hearing Disorders (3rd ed). Boston: Allyn & Bacon, 1996.

Pickles JO. An Introduction to the Physiology of Hearing (2nd ed). London: Academic, 1988.

Popelka GR (ed). Association for Research in Otolaryngology. St. Petersburg Beach, FL: Association for Research in Otolaryngology, 1994;17, 49.

Pulec JL. Meniere's Disease. In J Northern (ed), Hearing Disorders (3rd ed). Boston: Allyn & Bacon, 1996;165–176.

Reynolds DW, Stagno S, Stubbs G, et al. Inapparent congenital cytomegalovirus infection with elevated cord IgM levels: causal relationships with auditory and mental deficiency. N Engl J Med 1974;290:291–296.

Roeser RJ, Downs MP. Auditory Disorders in School Children (3rd ed). New York: Thieme, 1995.

Roland PS. Medical Aspects of Disorders of the Auditory System. In RJ Roeser, MP Downs (eds), Auditory Disorders in School Children (3rd ed). New York: Thieme, 1995.

Royster JD. Noise-Induced Hearing Loss. In J Northern (ed), Hearing Disorders (3rd ed). Boston: Allyn & Bacon, 1996;177–188.

Schow RL, Nerbonne MA. Overview of Audiological Rehabilitation. In RL Schow, MA Nerbonne (eds), Introduction to Audiologic Rehabilitation (3rd ed). Boston: Allyn & Bacon, 1996;2–26.

Schuknecht HF. Pathology of the Ear. Cambridge, MA: Harvard University Press, 1974.

Schuknecht HF. Presbycusis. Laryngoscope 1955;65:402–419.

Scott D. Sickle-Cell Anemia and Hearing Loss. In FH Bess, BS Clark, HR Mitchell (eds), Concerns for Minority Groups in Communication

Disorders [ASHA reports, 16]. Rockville, MD: American Speech-Language-Hearing Association, 1986;69–73.

Shewan CM. Incidence and Prevalence of Communication Disorders. In R Lubinski, C Frattali (eds), Professional Issues in Speech-Language Pathology and Audiology. Rockville, MD: American Speech-Language-Hearing Association, 1994;89–104.

Shulman A. Medical Methods, Drug Therapy and Tinnitus-Control Strategies. In A Shulman (ed), Tinnitus Diagnostic Treatment. Malvern, PA: Lea & Febiger, 1991.

Smith SD. Overview of genetic auditory syndromes. J Am Acad Audiol 1995;6:1–14.

Strasnick B, Jacobson J. Teratogenic hearing loss. J Am Acad Audiol 1995;6:28–38.

Chapter 11   Study Questions

1. Define a hearing disorder in terms of decibel levels and explain the differences that age and education impose.
2. List the principles and rationale behind the different formats of hearing assessment.
3. Contrast the effects of conductive, sensorineural, and central auditory disorders on the normal development of a young child versus an adult.
4. List the common causes and symptoms of a hearing loss.
5. Discuss medical and surgical intervention procedures for a conductive hearing impairment and sensorineural hearing impairment.

12   Hearing Assessment

Jane A. Baran

Chapter 11 presented information on the causes of hearing disorders. In this chapter, the discussion focuses on the measurement or assessment of the various types of hearing losses that accompany those hearing disorders. The presence of a hearing loss in a person has implications for the person's ability to communicate and function effectively in social situations. A hearing loss can often lead to social isolation, loss of self-esteem, and, in the case of young children, the inability to develop language in a normal fashion. The audiologist's role is, therefore, to determine the extent of the hearing loss and recommend intervention actions that will alleviate the problems encountered by the person. Because hearing disorders can result in a number of auditory manifestations, the audiologist should assess not only hearing sensitivity but also other auditory processes such as word recognition, dichotic listening, and perception of pattern sequences.

Prevalence of Hearing Loss

Hearing loss is the most prevalent of all communication disorders. Adams and Benson (1992) reported the prevalence of hearing impairment in the United States to be 9.1%. In other words, an estimated 22.6 million Americans have a significant hearing loss. However, the prevalence of hearing loss may be even greater, as the data reported by Adams and Benson relied on self-report of hearing loss in a sample of 100,000 households. Often, people deny the presence of a hearing loss for a number of reasons, or they are not aware of the presence of a hearing loss in themselves or a family member. Fluctuating conductive hearing losses due to recurrent otitis media are likely to go unreported, as are hearing impairments related to subtle forms of central auditory nervous system compromise. Many persons who have had strokes, demyelinating disease, and other frank neurologic conditions experience hearing difficulties in the absence of any significant loss of hearing sensitivity. In addition, many older adults who are undergoing normal aging processes experience some type of auditory nervous system compromise. These persons have problems understanding speech and processing speech in noisy environments, as well as other higher-level auditory problems, but not necessarily a loss of hearing sensitivity.

It is interesting to note the distribution of prevalence figures across age ranges (Table 12.1). The prevalence rate increases across the life span, with significant increases in people older than 65 years of age. Although these figures provide an estimate of hearing impairment in the United States, they may actually underestimate the prevalence of hearing impairments in most age ranges, especially in the youngest and oldest age groups. If fluctuating, conductive hearing losses were routinely included in the prevalence data, the rate of young children with hearing losses would increase noticeably. Also, if hearing impairments associated with central nervous system involvement or compromise were consistently included, the rate of older Americans with hearing impairments would increase significantly.

In addition to differences in the prevalence rates among persons in different age groups, differences are also noted in the prevalence of hearing loss in men and women. The prevalence of certain types of hearing loss are also more common among certain ethnic groups. There is evidence that women tend to have better hearing or experience hearing losses less frequently than men of the same age. There is also evidence that African-American men tend to have better hearing in the high-frequency range than white men of the same age (Buchanan et al. 1993; Post 1964; Roberts and Ahuja 1975; Royster et al. 1980a; Royster et al. 1980c; Royster and Thomas 1979). Differences between the two male groups are not as evident in younger men or in men matched by age for the lower hearing frequencies. For the most part, no significant differences have been reported between African-American and white females across the age ranges studied; however, when differences have been reported they have tended to show better high-frequency hearing in older African-American women than in older white women.

It is difficult to account for the differences noted in these prevalence rates; however, a few suggestions have been offered. The increase in the prevalence rate of hearing loss among men was initially believed to be due to the fact that the United States had become an industrialized nation, and that in our early history, many more men than women were employed in industry and exposed to high-noise levels (Bunch and Raiford 1931). More recent data suggest that when men and women are exposed to the same noise levels, women experience less hearing loss. Therefore, it appears that a biological factor renders women less susceptible to noise damage (Royster and Royster 1982; Royster and Thomas 1979). It has been

TABLE 12.1   Prevalence of Impairment per 100 Persons in the Civilian and Noninstitutionalized Population of the United States

Age (Years)	Prevalence (Percentage)
0–18	1.6
19–44	5.0
45–64	14.1
65–74	26.6
≥ 75	40.1
All ages	9.1

Source: Adapted from PF Adams, V Benson. Current Estimates from the National Health Interview Survey, 1991. Vital and Health Statistics [series 10 (184)]. Washington, DC: National Center for Health Statistics, Public Health Service. U.S. Government Printing Office, 1992.

suggested that the differences noted in African-American and white males can be accounted for by the presence of melanin (a biological polymer responsible for pigmentation) in African-Americans, which protects the inner ear from damage (Barrenäs and Lingren 1990; Garber et al. 1982; Tota and Bocci 1967).

Prevalence data are not available for other cultural and ethnic populations at large. However, there is some evidence (albeit limited) that suggests differences among the groups in the occurrence of certain types of otologic conditions and their associated hearing losses. Differences have been reported for a number of middle ear conditions. For example, the prevalence of otitis media is lower in African-American children than white children (Busch and Rabin 1980; Griffith 1979; Robinson and Allen 1984; Robinson et al. 1988; Shurin et al. 1979): The prevalence is higher among Pacific Islanders, Native Americans, and Hispanics (Giebink 1984; Lerner et al. 1989; Stewart 1986). Cholesteatoma, which can be a sequela to recurrent otitis media, is a relatively uncommon middle-ear condition, but its prevalence has been found to be greater among Native Americans and Eskimos than other ethnic groups (Buchanan et al. 1993; Nelson and Berry 1984). Otosclerosis is much more common in whites than in African-Americans (Guild 1944; Schuknecht 1974).

There are limited data on the prevalence of otologic conditions that affect the inner ear for various ethnic groups. A higher rate of occurrence of Meniere's disease has been reported for white adults than Asian adults (Black 1982). African-Americans show less-permanent threshold shift than whites following exposure to industrial noise (Royster et al. 1980b; Royster and Royster 1982; Royster and Royster 1988). On the other hand, hearing losses associated with sickle-cell disease are much more common among people of African descent than among people in any other ethnic group (Scott 1986). Hearing difficulties associated with sickle-cell disease can include losses of threshold hearing sensitivity, as well as various types of central auditory nervous system compromise (Berry 1975; Crawford et al. 1991; Friedman et al.

1980; Forman-Franco et al. 1982; Gould et al. 1991; Orchik and Dunn 1991; Sergeant et al. 1975; Sharp and Orchik 1978; Urban 1973).

Although there are no prevalence data for hearing difficulties related to central auditory nervous system compromise, there are data that show that the leading cause of neurologic impairment among African-Americans, Native Americans, and certain Asian-Pacific Americans is a cerebrovascular accident (i.e., stroke). If the stroke causes compromise of the auditory areas of the brain, hearing function is likely to be affected. Primary risk factors for stroke in these populations include hypertension, arteriosclerosis, sickle-cell anemia, and substance abuse (Wallace 1993). Additional information regarding the prevalence of hearing loss in various racial and ethnic groups can be found in Buchanan et al. (1993), Nuru (1993), and Royster et al. (1980c).

Pure-Tone Audiometry

Typically, one of the first questions that the audiologist is interested in answering is what is the patient's threshold hearing sensitivity. Threshold sensitivity is measured for a number of discrete sinusoidal sounds referred to as *pure tones*. The audiologist's task during pure-tone testing is to determine the lowest intensity level at which the person being tested can detect the presence of a pure-tone signal at least 50% of the time. The thresholds are typically recorded on a graph called an *audiogram* (Figure 12.1), which displays the test results at the octave frequencies between 125 or 250 Hz to 8,000 Hz.

Assessment Procedures

Threshold sensitivity can be measured by two different mechanisms: *air-conduction* testing and *bone-conduction* testing. In air-conduction testing, the patient wears headphones or inserts receivers that are capable of delivering the stimulus of interest to either the right or left ear of the patient. The stimulus, which begins as a sound wave and undergoes a number of energy transformations to end up as a neural impulse, travels from the earphone or receiver through the ear canal and middle ear into the cochlea and on to the central auditory pathways. This signal can also be presented through a bone vibrator, which causes the skull of the patient to vibrate and, in turn, directly stimulates the fluids in the inner ear (i.e., bone-conduction testing). The results are plotted on an audiogram similar to the one shown in Figure 12.1. Since the two ears are not completely separated, it may be necessary to introduce a masking noise (i.e., a narrow band of noise centered at the test frequency) into the nontest ear to ensure that it is not responding to the stimulus. This type of *cross hearing* is possible when the level of a pure-tone, air-conduction signal at a given test frequency exceeds the bone-conduction threshold of the nontest ear at the same frequency by 40–50 dB, as

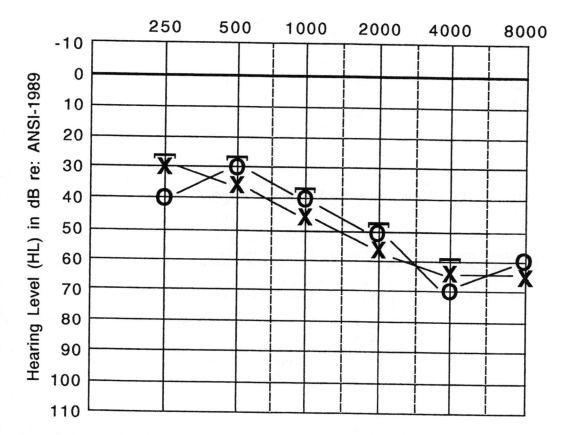

FIGURE 12.1 *Audiogram for a 70-year-old man with a bilateral sensorineural hearing loss. O represents right-ear thresholds. X represents left-ear thresholds. — represents the thresh-olds of the more sensitive cochlea (i.e., the better bone threshold).*

this level can be high enough to cause the entire skull to vibrate and a bone-conduction response to be generated in the nontest ear. During bone-conduction testing, the possibility of cross hearing occurs any time there is a difference in the bone conduction thresholds of the two ears. Therefore, masking of the nontest ear is frequently indicated.

Audiometric Interpretation

The pure-tone audiogram indicates a number of important things about the person's hearing loss. These include information about the nature, extent, and configuration of the hearing loss.

Degree of Hearing Loss

The abscissa or *x* axis of the audiogram represents the audiometric test frequencies ranging from 125 to 8,000 Hz. The ordinate or *y* axis is

TABLE 12.2 Classification of Hearing Loss Based on Hearing Threshold Sensitivity

Classification	Range of Hearing Levels (dB HL)
Normal	−10 to 15
Slight	16 to 25
Mild	26 to 40
Moderate	41 to 55
Moderately severe	56 to 70
Severe	71 to 90
Profound	Above 90

Source: Adapted from J Clark. Uses and abuses of hearing-loss classification. ASHA 1981;23:493.

TABLE 12.3 Classification System Used to Classify Audiometric Configurations

Term	Specifications
Flat	Less than 5 dB rise or fall in the audiometric test results per octave
Gradually sloping	Pure-tone thresholds that decrease 5–12 dB per octave
Sharply sloping	Pure-tone thresholds that decrease by more than 13 dB per octave
Rising	5 dB or more increase per octave
Trough (or cookie bite)	20 dB or greater loss at 1,000 Hz, 2,000 Hz, or both than at 500 Hz and 4,000 Hz
Miscellaneous	An audiometric configuration that does not conform to any of the other specifications

Source: Adapted from H Kaplan, VS Gladstone, LL Lloyd. Audiometric Interpretation: A Manual of Basic Audiometry. Boston: Allyn & Bacon, 1993;13.

read as Hearing Level (HL) with the scale ranging from −10 dB HL through 110 dB HL. Hearing loss is described by convention according to a classification system similar to the one presented in Table 12.2.

Shape of Loss

Classification systems have also been developed to describe the shape of the hearing loss. These systems have been designed to provide information regarding the configuration of the hearing loss. Table 12.3 displays one commonly used classification system.

Nature of Loss

The audiogram provides information relative to the nature or type of hearing loss. If the bone-conduction thresholds are more sensitive than the air-conduction thresholds in a given ear, the person is said to have a *conductive hearing loss.* This type of hearing loss is common in pathologic conditions that affect the outer or middle ear. If the bone- and air-conduction thresholds interweave in an ear and the thresholds fall outside the range of normal, then the patient is said to have a *sensorineural hearing loss.* This type of loss originates in either the cochlea or the neural pathways that comprise the eighth cranial nerve and central auditory nervous system. Some persons can have a conductive and a sensorineural hearing loss at the same time. These patients have what is referred to as a *mixed hearing loss.*

The audiogram indicates whether the hearing loss is bilateral (i.e., present in both ears) or unilateral (i.e., present in only one ear). It also provides information relative to the similarity of the hearing thresholds in the two ears. In many patients, the hearing thresholds are symmetrical or similar across the audiometric test frequencies. In other patients, the hearing in the two ears is noticeably asymmetrical, or different across the audiometric test frequencies.

Speech Audiometry

Pure-tone audiometry provides the audiologist with information regarding the lowest intensity that a person can hear, but it does not tell us much about how well a person can understand speech. In speech audiometry, the audiologist is typically looking for the answer to one or more of the following questions: (1) What is the lowest intensity level that a person can begin to perceive the presence of a speech stimulus or recognize some easily understandable words? (2) How well can a person understand speech at comfortable listening levels? (3) At what intensity level does a person prefer to listen to ongoing speech? and (4) At what intensity level does speech become uncomfortably loud for a person? As suggested by these questions, these measures involve either threshold measures, as in the case of the first question, or suprathreshold (i.e., above threshold) measures, as in the remaining three questions.

Speech Recognition Threshold

The most commonly used stimuli to measure the *speech recognition threshold* (SRT) are spondee words, or two-syllable words with equal stress on each syllable (e.g., playground and schoolboy). These stimuli are selected because they are relatively homogeneous (i.e., similar) with respect to audibility. Typically, a small set of words is used, and the patient is asked to repeat the words perceived. By presenting the spondee words in a systematic way and by varying the intensity of the words presented, the audiologist can establish the threshold (i.e., at least 50% correct identification) for recognition of this limited set of stimuli. The audiologist compares the SRT with the *pure-tone average* (i.e., average of pure-tone test results at 500, 1,000, and 2,000 Hz) of the same ear to determine if agreement exists. If the SRT agrees with the pure-tone average to plus or minus 6 dB, the audiologist feels confident that the audiogram is a fairly accurate representation of the person's hearing sensitivity. If the two measures do not agree, the audiologist entertains other possibilities (e.g., equipment malfunction or lack of patient cooperation).

Speech Detection Threshold

The *speech detection threshold* (SDT) is also a threshold measure. It is different from the SRT in that the person being tested needs only to recognize that a speech stimulus has been presented. He or she does not need to identify and repeat the stimulus. The audiologist typically attempts to obtain an SRT whenever possible; however, some patients may be unwilling or incapable of responding to the SRT stimuli in any meaningful way (e.g., repeating the test words or pointing to pictorial representations of the test words) and an SDT may be derived. The SDT has also been referred to as the *speech awareness threshold*. Because the SDT does not require recognition of the stimulus, it is typically 5–10 dB lower (i.e., better) than the SRT.

Speech Recognition Testing

Speech recognition testing is undertaken in an attempt to determine the impact of a patient's hearing loss on his or her ability to understand speech. The information obtained can be used to assist in the proper selection of amplification. It can also help point to a site of lesion for the hearing loss. By convention, most audiologists use monosyllabic words to assess speech recognition ability at suprathreshold levels, although any type of speech material can, and has, been used. Patients with hearing losses originating in the cochlea and eighth cranial nerve typically show reduced scores on speech recognition tests. The more depressed the score, the greater the difficulty the patient is likely to encounter in processing speech in everyday situations.

On occasion, the audiologist chooses to test speech recognition ability at a number of different intensity levels to generate a *performance versus intensity function*. If this is done, persons with losses originating in the cochlea show reduced discrimination scores at levels that are expected to result in maximum performance. However, if testing is conducted at levels above these levels, the patients' scores do not decrease. An interesting phenomenon, known as *rollover*, is sometimes noted in patients with eighth cranial nerve involvement. These patients are also likely to show reduced scores when tested at levels that should result in maximum performance; however, when the intensity levels are raised above these intensity levels, performance drops noticeably.

Most Comfortable Loudness Level

Most comfortable loudness (MCL) level is a measure used to determine the hearing level that a patient finds most comfortable for listening to speech. In patients with normal hearing, the level tends to occur at 40–55 dB above their threshold for speech. MCL is typically assessed using a continuous discourse stimulus. During the discourse, the patient is asked to indicate whether the speech is too soft, too loud, or most comfortable.

MCLs are not typically assessed during each audiologic evaluation. They are more likely to be used if a hearing-aid fitting is being considered.

Uncomfortable Loudness Level

The audiologist can choose to determine the level of speech that becomes uncomfortably loud for a patient—that is, the *uncomfortable loudness level* (UCL). In persons with normal hearing, this level typically pushes the limit of the audiometer (i.e., 100–110 dB HL); however, in many persons with hearing losses, this level is much lower. Having a lower than normal UCL is a common occurrence in patients with sensory (i.e., cochlear in origin) hearing losses because of a phenomenon known as *recruitment*. Recruitment is the abnormally rapid growth of loudness perception as intensity increases. The determination of UCL is important for the patient with a hearing loss who is being fitted with an amplification device. It is used to ensure that the amplification provided by the instrument does not exceed the patient's UCL. If it does, the patient will not wear the device. UCL can be measured using continuous discourse. During discourse, the patient is asked to indicate when the speech reaches a listening level beyond which any additional increases in level would cause discomfort.

Immittance Audiometry

Acoustic immittance is a measure of how readily the middle-ear system accepts or passes energy or, inversely, how much impedance the middle-ear system offers to an auditory stimulus. For example, if the middle ear is free of any pathologic condition, the sound waves striking the eardrum are passed through the middle ear without any significant opposition and most of the energy reaching the middle ear is passed into the inner ear. If, on the other hand, the middle ear has a significant middle-ear pathologic condition (e.g., fluid in the ear), then much of the energy striking the eardrum will be reflected out of the ear canal and less energy will pass through the middle ear to the inner ear. Immittance can be measured by presenting sound to an ear canal that has been sealed hermetically (i.e., by placing a probe tip in the ear canal so that air cannot escape) and measuring the sound pressure that remains in the ear canal as the air pressure in the ear canal is varied. Based on the measures obtained, inferences are made regarding how compliant the vibratory system is. There are three major tests in the immittance battery: tympanometry, static compliance, and acoustic reflexes.

Tympanometry

Tympanometry is a measure of how the immittance of the eardrum changes as air pressure is varied in the ear canal. It is sensitive to any pathologic condition that affects the middle-ear structures and function. The middle-ear space is an air-filled cavity located behind the eardrum. The eardrum moves or vibrates most easily when the air pressure in the middle-ear space is equal to that in the ear canal. Under these conditions, sound that enters the ear canal causes the eardrum to vibrate, and energy flows readily from the ear canal to the middle-ear space. If there is a change in the middle-ear pressure relative to that in the ear canal, a pressure differential exists across the eardrum. This pressure differential results in a change in the immittance of the system, and the energy flow drops. Virtually any middle-ear abnormality reflects an obvious change in either the pressure or compliance test results as measured by tympanometry.

Figure 12.2 shows a number of tympanograms. Each of these tympanograms is associated with unique physical characteristics. *Type A* is the tympanogram that would be obtained from a normal ear. Both middle-ear pressure and compliance are within normal limits. *Type As* is representative of a tympanogram that could be seen with pathologic conditions that increase the stiffness of the middle-ear system but do not affect middle-ear pressure. The tympanogram reflects normal pressure and reduced compliance. One such pathologic condition is otosclerosis. A second pathology that affects compliance but not pressure is a disarticulation or break in the ossicular chain. This results in a *Type Ad* tympanogram with normal pressure but increased compliance. Other tympanogram types are indicative of changes in pressure or compliance within the system, or both. In a *Type C* tympanogram, a peak of maximum compliance can be identified, but it is displaced to a negative pressure value. This type of tympanogram is seen in a person with a blocked or malfunctioning eustachian tube. The final type of tympanogram is the *Type B* tympanogram. In this case, compliance is usually severely reduced with no point of maximum compliance noted at any of the pressure values offered by the instrumentation. This type of tympanogram is often noted in persons with otitis media.

Static Compliance

Static compliance is measured by comparing the immittance of the system when the eardrum is at its most compliant point (i.e., when the air pressure in the ear canal equals the middle-ear pressure) and when the air pressure in the ear canal is raised to + 200 decaPascals (daPa). When the air pressure is at + 200 daPa, the immittance measurement is equivalent to the volume of air in the enclosed ear canal. However, when the eardrum is placed in its most compliant condition, the volume measured is larger than in the + 200 daPa test condition, because the volume includes the contribution of the middle-ear vibratory system. The static compliance is the difference between the two volume measures and is typically expressed in cubic centimeters (cc). Values below 0.3 cc and above 2.5 cc are considered to be indicative of middle-ear disorder. There are, however, a number of middle-ear conditions in which

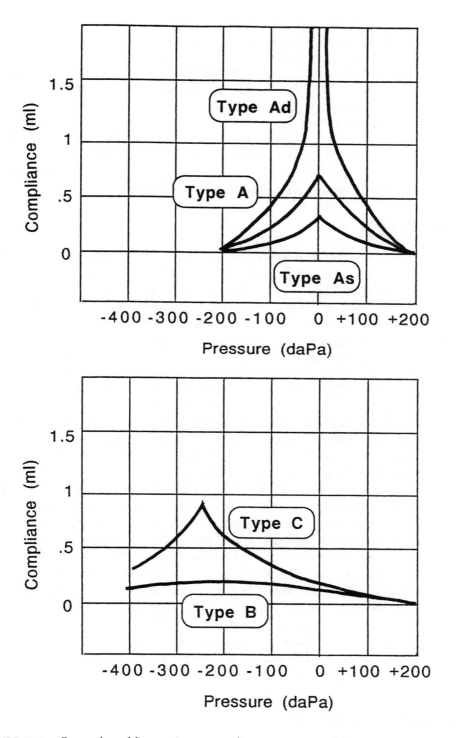

FIGURE 12.2 *Examples of five major types of tympanograms differentiated during immittance testing. (See text for details.)*

the results do not fall outside the normal range. This test procedure is most useful in the detection of a perforation of the eardrum or in the determination of the patency of a ventilating tube placed in the eardrum. If the ear canal is coupled to the middle ear, the first measurement (i.e., + 200 daPa) results in a volume measurement that is considerably larger than expected (i.e., 4.0–5.0 cc). Such a large volume measurement only occurs when the middle-ear space is directly contributing to the equivalent volume measurement. Therefore, the observation of a large equivalent volume measurement implicates the presence of a patent ventilating tube in the ear, or in the absence of a tube, the presence of a perforation in the eardrum.

Acoustic Reflexes

When an intense sound is presented to a normal ear, an acoustic reflex can often be elicited. Typically, acoustic stimuli (i.e., pure-tone signals, narrow-band noises, or broad-band noises) presented at 70–100 dB HL are sufficiently intense to cause the stapedius muscle in the middle ear to contract. When it contracts, the middle-ear vibratory system stiffens, and sound entering the ear cannot pass as readily through the middle ear to the inner ear. If the pressure in the ear canal is equal to that in the middle ear, this contraction can easily be detected as a change in the immittance of the middle-ear system—that is, less energy flows from the ear canal into the middle-ear system. By varying the intensity of the acoustic stimulus, the audiologist can determine the reflex threshold level. In a normal person, when an intense sound is presented to one or both ears, a consensual contraction is noted in both ears. Therefore, it is possible to measure both an ipsilateral and a contralateral acoustic reflex when a sufficiently intense sound is delivered to either ear. If the sound is delivered to the ear that is being monitored for changes in immittance, the reflex is referred to as an *ipsilateral acoustic reflex*. If the stimulus is delivered to the other ear, the audiologist is assessing what is referred to as a *contralateral acoustic reflex*. A discussion of the various types of abnormalities that can be detected with acoustic reflex testing is beyond the scope of this chapter. However, abnormalities are expected in ears with middle-ear pathologic conditions, cochlear hearing loss, and eighth cranial nerve or low brain stem involvement. Unique patterns of abnormalities are often noted for these various pathologic conditions and, when used in combination with other test data, can lead to a differential diagnosis among these conditions.

Otoacoustic Emissions

Otoacoustic emissions are a recent development in the field of audiology. The measurement of emissions involves the recording of sounds that emanate from the inner ear. This can be done by placing a miniature

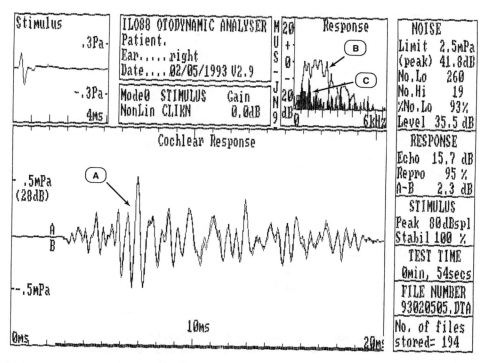

FIGURE 12.3 *A transient evoked otoacoustic emission derived from the right ear of a person with normal hearing. A represents the energy emitted from the cochlea over time. B represents the amplitude of the response. C represents the noise floor across the audiometric frequency range.*

microphone in an ear canal that has been sealed. The sensory cells within the cochlea expand and contract when stimulated. As the sensory cells respond to incoming sounds, they create sounds that can travel out from the cochlea through the middle ear and into the ear canal, where they can be detected by a miniature microphone. There are two major categories of otoacoustic emissions: *spontaneous otoacoustic emissions* and *evoked otoacoustic emissions*. In many persons, otoacoustic emissions can be measured in the absence of any eliciting stimulus (i.e., a spontaneous acoustic emission). It has been estimated that spontaneous emissions can be measured in about one-half of the population with normal hearing sensitivity (Kemp 1979).

The second category of emissions involves the presentation of a stimulus that elicits or evokes a response in a normal ear. These emissions can be evoked with either a click stimulus or a pair of tone bursts. If a click stimulus is used, the response is a click that represents sounds being generated over a large portion of the basilar membrane. The emission is spectrally analyzed to show the frequency distribution of the acoustic response (i.e., the emitted energy). This type of response is referred to as a *transient evoked otoacoustic emission*. An example of this type of emission is shown in Figure 12.3.

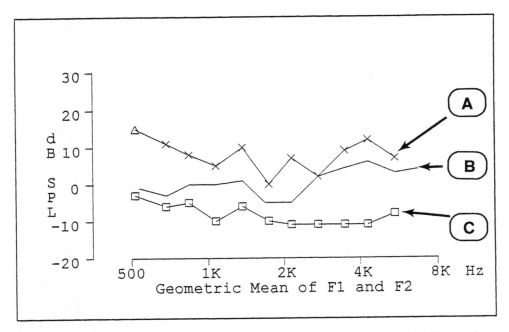

FIGURE 12.4 *A distortion product otoacoustic emission derived from the left ear of a person with normal hearing. A represents the amplitude of the cochlear response at 12 different distortion product frequencies. B represents the lower cutoff for normal results across the 12 distortion product test frequencies. C represents the amplitude of the noise measured at the 12 distortion product frequencies. (F1 = lower stimulus presented; F2 = higher stimulus presented.)*

Emissions can also be elicited by presenting tonal stimuli to the ear. This procedure involves the simultaneous presentation of two tone bursts that elicit distortion products (i.e., energy) that occur at frequencies different from the eliciting stimuli. The most robust response is typically observed at a frequency that is mathematically related to the two eliciting frequencies by the following formula: 2f1–f2, where f1 represents the lower stimulus presented and f2 represents the higher stimulus presented. To assess cochlear function across the audiometric frequency range, a number of stimulus pairs are presented over the frequency range from 500 to 8,000 Hz, with the relationship between the two tones in each presentation pair being maintained at a f2/f1 ratio of 1.2 to 1. This type of recording, called the *distortion product otoacoustic emission,* is displayed in Figure 12.4.

Otoacoustic emissions have been shown to be sensitive to the presence or absence of hearing loss related to cochlear involvement. To date, however, the clinical findings have not shown otoacoustic emissions to be useful in predicting the extent of hearing loss. In other words, otoacoustic emissions can be useful in determining if a person has a sensory hearing loss, but they do not provide a mechanism for establishing the extent of that loss (e.g., 30 dB HL or 50 dB HL). In spite of these limitations, otoacoustic emissions hold great promise for clinical use as a screening procedure for newborn infants and other difficult-to-test patients, because they are sensitive to abnormalities of the cochlea.

Electrophysiologic Testing

Electrophysiologic testing has become popular since the early 1970s. A number of responses or evoked potentials can be recorded during electrophysiologic testing. For all of the evoked potentials employed clinically, the underlying premise is that electrical potentials generated in the brain in response to auditory stimuli can be recorded, separated from the ongoing electrical activity of the brain, and measured. In each of the following procedures, an acoustic signal is delivered to one or both ears, and electrical potentials are measured at various sites on the scalp of the person being tested. There are a number of potentials that can be measured. Auditory brain stem response (ABR), middle latency response (MLR), and late auditory-evoked response (LAER) are three of the more popular evoked procedures.

Auditory Brain Stem Response

The *ABR* is a robust response that occurs within the first 10 milliseconds after stimulation in a normal person. As can be seen in Figure 12.5, a number of positive peaks occur in the waveform that represent synchronous firings of neural fibers at various sites along the eighth cranial nerve and in the brain stem. Typically, a number of waves are identified and their latencies (i.e., the time of occurrence post stimulation) are measured. In addition, the length of time that lapses between certain potentials is measured (i.e., the interwave latency) and represents transmission time along the central auditory nervous system pathways. Other measures of interest include the amplitude ratio of wave V to wave I and the latency difference of wave V in the right ear compared to the left ear (i.e., interaural latency difference). These measures are compared to normative data to determine if the response represents a normal or abnormal electrophysiologic response to the auditory stimulus.

The ABR has been shown to be highly sensitive to compromise of the eighth cranial nerve. Abnormalities have also been documented for a variety of disorders that have compromised the auditory areas of the lower brain stem (Hall 1992; Musiek et al. 1994).

Middle Latency Response

The *MLR* is evoked by either a click or tonal stimulus and occurs within 10–70 milliseconds after the stimulus. The response is the result of neural activity that is higher in the auditory system (subcortex and cortex). Typically, two negative potentials (i.e., Na and Nb) and two positive potentials (i.e., Pa and Pb) are seen (Figure 12.6). Abnormalities include

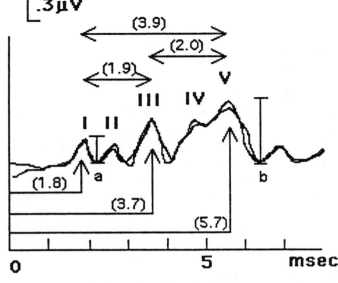

FIGURE 12.5 *A normal auditory brain stem response and its replication showing the presence of waves I through V. Latency measures for waves I, III, and V are indicated below the tracings, while the interwave latencies for waves I–III, III–V, and I–V are indicated by the arrows and the associated values above the tracings. The line markers above the letters a and b indicate the peak-to-trough measurements that are used to derive the amplitude of waves I and V, respectively. Note the actual amplitudes in μV are not specified. (Reprinted with permission from JA Baran, FE Musiek. Central Auditory Processing Disorders in Children and Adults. In LG Wall [ed], Hearing for the Speech-Language Pathologist and Health Care Professional. Boston: Butterworth–Heinemann, 1995;427.)*

(1) the absence of Pa, (2) an extended latency of Pa, (3) an amplitude difference for Na-Pa of greater than 50% for waveforms derived from one ear versus the other ear, and (4) an amplitude difference of greater than 50% for Na-Pa as measured from one hemisphere versus the other. Abnormalities have been demonstrated for patients with a variety of central nervous system disorders that compromise the subcortical or cortical auditory structures (Hall 1992; Musiek et al. 1994).

Late Auditory-Evoked Response

The *LAER* can be elicited by a number of auditory stimuli. The most commonly used stimulus is the pure-tone stimulus. The generator sites for these potentials are presumed to be cortical, and typically a negative potential (N1) and a positive potential (P2) are noted (Figure 12.7) in a person with normal auditory function. In addition to these potentials, an additional potential can be seen if the patient is required to attend to an occasional stimulus (rare), which differs from a common stimulus (frequent), in some readily apparent fashion. The stimuli are typically presented in an "oddball" paradigm, in which one stimulus is presented

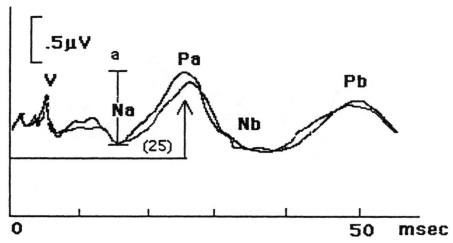

FIGURE 12.6 *A normal middle latency response and its replication showing the presence of two negative potentials (i.e., Na and Nb) and two positive potentials (i.e., Pa and Pb). Also shown in the tracings is wave V from the auditory brainstem response. The latency of Pa is indicated below the tracings, while the line marker below a indicates the peak-to-trough measurement that is used to derive the Pa-Na amplitude. Note the amplitude in μV is not specified. (Reprinted with permission from JA Baran, FE Musiek. Central Auditory Processing Disorders in Children and Adults. In LG Wall [ed], Hearing for the Speech-Language Pathologist and Health Care Professional. Boston: Butterworth–Heinemann, 1995;428.)*

frequently and a second stimulus is presently infrequently. The patient is instructed to ignore the frequent stimulus and keep track of the infrequent stimulus. The responses to the two different stimuli are then averaged in two different memory stores. The frequent tracing is the same as that described above (i.e., an N1 and P2 potential can be seen in a normal person). However, in the rare tracing, an additional positive (P3) and two negative (N2 and N3) potentials are recorded. To ensure recording of the late potentials and the P3, a time window of 800 milliseconds is needed.

The late auditory potential and the P3 have been shown to be abnormal in a number of persons with compromise of the higher auditory areas of the central auditory nervous system (Hall 1992; Musiek et al. 1994). These have included patients with frank involvement of the auditory areas of the cortex, and a number of psychological disorders, such as schizophrenia and dementia of the Alzheimer's type. Abnormalities have also been reported for some patients diagnosed with learning disabilities and in older adults who have presumably experienced some degenerative processes that have affected the central auditory nervous system.

Behavioral Tests of Central Auditory Function

There are many persons who experience hearing problems that arise from compromise or dysfunction of the central auditory nervous

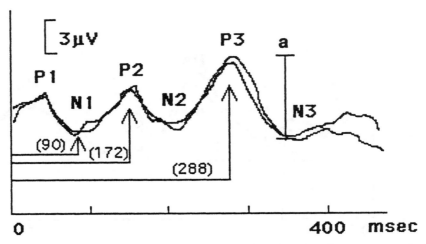

FIGURE 12.7 *A normal late auditory-evoked potential and P3 response depicting a rare tracing and its replication. Three positive peaks (i.e., P1, P2, and P3) are noted, as well as three negative peaks (i.e., N1, N2, and N3). Latency measures are indicated below the tracings for N1, P2, and P3. The line marker below* a *indicates the peak-to-trough measurement that is used to derive the amplitude of P3. Note the actual amplitude in μV is not specified. (Reprinted with permission from JA Baran, FE Musiek. Central Auditory Processing Disorders in Children and Adults. In LG Wall [ed], Hearing for the Speech-Language Pathologist and Health Care Professional. Boston: Butterworth–Heinemann, 1995;429.)*

system. Most of these persons show little or no deficit during pure-tone testing and routine speech audiometric testing. However, when the speech signal is degraded, deficits often appear. Additionally, many persons who do not show deficits in their ability to hear sounds have difficulties if asked to perform other auditory tasks, such as processing sequences of tonal stimuli. The audiologist has a number of tests to assist in the assessment of these types of deficits. The electrophysiologic tests presented above can be useful in the assessment of the person with central auditory nervous system compromise. However, many behavioral tests are available for assessment of these persons that can be more sensitive for certain lesion sites than the electrophysiologic tests available. The behavioral tests can be divided into four major categories: binaural interaction tests, monaural low redundancy speech tests, dichotic speech tests, and temporal patterning tests.

Binaural Interaction Tests

Binaural interaction tests are particularly sensitive to compromise at the level of the brain stem. They involve the use of speech materials or pure tones as the test stimuli. One of the more sensitive tests in this category is the *masking level difference* (MLD) test (Olsen et al. 1976). In this test, either a pulsed pure-tone stimulus (typically a 500 Hz stimulus) or speech stimuli (i.e., spondee words) are presented to the two ears at the same time that a broad band noise is presented to both ears. The noise level is set at one level and is held constant throughout the test, while the intensity of the test stimuli is varied until a threshold is determined. The patient is tested under two conditions. One is a homophasic condition, in which the stimuli and the noise are in phase between the two ears. The second is an antiphasic condition, in which one of the stimuli is held in phase while the second stimulus is presented at 180 degrees out of phase. A threshold is established in both conditions. The threshold obtained in the second condition is subtracted from the threshold obtained in the first condition to determine the amount of release from masking. It is important to note that this test requires normal and bilaterally symmetric hearing for administration and interpretation. The MLD test, as well as other tests in this category, is sensitive to compromise in the auditory areas of the brain stem; however, as a group these tests are only moderately sensitive to compromise of the brain stem structures (Baran and Musiek 1991).

Monaural Low-Redundancy Speech Tests

Monaural low-redundancy speech tests use speech materials as test stimuli. These materials are degraded or distorted in some fashion. The distortion can be either temporal or spectral. For example, in the *low-pass filtered speech test*, monosyllabic words are passed through a filter with a cut-off frequency of 500 Hz and an 18 dB–per-octave rejection rate (Willeford 1976). In one version of the test, 50 words are presented monaurally (i.e., to one ear), and the patient is asked to repeat all the words perceived. A percentage correct score is determined for each ear and compared to normative data to assess whether the scores derived represent normal or abnormal performance. These types of tests have been shown to be moderately sensitive to compromise of the auditory areas of the cerebrum, but they also can be affected by compromise of the auditory periphery or lower centers of the auditory nervous system (Baran and Musiek 1991).

Dichotic Speech Tests

The test stimuli of dichotic speech tests also include speech materials. For these tests, however, different speech materials are presented to the two ears at the same time. An example of this test is the *dichotic digits test* (Musiek 1983). The patient is presented four digits (two in each ear) in an overlapping fashion and is asked to repeat all digits perceived. For this test, only the digits from one to ten (but not seven) are used. Percentage correct scores are derived for each ear and compared to normative data. The dichotic digits test, as well as other dichotic speech tests, is sensitive to compromise of the auditory cerebrum, as well as the interhemispheric auditory fibers (Baran and Musiek 1991). As with any test for higher auditory function, compromise or involvement of the auditory periphery and auditory regions of the brain stem can affect performance.

Temporal Patterning Tests

In temporal patterning tests, nonspeech signals are used as test stimuli and are presented in a pattern that the patient processes. The patient then indicates what is perceived. One of the more popular tests in this category is the *frequency patterns sequences test* (Pinheiro 1977). It consists of test sequences that can be presented either to one ear at a time, dichotically (i.e., to two ears simultaneously), or in the soundfield. Each test sequence contains three tone bursts that are composed of high (i.e., 1,122 Hz) and low (i.e., 880 Hz) frequencies. The sequences are constructed so that in each sequence one of the tone bursts differs in frequency from the other two frequencies. This allows the generation of six possible sequences (i.e., HHL, HLH, LHH, LLH, LHL, and HLL). The patient is asked to verbally describe the sequences, as this assesses processing in both hemispheres, as well as in the interhemispheric fibers. If a patient is unable to verbally describe the sequences, he or she can be asked to hum the responses. However, if a humming response is used, one cannot assume that processing in both hemispheres is being assessed. Temporal patterning tests are sensitive to compromise of the auditory areas of the cerebrum and the interhemispheric fibers. As with the other behavioral tests, they can be affected by lesions lower in the central auditory nervous system (Musiek et al. 1994).

Factors That Influence Test Selection

As shown in the preceding section, behavioral tests can be useful in the assessment of central auditory nervous system involvement. In this chapter, only one representative test within each of the four major categories has been presented. There are, in fact, several tests available in each category that the audiologist can choose from. Not every patient is given every test or even one test from every category. The audiologist typically selects a battery of tests based on a number of considerations, which include (1) the age of the patient; (2) the patient's native language, language skills, or both; (3) the suspected site of lesion; and (4) the presence or absence of a peripheral hearing loss. The audiologist must select only those tests to which a given patient is able to respond. For instance, a test that requires a written response would not be appropriate for a young child or a patient with motor involvement of the upper extremities. Some tests require that the patient be able to read a list of possible responses. This would limit applicability of these tests to patients who are able to perform the task. If language differences are a consideration, tests such as the dichotic digits test and many of the temporal patterning tests should be considered. The vocabulary needed to perform the digits test is limited to the numbers from one to ten. In the case of the patterning tests, the vocabulary is frequently limited to two words (e.g., *short* and *long* or *high* and *low*). If the person being tested is not familiar with these words, often the audiologist can learn the two foreign words required for each test, thus permitting the patient to respond in his or her native language. Some of the tests are less affected by the presence of a peripheral hearing loss. These tests should be chosen when a patient suspected of having central auditory nervous system compromise is also known to have a peripheral hearing impairment. Finally, the audiologist attempts to select tests based on the suspected site of lesion. If a brain stem lesion is suspected, the audiologist can choose to perform an ABR, the MLD test, or both. If a cerebral lesion is suspected, the audiologist can rely on some of the behavioral tests, such as dichotic speech tests and temporal patterning tests. Additional information regarding these issues, as well as descriptions of other behavioral tests that fall into each of the four major categories, can be found in Baran and Musiek (1991; 1995).

Conclusion

Hearing problems are found in persons of all ages, racial and ethnic backgrounds, and socioeconomic status. When the problems are severe, as in the case of profound hearing loss, they are likely to be noticed. However, when the impairments are more subtle, as in the case of mild peripheral hearing loss, or when the deficits affect the central auditory nervous system, the problems can remain undetected. These hearing impairments, however, are real and can impact the person's quality of life. A toddler with a recurrent middle-ear condition and a fluctuating hearing loss can fail to develop speech and language in a normal fashion. The school-age child with a mild loss can encounter academic difficulties, because he or she is unable to follow his or her teacher's presentations and instructions. The adult with a central auditory nervous system disorder can encounter difficulties in the workplace. The older person with a hearing loss can suffer isolation and a hesitancy to participate in social activities, because he or she cannot participate fully in conversations and social interchanges. For all of these reasons, an aggressive approach to the assessment of auditory function is recommended. Once a hearing loss is identified, an intervention program can be designed to meet the individual needs of each patient and hopefully avert some of these negative outcomes. Chapter 13 addresses this important aspect (i.e., intervention) in the provision of services to the person with a hearing impairment.

References

Adams PF, Benson V. Current Estimates from the National Health Interview Survey, 1991. Vital and Health Statistics [series 10 (184)]. National Center for Health Statistics, Public Health Service. Washington, DC: U.S. Government Printing Office, 1992.

Baran JA, Musiek FE. Behavioral Assessment of the Central Nervous System. In WF Rintelmann (ed), Hearing Assessment (2nd ed). Boston: Allyn & Bacon, 1991;549–602.

Baran JA, Musiek FE. Central Auditory Processing Disorders in Children and Adults. In LG Wall (ed), Hearing for the Speech-Language Pathologist and Health Care Professional. Boston: Butterworth–Heinemann, 1995;415–440.

Barrenäs ML, Lingren F. The influence of inner ear melanin on susceptibility to TTS in humans. Scand Audiol 1990;19:97–102.

Berry RA. Sickle-cell anemia: audiological findings. J Am Audiol Soc 1975;1:61–63.

Black FO. Vestibular function assessment in patients with Meniere's disease: the vestibulospinal system. Laryngoscope 1982;92:1419–1436.

Buchanan LH, Moore EJ, Counter SA. Hearing Disorders and Auditory Assessment. In DE Battle (ed), Communication Disorders in Multicultural Populations. Boston: Butterworth–Heinemann, 1993;256–286.

Bunch CC, Raiford TS. Race and sex variations in auditory acuity. Arch Otolaryngol 1931;13:423–434.

Busch PJ, Rabin DL. Racial differences in encounter rates for otitis media. Pediatr Res 1980;14:115–117.

Crawford MR, Gould HJ, Smith WR, et al. Prevalence of hearing loss in adults with sickle-cell disease. Ear Hear 1991;12:349–351.

Forman-Franco B, Karayalcin G, Mandel D, Abramson AL. The evaluation of auditory function in homozygous sickle-cell disease. Otolaryngol Head Neck Surg 1982;90:850–856.

Friedman EM, Luban NLC, Herer GR, Williams I. Sickle-cell anemia and hearing. Ann Otol Rhinol Laryngol 1980;89:342–347.

Garber SR, Turner CW, Creel D, Witkop CJ. Auditory system abnormalities in human albinos. Ear Hear 1982;3:207–210.

Giebink GS. Epidemiology and Natural History of Otitis Media. In DJ Lim, CD Bluestone, JO Klein, et al. (eds), Recent Advances in Otitis Media with Effusion. Philadelphia: BC Decker, 1984;5–9.

Gould HJ, Crawford MR, Smith WR, et al. Hearing disorders in sickle-cell disease: cochlear and retrocochlear findings. Ear Hear 1991;12:352–354.

Griffith TE. Epidemiology of otitis media: an interracial study. Laryngoscope 1979;89:22–30.

Guild S. Histologic otosclerosis. Ann Otol 1944;53:246–266.

Hall JW. Handbook of Auditory Evoked Responses. Boston: Allyn & Bacon, 1992.

Kemp DT. Evidence of mechanical non linearity and selective wave amplification in the cochlea. Arch Otorhinolaryngol 1979;224:37–45.

Lerner M, Fujikawa S, Adams WH. Hearing loss and middle-ear abnormalities in a group of Marshallese children. Hear J 1989;41:21–24.

Musiek FE. Assessment of central auditory dysfunction: the dichotic digits test revisited. Ear Hear 1983;4:79–83.

Musiek FE, Baran JA, Pinheiro ML. Neuroaudiology: Case Studies. San Diego: Singular Publishing, 1994.

Nelson SM, Berry RI. Ear disease and hearing loss among Navajo children: a mass survey. Laryngoscope 1984;94:316–323.

Nuru N. Multicultural Aspects of Deafness. In DE Battle (ed), Communication Disorders in Multicultural Populations. Boston: Butterworth–Heinemann, 1993;287–305.

Olsen WO, Noffsinger D, Carhart R. Masking level differences encountered in clinical populations. Audiology 1976;15:287–301.

Orchik DJ, Dunn JW. Sickle-cell anemia and sudden deafness. Ear Hear 1991;103:369–370.

Pinheiro ML. Tests of Central Auditory Function in Children with Learning Disabilities. In R Keith (ed), Central Auditory Dysfunction. New York: Grune & Stratton, 177;223–256.

Post RH. Hearing acuity variation among Negroes and whites. Eugen Quart 1964;11:65–81.

Roberts J, Ahuja EM. Hearing Levels of Youths 12–17 Years. United States National Center for Health Statistics, Series 11, No. 145. Washington, DC: U.S. Department of Health, Education and Welfare, 1975.

Robinson DO, Allen DC. Racial differences in tympanometric results. J Speech Hear Disord 1984;49:140–144.

Robinson DO, Allen DV, Root LP. Infant tympanometry: differential results by race. J Speech Hear Disord 1988;53:341–346.

Royster LH, Driscoll DP, Thomas WG, Royster JD. Age effect hearing levels for a black nonindustrialized noise exposed population (ninep). Am Ind Hyg Assoc J 1980a;41:113–119.

Royster LH, Lilley DT, Thomas WG. Recommended criteria for evaluating the effectiveness of hearing conservation programs. Am Ind Hyg Assoc J 1980b;41:40–48.

Royster LH, Royster JD. Getting Started in Audiometric Data Base Analysis. In W Melnick (ed), Seminars in Hearing: Noise and Hearing. New York: Thieme, 1988;325–337.

Royster LH, Royster JD. Methods of Evaluating Hearing Conservation Audiometric Data Bases. In PW Alberti (ed), Personal Hearing Protection in Industry. New York: Raven, 1982;511–529.

Royster LH, Royster JD, Thomas WG. Representative hearing levels by race and sex in North Carolina industry. J Acoust Soc Am 1980c;68:551–566.

Royster LH, Thomas WG. Age effect hearing levels for a white nonindustrial noise exposed population (ninep) and their use in evaluating hearing conservation programs. Am Ind Hyg Assoc J 1979;40:504–511.

Schuknecht HF. Pathology of the Ear. Cambridge, MA: Harvard University Press, 1974.

Scott D. Sickle-Cell Anemia and Hearing Loss. In FH Bess, BS Clark, HR Mitchell (eds), Concerns for Minority Groups in Communication Disorders [report no. 16]. Rockville, MD: American Speech-Language-Hearing Association, 1986;69–73.

Sergeant GR, Norman W, Todd GB. The internal auditory canal and sensorineural hearing loss in homozygous sickle-cell disease. J Laryngol Otol 1975;98:453–455.

Sharp M, Orchik DJ. Auditory function in sickle cell anemia. Arch Otolaryngol 1978;104:322–324.

Shurin PA, Pelton SI, Donner A, Klein JO. Persistence of middle-ear effusion after acute otitis media in children. N Engl J Med 1979;300:1121–1123.

Stewart J. Hearing Disorders Among the Indigenous People of North American and the Pacific Basin. In OL Taylor (ed), Nature of Communication

Disorders in Culturally and Linguistically Diverse Populations. San Diego: College Hill Press, 1986;237–376.

Tota G, Bocci G. The importance of the color of the iris on the evaluation of resistance to auditory fatigue. Revue D'Oto-Neuro-Ophtalmologie 1967;42:183–192.

Urban G. Reversible sensorineural hearing loss associated with sickle-cell crises. Laryngoscope 1973;5:633–638.

Wallace GL. Adult Neurogenic Disorders. In DE Battle (ed), Communication Disorders in Multicultural Populations. Boston: Butterworth–Heinemann, 1993;239–255.

Willeford J. Differential Diagnosis of Central Auditory Dysfunction. In L Bradford (ed), Audiology: An Audio Journal for Continuing Education (Vol 2). New York: Grune & Stratton, 1976.

Chapter 12 Study Questions

1. Differentiate among a conductive hearing loss, a sensorineural hearing loss, and a mixed hearing loss.
2. Define the relationship between the speech recognition threshold and the pure-tone test results.
3. Identify five major types of tympanograms and discuss the characteristics of each.
4. Differentiate between the peripheral and central auditory systems and identify which tests are sensitive to compromise in each system.
5. Identify the tests discussed in this chapter that should not be affected by language, dialectical differences, or both.

13   Hearing Rehabilitation

Karen S. Helfer

What is Hearing Rehabilitation?

Hearing loss often cannot be corrected using medical means. Hearing rehabilitation, which is also called *aural rehabilitation*, refers to the nonmedical remediation of hearing loss. The goal of hearing rehabilitation is to improve the communication ability of hearing-impaired persons.

Two types of activities make up hearing rehabilitation. The first category is the use of technology to assist hearing-impaired people. This technology includes hearing aids and other devices used to enhance hearing ability, draw a person's attention to signals in the environment, or take advantage of another sense (e.g., vision) to communicate an auditory message. The second aspect of hearing rehabilitation focuses on behavioral strategies and techniques designed to improve communication. These activities are necessary because of the noncorrective nature of hearing aids and other devices. Even though hearing aid technology has improved greatly, hearing aids cannot correct hearing loss in the way that glasses correct vision. Therefore, many hearing-impaired people experience significant communication difficulty, even when they are fit with appropriate hearing aids. Hence, an important part of hearing rehabilitation is helping hearing-impaired people use auditory and visual speech information to their best advantage.

Who are the professionals performing hearing rehabilitation? Hearing rehabilitation is within the scope of practice of both speech-language pathology and audiology (see Chapter 3). Intervention with children, especially school-age children, often is done by speech-language pathologists, because they are more likely to be working in school systems. Many audiologists dispense hearing aids and other hearing technology. Approximately 28–40% of audiologists conduct speechreading, auditory training activities, or both (Audiology Update 1991). Another type of practitioner involved in hearing rehabilitation is the hearing aid dealer. The credentials required to sell hearing aids vary by state, but in no state is a degree in audiology necessary to sell hearing aids. Approximately 49% of hearing aids are dispensed by audiologists. Most of the remaining devices are sold by hearing aid dealers (Kochkin 1996). The level of expertise, experience, and training of hearing aid dealers varies widely.

This chapter includes information on both aspects of hearing rehabilitation: technology and communication strategies. Intervention with adults and children are covered separately, because the needs and abilities of hearing-impaired persons depend strongly on age.

Technology for Hearing-Impaired People

Hearing Aids

Types of Hearing Aids

Hearing aids are small electrical devices that amplify auditory signals. A trend toward miniaturization has greatly altered the appearance and function of hearing aids. About 78% of hearing aid fittings are the in-the-ear (ITE) type (Kirkwood 1996). Within the class of ITE aids are smaller versions, the in-the-canal and completely in-the-canal hearing aids. At the end of 1995, almost 11% of all hearing devices sold in this country were completely in-the-canal hearing aids (Kirkwood 1996) (Figure 13.1).

Behind-the-ear (BTE) hearing aids constitute slightly more than 20% of all hearing aid fittings (Kirkwood 1996). This type of hearing aid sits behind the pinna and is coupled to the ear via an earmold. One benefit of BTE hearing aids is that their relatively large size allows for the incorporation of a variety of options that the audiologist can adjust to modify the signal.

The oldest type of hearing aid is a body aid. Body aids consist of both body-worn and ear-level components, which are connected by a cord. Body aids continue to be used by people with severe and profound hearing loss, especially children.

Eyeglass hearing aids once were popular with adult hearing aid users. A hearing aid was built into the temple portion of the eyeglass frame, eliminating the problem of fitting both a hearing aid and an eyeglass frame behind the ear. The relatively small size of today's BTE hearing aids, the inconvenience of losing the use of both eyeglasses and hearing aid when one or the other malfunctions, and the prevalence of ITE hearing aid fittings have effectively eliminated the use of eyeglass hearing aids.

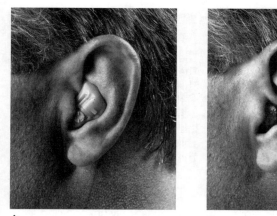
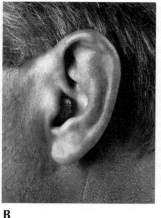
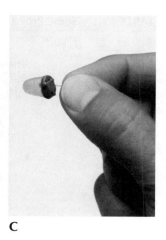

A   B   C

FIGURE 13.1   *Types of in-the-ear hearing aids. A. A conventional in-the-ear hearing aid. B. An in-the-canal hearing aid. C. A completely in-the-canal hearing aid. (Reprinted with permission from Starkey Labs, Inc., Eden Prairie, MN.)*

Table 13.1 summarizes the advantages and disadvantages of the three most commonly fit types of hearing aids.

Basic Components of Hearing Aids

All hearing aids amplify the auditory signal. The basic components of a hearing aid are shown in Figure 13.2. A microphone changes the acoustic signal (sound waves) into an electrical signal. Hearing aid microphones can be omnidirectional (i.e., picking up sounds from all around) or directional. Directional hearing aids are designed to reduce the amplification of sounds arriving from the rear. Directional microphones have been found superior for listening in noisy environments (Hawkins and Yacullo 1984).

The amplifier in a hearing aid increases the size of the electrical signal. Amplifiers used in hearing aids are considered wide band—that is, they amplify a signal in a wide frequency range, typically from 200 Hz to 7,000 Hz. Most hearing aids have a manual volume control, also referred to as a *gain control*, that allows the user to change the amount of amplification. This feature works similarly to the volume control on other electronic devices (e.g., radios). Some newer hearing aids incorporate an automatic gain control that eliminates the need for user adjustment of volume. Other devices require that the user carry a remote control to adjust volume.

The receiver is the component that transduces the electrical signal back into acoustic energy (i.e., sound waves). In BTE and ITE hearing aids, the receiver is inside the case of the aid. In body aids, the receiver is at the end of the cord that connects the ear-level components with the body-worn components.

TABLE 13.1   Some Pros and Cons of Three Types of Hearing Aids

Type of Hearing Aid	Pros	Cons
Body	The large size allows more power. Because of the distance between the microphone and the ear, amplification is possible without feedback. The large controls are helpful for persons with poor dexterity.	The cord is prone to breaking. There is no true binaural fitting. The microphone is on the body; thus, the patient cannot take advantage of pinna effects. It is cosmetically unappealing to some persons.
Behind-the-ear	The relatively large size allows for a number of options (e.g., tone control, gain control, and direct audio input). It is appropriate for a wide range of hearing losses.	The microphone is on top of the ear; therefore, the patient cannot take advantage of pinna effects. It is cosmetically unappealing to some persons.
In-the-ear	The microphone is in the ear; therefore, the patient can take advantage of pinna effects. It is cosmetically appealing to many persons.	Because of the proximity of the microphone and ear canal, the risk of feedback is greater. There is little room for options (e.g., tone control, gain control, and direct audio input). The small controls can pose problems for persons with poor dexterity.

As with other electrical devices, batteries are used to supply power to hearing aids. Most hearing aids use small batteries that produce between 1.3 volts and 1.5 volts. The preferred type of battery for hearing aids is the zinc-air battery. Hearing aid batteries are available in several sizes, so it is important that the new hearing aid user be counseled regarding the battery size that is required by his or her hearing aid(s).

Earmolds

All hearing aids are coupled to a person's ear using an earmold. The earmold is connected to a BTE aid via a piece of plastic tubing. On a body aid, the earmold snaps onto the receiver. ITE hearing aids use an earmold that is molded onto the hearing aid. In most cases, earmolds are custom-made after an impression is taken of the user's external ear.

Several styles of earmolds are available. Generally, the more powerful the hearing aid, the more occluding (or solid) the earmold needs to be. This is because of the risk of feedback (i.e., a high-pitched squeal that is caused by sound reamplification by the microphone). More occluding earmolds reduce the risk of feedback and, therefore, are used when greater amounts of amplification are necessary. The most commonly used earmold materials are hard lucite and soft acrylic.

In addition to delivering sound to a user's ear canal, the earmold can modify the signal. For example, a vent can be drilled into the earmold. This vent reduces the amount of low-frequency amplification, which is

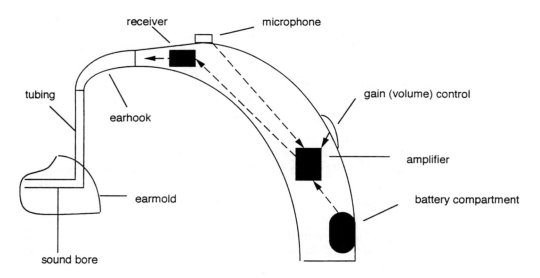

FIGURE 13.2 *A schematic of a basic behind-the-ear hearing aid. Internal components are represented by shaded boxes.*

advantageous because many hearing aid users have normal or near-normal low-frequency hearing. A stepped-bore (or high-frequency) ear-mold can be constructed, in which the sound bore has a graduated diameter. This modification shifts some amplification to a higher frequency region. Finally, dampers can be placed in the earmold or tubing to smooth out the frequency response (i.e., the amount of amplification across different frequencies).

Hearing Aid Controls

Most hearing aids have one or more controls that the person fitting the hearing aid can adjust. The tone control changes the frequency response of the hearing aid, usually by altering the amount of low-frequency amplification. The output, or saturation sound pressure level (SSPL), control determines at what level the hearing aid stops amplifying. All hearing aids have some mechanism (called an *output limiting system*) that prevents loud sounds from being amplified to a level that is uncomfortable to the user. As mentioned earlier under "Basic Components of Hearing Aids," the majority of hearing aids have a volume (or gain) control that allows the user to adjust the loudness of the amplified signal.

Binaural Versus Monaural Amplification

Although most people fit with hearing aids have bilateral hearing loss, approximately 45% of hearing aid fittings in this country are monaural, or fit to only one ear (Grahl 1993). Many people think that they can get by with just one hearing aid and, thus, are hesitant to pay extra for a binaural fitting.

There are a number of reasons why binaural fittings are preferable in most cases of binaural hearing loss. People who use only one hearing aid are at a disadvantage when trying to hear sounds coming from the side without the hearing aid. This situation is called *head shadow*: The head literally casts a shadow on the ear with the hearing aid. The use of binaural amplification eliminates problems associated with head shadow. Binaural hearing aids can improve the ability to localize sounds (Markides 1977; Schreurs and Olsen 1985), as well as the understanding of speech in noisy situations (Markides 1977; Cox et al. 1981; Naidoo 1993). The fact that sounds appear louder when presented to both ears (or loudness summation) allows a hearing aid wearer to use a lower volume-control setting on each hearing aid, thereby reducing the chance of feedback. Many hearing aid users report that binaural amplification sounds more natural or balanced than monaural amplification (Erdman and Sedge 1981). Finally, binaural hearing, when compared to monaural hearing, is reported to make listening easier (Feurstein 1992).

Hearing Aid Measurement and Standards

The measurement and performance of hearing aids is specified by the American National Standards Institute (ANSI) (BSR S3.22). The current standards require the measurement of hearing aids using a hearing aid test-box system. This device plays specific, calibrated sounds into a chamber in which the hearing aid is placed. The output of the hearing aid is measured in response to these calibrated sounds. Results of this assessment can be compared to a specification sheet (commonly called a *spec sheet*), which manufacturers supply with hearing aids. The ANSI document states the allowable tolerances for hearing aid performance. For example, hearing aids should stop amplifying after a certain level of input sound, and very loud sounds should not be amplified, because they are uncomfortable to the hearing aid user. One measure specified by ANSI is SSPL, which is the maximum amount of output from a hearing aid. ANSI specifies that the maximum SSPL value measured from a hearing aid should be within 3 dB of the manufacturer's specifications.

Fitting and Dispensing Hearing Aids

Dispensing procedures for hearing aids have changed significantly since the 1980s. Most hearing aids were previously selected using a comparative evaluation, in which speech perception was measured while the client tried a number of different hearing aids or hearing aid settings. This method of hearing aid dispensing has fallen out of practice for several reasons. First, significant differences in performance are often not obtained among various hearing aids or settings. Second, most persons opt for ITE hearing aids, for which a comparative evaluation is not possible, because these hearing aids are custom made.

Many audiologists use a prescriptive method to determine the desired hearing aid characteristics. A number of prescriptive formulae

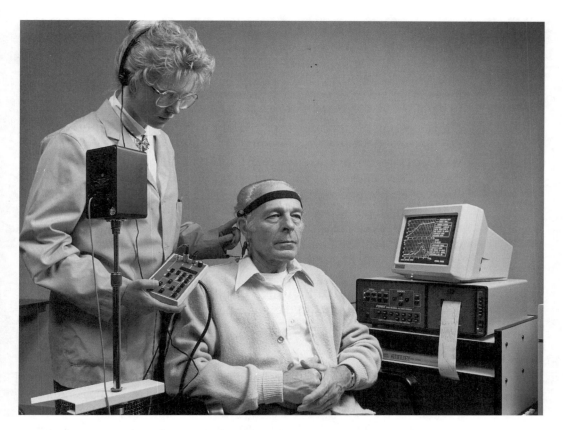

FIGURE 13.3 *A real-ear hearing aid measurement system. (Reprinted with permission from Frye Electronics, Inc., Tigard, OR.)*

are available that use audiometric data (most commonly pure-tone thresholds) to arrive at how much amplification should be supplied at various frequencies. An example of this is the NAL-R procedure (Byrne and Dillon 1986), which was developed at the National Acoustic Laboratories in Australia. Because they involve a large number of calculations, these formulae often are calculated using a computer program or in conjunction with a real-ear measurement system. An example of this type of system is shown in Figure 13.3. Real-ear systems are devices that allow the measurement of the hearing aid while it is worn by the user. A soft, flexible tube is inserted into the user's ear canal. This tube leads to a microphone, which measures the sound pressure level near the tympanic membrane. Measurements are made both with and without the person wearing a hearing aid. Thus, the amount of amplification (or gain) can be determined by comparing the sound pressure level in the ear canal without a hearing aid to that with a hearing aid. Most real-ear systems have software that automatically calculates targets based on prescriptive formulae. The audiologist enters pure-tone thresholds or other audiometric data, which the software converts to targets, or desired amounts of amplification across frequency. The audiologist then measures the real-ear response of the hearing aid to determine whether the targets have been met. Real-ear measurement systems also allow for rapid examination of the effects of modifications made to the hearing aid (e.g., venting or changing the tone control).

Even if a prescriptive formula is used to select a hearing aid, the client's subjective performance (i.e., how well he or she perceives the hearing aid to be working) and objective performance (i.e., how well he or she performs on tests of auditory perception while wearing the device) must be determined. Objective performance measures often include assessing speech perception ability with and without the hearing aid to assure that the client receives benefit. Subjective performance can be as unstructured as asking the client's opinion of how the hearing aid sounds. The client might also be asked to complete a questionnaire judging how well he or she functions while using the hearing aid(s). Two questionnaires designed for this purpose are the Abbreviated Profile of Hearing Aid Benefit (Cox and Alexander 1995) and the Hearing Aid Performance Inventory (Walden et al. 1984).

Hearing Aid Orientation

An important part of hearing rehabilitation is counseling the hearing aid user about how to take care of and use the hearing aid. This is often referred to as *hearing aid orientation* (Table 13.2). It is particularly important to counsel the new hearing aid user that it often takes time, patience, and practice to obtain optimum benefit from a hearing aid.

The most important aspect of hearing aid orientation occurs before the hearing aids are fit. Clients must have realistic expectations about the hearing aids. Misleading advertising by a number of hearing aid companies has led many persons to believe that a hearing aid should solve their communication problems, especially in noisy situations. Prospective hearing aid users must be advised about the limitations, as well as potential benefits, of these devices.

When the hearing-impaired person is a young child, the parents must be taught the limitations, use, and care of the hearing aids. This includes discussing the importance of consistent use of amplification. Many young children resist using hearing aids at first, and often it is necessary to set up a wearing schedule in which the child uses the aids for 15 minutes the first day, 30 minutes the second day, and so on, until full-time use during waking hours is obtained.

Recent Developments in Hearing Aid Technology

The technology of hearing aids has advanced dramatically. It is likely that the hearing aids sold in the future will be different from those currently on the market. Most of the recent developments have been made possible with the advent of digital technology. Many of today's hearing aids use some kind of digital circuitry, incorporating one or more com-

TABLE 13.2   Components of Hearing Aid Orientation

I. Benefits and limitations of hearing aids
II. Mechanical information
   A. Parts of the hearing aid and how they work
   B. Insertion and removal of hearing aid: demonstration and practice
   C. Manipulation of the volume control and other controls: demonstration and practice
   D. Batteries
      1. Size and type, where to purchase, how to dispose of
      2. Approximate battery life
      3. Insertion and removal: demonstration and practice
   E. Make, model number, and warranty information
III. Care of the hearing aid
   A. Cleaning the hearing aid and earmold
   B. How to treat a hearing aid (e.g., keep dry and avoid intense heat)
IV. Troubleshooting
   A. Normal and abnormal feedback
   B. What to do when the hearing aid is not working properly
V. Initial hearing aid use
   A. Easy and difficult listening situations: beginning with easy and gradually working up to difficult
   B. Patience and practice

puter chips. These chips allow processing of the incoming signal and, theoretically, can improve the quality or intelligibility of speech.

The digital technology can be seen in hearing aids that are sometimes considered "noise reduction." Some "noise reduction" hearing aids adjust the amount of low-frequency amplification depending on the incoming signal. Other devices, such as the K-Amp Circuit (Etymotic Research, Inc., Elk Grove Village, IL), which is used in a number of manufacturers' hearing aids, amplify only quiet sounds and let loud sounds pass through the hearing aid unamplified.

Digital technology has also brought about programmable hearing aids. Many manufacturers offer hearing devices in which the frequency response, output limiting characteristics, or both can be programmed an infinite number of times. This allows the audiologist to easily alter the hearing aid's response, which makes it very adaptable. Some of these devices have more than one program or memory. For example, the 3M Multipro (Sonar Hearing Health, Eagan, MN) has eight memory banks into which eight different hearing aid programs can be stored. The philosophy behind this technology is that one set of hearing aid characteristics is not ideal for all listening situations (e.g., less low-frequency gain is desired in noisy situations). These hearing aids allow the user to change the amplification with the push of a button.

Several problems have arisen because of the new hearing aid technology. Some of these devices (especially programmable hearing aids) are considerably more expensive than conventional devices. Many hearing aid users are reluctant to pay more than the cost of a conventional hearing aid. Additionally, fitting practices have not caught up with the new technology. For example, the prescriptive formulae used for conventional hearing aids are not appropriate when fitting some newer devices. Finally, manufacturers have not demonstrated convincingly that this new technology benefits hearing-impaired persons. In fact, in 1993 the U.S. Food and Drug Administration charged several manufacturers with deceptive advertising, because claims of improved speech perception with noise reduction devices were not substantiated by research data. As a result, hearing aid manufacturers must follow stringent guidelines that specify the research data they must collect to support claims about their devices.

Assistive Devices

Hearing aids are not the only type of technology available to hearing-impaired persons. An array of devices, known as *assistive devices*, are available to enhance hearing-impaired persons' communication and safety.

Several assistive devices are not specifically designed for hearing-impaired persons but can be used for communication purposes. One example of this is a FAX machine, which employs a visual form of communication. A second example is communication between computers equipped with modems.

The use of assistive devices is expected to become more prevalent because of the passing of the Americans with Disabilities Act in 1990. This act includes the requirement that employers make "reasonable accommodations" for their hearing-impaired employees, such as installing specialized telephone equipment. It also specifies that communication access must be assured in public buildings. For example, theaters must provide listening devices, and hotels must have rooms equipped with text telephones.

Listening Devices

Listening devices are useful because of the difficulty many hearing-impaired persons have communicating in rooms that are noisy, reverberant, or large. Assistive listening devices are found in classrooms, theaters, and houses of worship. They are also helpful for one-to-one communication in difficult listening situations (e.g., cars and restaurants).

The idea behind listening devices is to improve the signal-to-noise ratio (i.e., the intensity of what the person wants to hear versus the intensity of background noise). This is done by placing a microphone close to the speaker's mouth, thereby reducing the effect of noise and distance between the speaker and listener.

Assistive listening devices differ in how they transmit the signal from the speaker to the listener. The first such devices were hard-wire, meaning that the microphone was attached to an amplifier via a wire, which was in turn attached to a set of headphones via wires. These hard-wire devices are now used infrequently. Many listening devices used today are wireless.

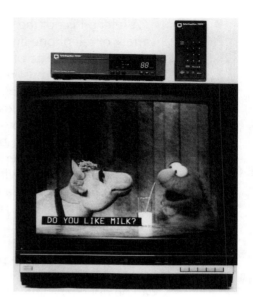

FIGURE 13.4 *An example of a television program with closed captions. (Reprinted with permission from the National Captioning Institute, Vienna, VA.)*

Infrared listening systems transmit the speech signal using invisible light. The listener wears a receiver that picks up the light signal and converts it into an auditory signal. In induction loop systems, a coil (or loop) of wire is placed around the perimeter of a room (or around a chair in which the hearing-impaired person sits). When amplified sound from the speaker's microphone is sent through the loop, electromagnetic energy radiates from the wire. This electromagnetic energy can be picked up by a telecoil (i.e., an induction coil placed in a hearing aid) or an external induction receiver. Another type of assistive listening device is an FM system, which essentially sets up a small radio station that transmits the signal via FM radio waves. The speaker's microphone is attached to a transmitter, and the listener uses a receiver coupled to headphones or to the hearing aid.

Many hearing-impaired people use these devices for television listening by placing the microphone near the speaker on the television. Other hearing-impaired persons benefit from closed captioning, in which printed captions appear on the screen. Figure 13.4 shows a television program with captions. A special decoder is needed to see these captions, although, as of 1993, all televisions sold in the United States must have a built-in decoder.

Telephone Devices

Telephone devices are necessary for many hearing-impaired persons. As mentioned above, hearing aids can be fabricated to include a telecoil. This transducer picks up electromagnetic energy, which is leaked from many telephones. When the telecoil is activated, the microphone is deactivated. Thus, a telecoil user can hear a telephone conversation without picking up extraneous room noise and without interference from feedback.

A telecoil is not the only option for telephone communication. A variety of telephone amplifiers are available, as are devices that alter or increase the volume of the ring of the telephone.

Some persons must rely on visual signals instead of auditory signals when using the telephone. A telephone device for the deaf (TDD), which is also called a *text telephone* or *teletypewriter*, allows a hearing-impaired person to see a visual, written display of a message and, in turn, type a message back. In the past, persons who used a TDD were limited in that they could only communicate with other TDD users. The Americans with Disabilities Act mandated that, as of 1993, all states must provide a relay service. This service allows a non-TDD user to contact a TDD user via an operator, and vice versa.

Warning Devices

Warning devices help a person identify warning sounds in the environment (e.g., smoke alarms, alarm clocks, doorbells, or a baby's cry). This can be done by using any combination of the following: (1) an enhanced auditory signal (in which the intensity of the warning sound is increased or the pitch is changed), (2) a visual signal (e.g., a device that causes a lamp to flash when the doorbell rings), and (3) a tactile signal (e.g., a bed shaker that is used in place of an auditory alarm clock).

Cochlear Implants

The development of cochlear implants has given deaf persons a new option for help in communicating. A cochlear implant is a device that essentially bypasses an impaired cochlea and directly stimulates the eighth cranial nerve. An example of a cochlear implant system is shown in Figure 13.5. Cochlear implants consist of a surgically implanted electrode array and receiver, and an externally worn microphone and speech processor. All implants used today are multichannel, meaning that more than one electrode is used to stimulate neurons.

Cochlear implants are appropriate only for persons who receive little or no benefit from conventional hearing aids. Cochlear implants are more successful in persons who are postlinguistically deaf (i.e., those who had some language before losing their hearing), although prelinguistically deaf children and adults are implanted.

One difficulty involved in the use of cochlear implants is the amount of variability in performance among users of these devices. Some implant users recognize speech over the telephone, whereas others can identify only environmental sounds. Problems associated with the use of cochlear implants include the unknown effects of long-term electrical stimulation and resistance from the Deaf community. (The term *Deaf* with a capital *D* refers to deafness as a cultural identity rather than a disability.) These potential drawbacks are mitigated by the fact that many cochlear implant users are able to recognize auditory sounds better through their implant than with hearing aids.

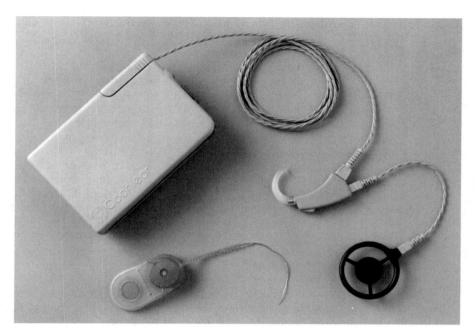

FIGURE 13.5 *The Nucleus 22-channel cochlear implant system. Clockwise from bottom left, the components are the implanted receiver and electrode array, the body-worn speech processor, the ear-level microphone, and the external transmitter. (Reprinted with permission from Cochlear Corporation, Englewood, CO.)*

Tactile Aids

Some hearing-impaired persons use tactile aids to help understand speech cues. These devices transduce an auditory signal into a vibro-tactile or electrotactile signal, which is presented to the skin via one or more stimulators. The stimulators often are worn on the wrist or on the chest. Tactile aids can convey only limited types of speech information, such as syllable stress and number, voicing, and duration. Practice often is necessary before a person can benefit from a tactile aid. Because of these limitations, tactile aids primarily are used to supplement lipreading.

Hearing Rehabilitation in Adults

Many persons develop presbycusis, a loss of hearing that often accompanies aging. Others experience hearing loss from viral infections, ototoxic drugs, or long-term exposure to intense noise (see Chapter 12 for additional information about hearing disorders). The influence of hearing loss on a person's life depends on many factors (Table 13.3). Some of these factors relate to the hearing loss itself. Other variables involve nonaudiometric characteristics or the communication partner. Because

TABLE 13.3   Variables That Affect the Impact of Hearing Loss on a Person's Life*

	Helpful Factors	Nonhelpful Factors
Speaker	Uses clear speech with slightly increased volume Uses slightly slowed rate of speech Faces the listener Is familiar to listener Is patient and persistent Uses messages with appropriate contextual information Rephrases as necessary	Speaks rapidly Has unfamiliar accent or dialect Speaks with low vocal intensity Is not facing listener or speaks from another room Eats, smokes, or obscures face while speaking Uses complex or lengthy sentences Uses unfamiliar vocabulary Changes topics abruptly
Environment	Appropriate lighting Optimal distance Minimal noise Minimal reverberation High-quality public address system	Dim lighting or light directly in listener's eyes Distance between listener and speaker too close or too far Excessive noise, reverberation, or both Poor-quality public address system or no public address system
Listener	Uses appropriate hearing aid(s), assistive devices, or both Has a positive attitude toward communication Is an assertive communicator Uses contextual information well Synthesizes auditory and visual information Has supportive network of communicators	Refuses to use hearing aids or assistive devices Uses inappropriate or malfunctioning hearing aid Is a passive or aggressive communicator Has cognitive or central auditory system disorder Has low vision Uses poor listening strategies

*Variables can be either helpful (meaning that they help minimize the impact of the hearing loss) or nonhelpful (those that exacerbate the impact of the hearing loss).
Source: Adapted from DA Sanders. Aural Rehabilitation. Englewood Cliffs, NJ: Prentice-Hall, 1971.

the audiogram only conveys information about hearing ability, the impact of the hearing loss on a person's life (i.e., the degree of hearing handicap experienced) cannot be predicted simply by looking at audiologic test results.

Hearing loss has the potential to affect all areas of a person's life: how he or she functions at work, his or her relationship with others, and even self-concept. If hearing aids were corrective, in theory, a person could be fit with amplification and hearing problems would be solved. As mentioned earlier, however, hearing aids are not corrective, and many persons fit with appropriate amplification still experience significant communication difficulty. Hearing rehabilitation is designed to address the problems brought about by the hearing loss. The goal is to assist the client in developing skills, strategies, and an information base to help him or her accept responsibility for improving communication.

Hearing rehabilitation with adults takes many forms, depending on the clinician providing the intervention. A hearing rehabilitation program can consist of either individual sessions, group sessions (with more than one client), or a combination of the two. Group sessions are valuable for several reasons: (1) hearing-impaired people can benefit from the expertise and support of other hearing-impaired people, (2) hearing-impaired people can practice newly learned skills in a safe environment, (3) hearing-impaired people can benefit from helping other hearing-impaired people, and (4) group sessions are cost effective for the clinician. On the other hand, individual hearing rehabilitation allows the clinician to address a client's specific problems. Regardless of the form of the program, the participation of the hearing-impaired client's primary communication partner (typically a spouse or a close friend) often is encouraged.

Hearing rehabilitation programs also vary in their content. Some programs are primarily information based: Their purpose is to convey information (e.g., about hearing aids and assistive devices) to hearing-impaired people. Other programs contain strong skill-based components, in which the client learns and practices activities designed to enhance his or her ability to communicate. With skill-based programs, pre- and postintervention assessment of communication skills (e.g., lipreading and the amount of perceived hearing handicap) often is completed in an attempt to document improvement.

Communication Skill Training

Speechreading

Much information about a speech signal is conveyed through vision. The term *lipreading* refers to using the visual aspects of the movement of the articulators to augment speech understanding. The term *speechreading* includes not only lipreading but also the use of visual cues from gestures, facial expressions, postures, and the environment.

Many people have the incorrect notion that lipreading can be substituted for hearing. Even the best lipreader cannot get all of a message through visual cues because of several limiting factors. First, sounds produced in the back of the mouth (e.g., /k/, /g/, /h/) are not visible. Moreover, some sounds are produced almost identically and, therefore, look alike on the lips. For example, the words *fat* and *vat* are difficult to distinguish visually. Groups of similar-looking sounds are referred to as *homophenous categories*. Other limitations are related to variability of sound production. Sounds are produced differently depending on their neighboring sounds (coarticulation), and not everyone produces sounds identically (in part because of dialects and accents).

Some people are better at lipreading than others. In fact, research suggests that lipreading is related to neurologic factors that cannot be changed (Samar and Sims 1983). On the other hand, other data suggest that lipreading can be improved with training (Walden et al. 1981).

Even if lipreading cannot be trained, the ability to use linguistic information can be improved. One example of this occurs when a hearing-impaired person misses a word auditorily but can use lipreading to narrow down the choices to several words that look alike on the lips (e.g., *ban, pan,* and *man*). The client can be trained to use sentence context to figure out what is said. For example, if the client hears the sentence "He put the fish in the … .", he or she could determine that the missing word must be *pan* based on the sentence context. This is referred to as a *synthetic speechreading activity.*

Synthetic speechreading activities work on comprehension via skills such as the use of context and identification of key words. Analytic speechreading activities consist of familiarizing the client with homophenous categories and how individual sounds appear on the lips. Many hearing rehabilitation programs use a combination of synthetic and analytic activities.

Auditory and Auditory-Visual Training

In the majority of communication situations, persons use both auditory and visual speech cues to facilitate understanding. Hence, many audiologists believe that, at least with adults, hearing rehabilitation should focus on a combination of auditory and visual information. This is referred to as *auditory-visual (AV) training.* Clinicians often use either a low vocal intensity or tape-recorded background noise when doing AV training to make it both more realistic and more challenging.

There are situations, however, in which auditory (A) training is conducted with adults. In A training, the client is given only auditory cues: The mouth is covered or obscured to prevent the client from lipreading. This is beneficial, for example, with new hearing aid users who need assistance learning to identify hearing aid–processed speech sounds. Another example of an A training activity is telephone training, during which clients learn strategies for communicating via the telephone.

Activities for A and AV training range from those using syllable-level stimuli to exercises using conversations. For example, a client may be asked to discriminate one of three choices of syllables (e.g., /fa/, /da/, /ga/) using either an A or AV presentation. At a more advanced level, a clinician might say a sentence that offers contextual information, using low vocal intensity on the last word. For example, the clinician might say, "We bought the coat in that store." The word *store* would be said with low vocal intensity. The client must use sentence context, in addition to the auditory and visual message, to discern the final word. Similarly, the clinician may give a topic (e.g., shopping) and say sentences related to that topic in a manner that makes it difficult for the client to hear (e.g., by using a tape recording of background noise). The client must use the topic-related context to help understand the sentences.

A training technique that is used widely for both A and AV training is tracking, which was developed by DeFilippo and Scott (1978). In tracking, the clinician reads a story or article phrase by phrase, and the client must repeat back each phrase verbatim. The client must ask for a

TABLE 13.4 Communication Repair Strategies: Requests That a Hearing-Impaired Person May Make of His or Her Communication Partner(s)

Speak slower
Speak louder
Repeat the last word
Face me when you are speaking
Use that word in a sentence
Spell the word using code words (e.g., *b* as in *b*all, *o* as in *o*range, *y* as in *y*ellow)
Say that in a different way
Spell that word
Write that word

repair strategy if he or she misses part or all of a phrase. Repair strategies are specific requests that a hearing-impaired person uses to help understand a message (Table 13.4). In this way, the client takes control of the situation by asking the clinician what is needed to help him or her understand. At the end of the tracking activity, a word-per-minute score is calculated from the number of words tracked over a given period of time. Although there are problems associated with tracking (e.g., finding material from various sources that is of a similar level of difficulty), many clinicians use this technique because it works not only on A or AV reception but also on assertiveness.

Another example of hearing rehabilitation activities is the conversational approach, developed by Erber (1988). This approach simulates real-life communication, in which the hearing-impaired person may or may not be the initiator of the conversation. For example, there are activities that help the client realize that some types of questions lead to more predictable (therefore more easily understood) answers than others. Other activities work on training the hearing-impaired person's communication partner to use strategies that might increase the probability that he or she will be understood.

Coping Strategies

Some hearing rehabilitation activities are designed to improve a person's ability to cope in real-life listening situations. A number of these activities are based on the concept of stage management. Stage management refers to the act of setting up a communication environment to one's best advantage.

What is the ideal communication environment? First, a good listening situation has minimal noise and little reverberation. The lighting should be bright enough for a person to be able to speechread, but the source of the light should not be in the speechreader's eyes. A distance of approximately 6 feet between the communication partners allows the hearing-impaired person to see cues necessary for speechreading. This distance is also close enough for much of the sound to be picked up directly by the hearing aid microphone. An angle of 0–45 degrees is ideal for speechreading and getting sound directly to the microphone. The communication partner should not obscure his or her mouth or articulatory gestures in any way (e.g., by chewing gum or yawning while speaking). If there is noise in the room, the hearing-impaired person should be as far away from the noise source as possible. For those who use only one hearing aid, the ear with the hearing aid should be directed toward the person speaking.

Many activities can be devised to demonstrate these factors and how to use stage management to improve the communication environment. One prerequisite to some of these activities is assertiveness. The client must be willing to speak up and request that something be done when the listening situation is not ideal. He or she may need to ask that his or her table be moved in a restaurant or that a person face him or her when speaking. He or she also may need to use a repair strategy to help clarify a message (see Table 13.4). Hence, for some clients assertiveness training, as well as help in recognizing the differences between passive, assertive, and aggressive behaviors, is a valuable component of hearing rehabilitation.

An excellent method for working on stage management and assertiveness is role playing. In role playing, the clinician or the client's significant other plays the role of someone who makes communication difficult. The client then uses stage management and repair strategies to understand the message. For example, a role play might be devised in which the client must obtain specific information about a cruise from a travel agent. The clinician or significant other acts as the travel agent who makes communication difficult (e.g., by covering his or her mouth or speaking with his or her back turned). An important component of role playing is discussing strategies that did and did not work after the role play is concluded.

It is helpful to use situations in hearing rehabilitation that actually cause difficulty for the hearing-impaired person. One means of determining problem areas in the client's real life is through the use of hearing handicap scales. These are questionnaires that probe situations of difficulty and reactions to hearing loss. Hearing handicap scales are available for many subpopulations (e.g., elderly, children, and those with severe or profound hearing loss). These scales can yield valuable information about specific situations of difficulty. Audiologists also use hearing handicap scales to help determine candidacy for hearing rehabilitation. Some scales can also signal when a client is having difficulty adjusting to the hearing impairment and possibly needs counseling.

Counseling

Two forms of counseling are conducted during hearing rehabilitation. The first type is informational, in which information is conveyed to the client. An example of this is talking to the client about assistive devices. The second type of counseling is emotional. Emotional-type counseling deals with the client's, as well as his or her family's, feelings about and acceptance of the hearing loss. Emotional-type counseling often is not a planned activity, rather, it arises from the relationship that develops between a client and a clinician.

The amount of emotional-type counseling a clinician performs depends on his or her comfort level in dealing with clients' feelings. Many speech-language pathologists and audiologists do not feel comfortable delving into counseling, because they often do not have formal training in this area. However, audiologists know the most about hearing loss and its potential impact on a person's life. When the focus of counseling shifts to problems or reactions that are unrelated to the hearing loss, clinicians should recognize that it is time to refer the person to a qualified mental health professional. For information on counseling in hearing rehabilitation, see Luterman (1991).

Hearing Habilitation and Rehabilitation with Children

Hearing loss can impact every facet of a child's life, including speech and language development, educational achievement, relationships with parents and others, and self-image. The negative effects of hearing loss can be reduced, to some extent, by early intervention, which should begin as soon as the hearing loss is identified.

Age of onset is an important factor in determining the impact of the hearing loss (see Chapter 12). Hearing loss that occurs before a language base has been established is referred to as *prelinguistic hearing loss*. Hearing impairment that begins after language development is referred to as *postlinguistic hearing loss*. In general, a prelinguistic hearing loss has a greater effect on speech and language development.

The diagnosis of a significant hearing loss in a child often has profound effects on the child's parents. Many parents experience feelings such as denial, guilt, anger, and inadequacy (Luterman 1991). As professionals, clinicians best serve parents by being empathetic listeners, thereby giving them the opportunity to express these feeling. Clinicians should avoid overwhelming parents with too much information immediately after the diagnosis. Luterman (1991) suggests letting parents ask for the information they need as it is needed. In this way, the parents get only the information they can handle. Clinicians also should make sure that the intervention is designed to empower the parents. Parents should realize that what they do can and does make a difference in their child's life. One way of empowering parents is by involving them in the intervention process.

Intervention with prelinguistically hearing-impaired children is often referred to as *hearing habilitation* rather than hearing rehabilitation, because one cannot rehabilitate what was never there. Hearing habilitation and hearing rehabilitation with children differs from intervention with adults in a number of ways. Concerns are somewhat different: In young children, attention must be paid to psychosocial development, language development, and educational development. Moreover, hearing habilitation should be a team effort. The clinician works in conjunction with the family, the teacher, and, perhaps, other health care professionals (especially if the child has other disabling conditions).

Communication Methods

Parents of young children with severe or profound hearing loss face the often difficult decision of how to communicate with their child. It is the clinician's job to present unbiased information about the various options for communication methods. The parents must be given the opportunity to decide which avenue to pursue. The controversy regarding how to communicate with hearing-impaired children has been going on since the 1700s. The two major camps are oral communication methods and manual communication methods.

Proponents of oral methods think that every child should be given the opportunity to communicate using speech. They believe that, because this is essentially an oral world, oral communication is less limiting in terms of the child's eventual educational and vocational options. With oral methods, the child is trained to use his or her residual hearing (often in conjunction with speechreading) to receive speech and, in turn, is taught to speak. The use of sign language is prohibited in most oral programs. It should be pointed out that oral communication is very difficult for many children with severe or profound hearing impairment and requires years of hard work. Even with the best intervention, some prelinguistically hearing-impaired children are not able to achieve intelligible speech. On the other hand, many children with severe or profound hearing loss become effective oral communicators who are full participants in the hearing world.

The second category of communication methods is manual, which usually refers to the use of American Sign Language (ASL). ASL is a true language that differs from oral English in grammatical structure. Proponents of this method believe that oral communication is insufficient for the psychosocial development of young children, because it often leads to frustrated, difficult communication between a child and his or her parents. Advocates of manual methods point to the fact that ASL is the preferred language of many deaf adults. Furthermore, proponents of manual methods believe that the use of signs allows better language development, because after the child learns the signs, he or she understands the message. An educational movement is under way in which children are raised using ASL as their first language and learn oral English as a second language.

Many children are educated using a combination of oral and manual methods. The most common example of this is total communication (TC). TC is a philosophy that advocates the use of all possible cues (oral and manual) to help the child learn language. Children educated with TC use their residual hearing, speechreading, and a signed form of oral English (often Signed English) that incorporates ASL vocabulary in English word order.

Another example of the combined approach is cued speech. Cued speech was developed to help overcome the problems associated with speechreading homophenous sounds. In cued speech, eight different hand positions represent the consonants. These are placed in one of several sites around the face to signify the vowels (Figure 13.6).

Intervention with Hearing-Impaired Infants and Preschoolers

As mentioned earlier in this chapter, intervention should begin as soon as the hearing loss is identified. Hearing habilitation programs for hearing-impaired infants often are parent-centered, meaning that the clinician is actually training the parent to do the intervention. This type of program is ideal because the parents spend the majority of the time with the infant. Furthermore, parent-centered programs empower the parents, helping them to realize that they are capable of handling the task of raising a hearing-impaired child.

Some parent-centered programs rely on visits by the practitioner, in which a clinician sees the family (either in their home or at a clinic) on an occasional basis. Correspondence courses (such as that offered by the John Tracy Clinic) are available in which the parent sends reports to the facility and, in return, is given future work by mail. It should be pointed out that parent-centered programs are not always feasible. Because of the financial situation of many contemporary families, having a parent out of the workforce is a luxury that cannot be afforded. Single parents who must work also may be unable to expend the time necessary for intervention in the home. Moreover, parent-centered programs are difficult to implement successfully in families in which English is not the primary language spoken at home.

In hearing habilitation with infants, parents often modify everyday activities to increase auditory and language stimulation. Efforts are made to bring the infant's attention to sounds in the environment and actions provoked by the sounds (e.g., answering the door when the doorbell rings). Parents also play a key role in keeping logs of the infant's expressive and receptive vocabulary and his or her reaction to sounds.

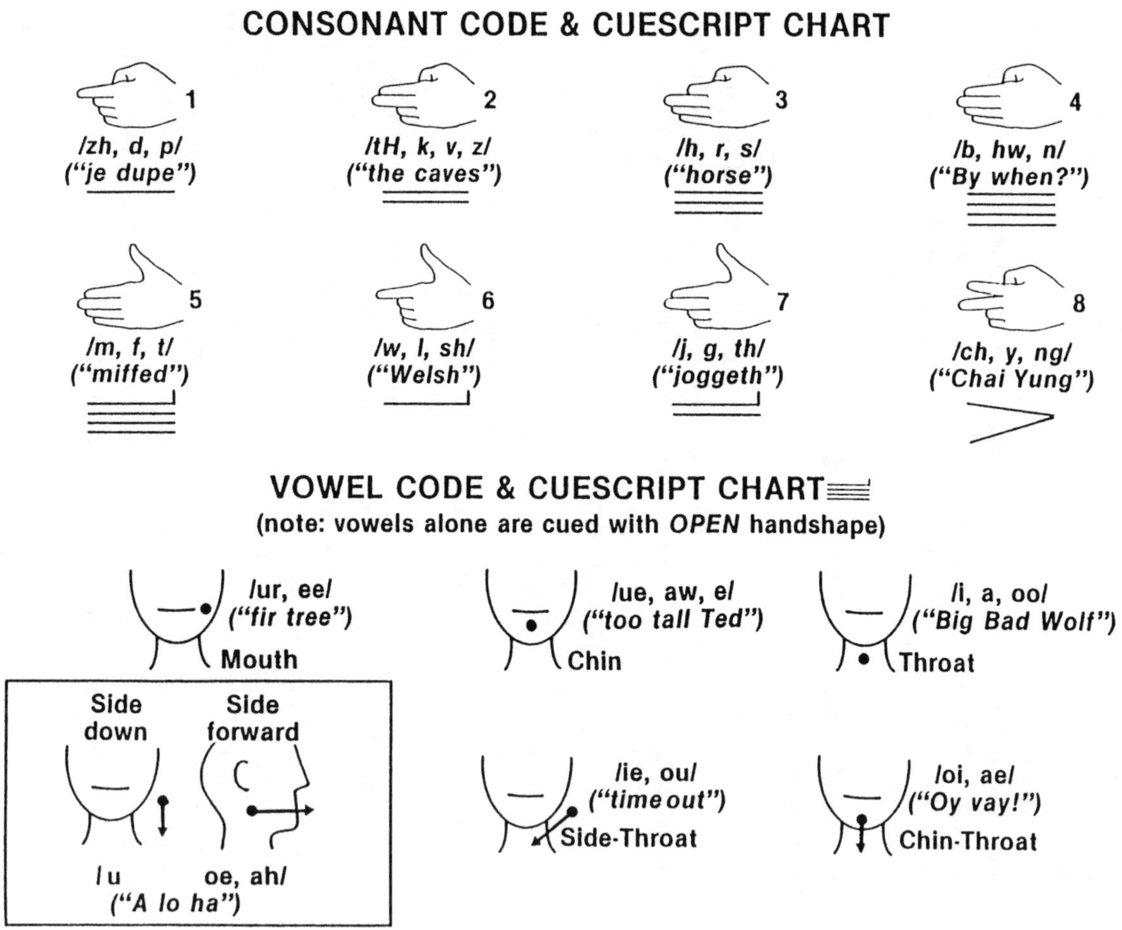

CONSONANT CODE & CUESCRIPT CHART

1
/zh, d, p/
("je dupe")

2
/tH, k, v, z/
("the caves")

3
/h, r, s/
("horse")

4
/b, hw, n/
("By when?")

5
/m, f, t/
("miffed")

6
/w, l, sh/
("Welsh")

7
/j, g, th/
("joggeth")

8
/ch, y, ng/
("Chai Yung")

VOWEL CODE & CUESCRIPT CHART
(note: vowels alone are cued with OPEN handshape)

/ur, ee/
("fir tree")
Mouth

/ue, aw, e/
("too tall Ted")
Chin

/i, a, oo/
("Big Bad Wolf")
Throat

Side down

Side forward

/u oe, ah/
("A lo ha")

/ie, ou/
("time out")
Side-Throat

/oi, ae/
("Oy vay!")
Chin-Throat

FIGURE 13.6 *Hand configurations and placements used in cued speech. (Reprinted with permission from Gallaudet University, Washington, DC.)*

Clinicians must be sensitive to potential cultural differences that can come into play when working with families. For example, most early intervention programs stress the importance of eye contact when communicating with hearing-impaired infants. In Japanese and Native American cultures, however, extended eye contact is considered rude, and children traditionally are taught to show respect by bowing their head and using little or no eye contact (Yacobacci-Tam 1987). Another example involves the roles of the parents in traditional Hispanic families. Clinicians should consider that in such families the father is often the decision maker; hence, the clinician should turn to the father to answer questions regarding parental decisions (Rodriguez and Santiviago 1991).

As the child approaches preschool age, activities are designed to enhance cognitive development and educational readiness, as well as language development. Intervention with children in the preschool years usually takes the form of structured play. Attention is given to concepts necessary for future learning (e.g., numbers, letters, colors, shapes, and sorting). As the child approaches 3 years of age, it becomes more likely that he or she will be placed in some type of out-of-home preschool program.

Intervention with School-Age Children

Children's language needs increase as they get older, as do the demands that school learning places on language abilities. An important decision must be made concerning the environment of the child's education. Options for the child include attending a school for the deaf, being placed in a self-contained classroom with other hearing-impaired (or variously disabled) children, and being mainstreamed in a regular classroom. Most hearing-impaired children who are mainstreamed receive some type of special help, such as speech-language intervention, a classroom interpreter, resource room services, or any combination of these.

The classroom represents a difficult listening environment for all children, especially those with hearing impairments. Noise sources in typical classrooms include moving chairs, slamming desk tops, ventilation systems, and children's voices. The audiologist or speech-language pathologist working with a hearing-impaired child should conduct at least one classroom visitation to determine ideas for improving the child's listening environment. Many hearing-impaired children use some type of classroom assistive device (most often an FM system) to help improve the signal-to-noise ratio. Some school systems have sound-field FM systems. With this type of system, the teacher's voice is amplified and delivered to one or more loudspeakers. All children benefit from the enhanced speech signal, especially those who have mild-to-moderate hearing loss from recurrent otitis media (Flexer 1993).

By the time the child is of school age, attention usually is given to both speech and language development. The reader is referred to Ling (1976) for a detailed program of speech intervention with hearing-impaired children. Intervention for language disorder or delay often is similar to that done with normal-hearing children. However, many hearing-impaired children need extra help learning new material that is presented in the classroom. Language activities can include pretutoring of vocabulary that is used in subsequent classes.

Attention also must be given to the development of auditory skills in hearing-impaired children. On a basic level, this includes localization and discrimination of both nonspeech and speech sounds (e.g., auditory training of the difference between voiced and unvoiced sounds, such as /pa/ versus /ba/). Improvement of higher-level skills, such as auditory memory and auditory sequencing, may be goals of later intervention.

One important component of working with hearing-impaired children is training the classroom teacher. Many teachers have little exposure to hearing-impaired people; hence, they need specific information about how to help the hearing-impaired student. Teachers should first receive a detailed report specifying the child's strengths and anticipated problem areas in classroom learning situations. Teachers also need concrete information regarding the use of hearing aids or classroom listening devices and the optimization of communication with the hearing-impaired student. Finally, teachers can help socialize the hearing-impaired child within the classroom. Time can be devoted to explaining hearing, hearing loss, and hearing aids to the class, fostering the attitude that the hearing impairment is an interesting (instead of stigmatizing) aspect of the child's life.

Multicultural Perspectives

Clinicians must be sensitive to cultural differences that influence intervention. For example, in some traditional Hispanic cultures, it is considered rude to start the business at hand without first participating in some small talk (Rodriguez and Santiviago 1991). Hence, clinicians working with Hispanic clients should devote the beginning of sessions to discussing topics unrelated to hearing rehabilitation. Persons from several cultures (e.g., Mediterranean, Middle Eastern, and Asian cultures) consider intense questioning rude (Condon and Yousef 1985). These persons may be offended when the clinician attempts to complete a hearing handicap scale. In such situations, it is recommended that the clinician spend time explaining the importance of these questionnaires.

Language barriers also can limit access to hearing rehabilitation programs. The paucity of speech-language pathologists and audiologists who are fluent in languages other than English restricts the number of patients who can receive hearing rehabilitation services. One possible remedy to this problem is to train peer counselors to provide rudimentary information about hearing loss and hearing rehabilitation. The ideal solution, however, is to recruit more bilingual persons to become communication disorders professionals. On a positive note, hearing aid companies are beginning to recognize that many of their consumers are not fluent in English and are producing their hearing aid instruction manuals in other languages.

Conclusion

Hearing rehabilitation consists of many types of activities, all with a common goal of improving the communication ability of hearing-impaired persons. The audiologist or speech-language pathologist can use both technology and behavioral activities to meet this goal. Both strategies are important, because available technology cannot cure hearing loss. The clinician also must keep in mind that communication inherently involves more than one person. A successful hearing rehabilitation program should include not only the person with hearing loss but also those with whom he or she communicates.

References

Audiology Update. Rockville, MD: American Speech-Language-Hearing Association, 1991.

Byrne D, Dillon H. The National Acoustic Laboratories' new procedure for selecting the gain and frequency response of a hearing aid. Ear Hear 1986;7:257–265.

Condon JC, Yousef FS. An Introduction to Intercultural Communication. New York: Macmillan, 1985.

Cox R, Alexander GC. The abbreviated profile of hearing aid benefit. Ear Hear 1995;16:176–186.

Cox R, DeChicchis AR, Wark DJ. Demonstration of binaural advantage in audiometric test rooms. Ear Hear 1981;2:194–201.

DeFilippo CL, Scott BL. A method for training and evaluating the reception on ongoing speech. J Acoust Soc Am 1978;63:1186–1192.

Erber NP. Communication Therapy for Hearing-Impaired Adults. Washington, DC: Alexander Graham Bell Association for the Deaf, 1988.

Erdman SA, Sedge RK. Subjective comparisons of binaural versus monaural amplification. Ear Hear 1981;2:225–229.

Feurstein JF. Monaural versus binaural hearing: ease of listening, word recognition and attentional effort. Ear Hear 1992;13:80–86.

Flexer C. Management of hearing in an educational setting. In JC Alpiner, PA McCarthy (eds), Rehabilitative Audiology: Children and Adults (2nd ed). Baltimore: Williams & Wilkins, 1993.

Grahl C. A dispenser yardstick: how to measure your 1992 performance. Hearing Instruments 1993;44:4–13.

Hawkins DB, Yacullo W. Signal-to-noise ratio advantage of binaural hearing aids and directional microphones under different levels of reverberation. J Speech Hear Disord 1984;49:278–286.

Kirkwood DH. Resurgent hearing aid market nearing record-high level. Hear J 1996;46:7–14.

Kochkin S. MarkeTrak IV: 10-year trends in the hearing aid market—has anything changed? Hear J 1996;49:23.

Ling D. Speech and the Hearing-Impaired Child: Theory and Practice. Washington, DC: Alexander Graham Bell Association for the Deaf, 1976.

Luterman DM. Counseling the Communicatively Disordered and Their Families. Austin, TX: PRO-ED, 1991.

Markides A. Binaural Hearing Aids. London: Academic, 1977.

Naidoo SV. Sound quality and speech intelligibility judgments with monaural and binaural hearing aids. Ph.D. diss., University of South Carolina. Ann Arbor, MI: University Microfilms, 1993.

Rodriguez O, Santiviago M. Hispanic deaf adolescents: a multicultural minority. Volta Rev 1991;93:89–97.

Samar V, Sims D. Visual evoked-response correlates of speechreading performance in normal-hearing adults: a replication and factory analytic extension. J Speech Hear Res 1983;26:2–9.

Schreurs KK, Olsen WO. Comparison of monaural and binaural hearing aid use on a trial period basis. Ear Hear 1985;6:198–202.

Walden B, Demorest M, Helpler E. Self-report approach to assessing benefit derived from amplification. J Speech Hear Res 1984;27:49–56.

Walden BE, Erdman SA, Montgomery AA, et al. Some effects of training on speech recognition by hearing-impaired adults. J Speech Hear Res 1981;24:207–216.

Yacobacci-Tam P. Interacting with the culturally different family. Volta Rev 1987;89:46–58.

Chapter 13   Study Questions

1. Describe the benefits and limitations of the various types of hearing aids.
2. What are the advantages of using binaural (versus monaural) hearing aids?
3. Describe the information conveyed to a hearing aid user during hearing aid orientation.
4. Discuss the ways in which assistive listening device systems can transmit the signal from the speaker to the listener.
5. Why can't lipreading be used as a substitute for hearing?
6. Describe several types of activities used during auditory and auditory-visual training.
7. Discuss the arguments for and against oral and manual communication methods.

Appendix A

Hints for Hearing-Impaired Persons

1. Use cues in the environment to help anticipate what will be said. For example, if you are in a bank, try to think of what kinds of messages are likely to occur in that situation.
2. Be willing to admit to others that you have a hearing loss and that you did not understand what they have said. Know which communication strategies work best for you (e.g., repeating, rephrasing, or spelling a word), so that you can direct your communication partner.
3. Set up the listening environment to your best advantage—that is,

   - Make sure the light shines on the speaker's face, not in your eyes.
   - Sit with the source of noise behind you.
   - Move to a quieter area or eliminate the noise source (e.g., turn down the television or radio, turn off the water).
   - Move closer to the person speaking.
   - Make sure the speaker is facing you.
   - Seat yourself so that all (or most) of the people with whom you are talking are on one side of you (e.g., do not sit between two people and try to carry on a conversation with both of them).

4. Use visual information when hearing is difficult. Be sure to observe expressions, gestures, and postures, in addition to lip movement. Try to integrate what is seen with what is heard.
5. Do not be concerned about understanding every word. It is much more important to grasp the idea of what is said. One way to make this easier is to determine the topic of the conversation as soon as possible or to have someone cue you in to the topic.
6. Confirm and feed back the information you have heard (e.g., say "… that was Friday, June 9th, at what time?") rather than asking for the entire message to be repeated.
7. Arrive early at meetings to seat yourself in the best place.
8. Keep informed about world, local, and personal events.
9. Be willing to guess about what is said but be flexible in your guessing. Incoming information can make you change your mind about what you think was said.
10. Understand that most normal-hearing people have had little contact with hearing-impaired persons. Educate them on how to be more effective communicators.

11. Be assertive, not aggressive or passive. You have every right to participate in conversations. Do not bluff or nod when you do not understand the message.
12. Use the appropriate hearing aids and assistive devices. Have your hearing (and hearing aids) checked annually.
13. Relax and have a sense of humor!

Appendix B

Hints for Families and Friends of Hearing-Impaired Persons

1. Speak slightly louder than normal and slightly slower than normal. Shouting often causes distortion, especially if the hearing-impaired person wears a hearing aid.
2. Do not try to speak to the hearing-impaired person from another room. Hearing aids are not very effective when the listener and speaker are far from one another. The ideal distance for communication is between 3 and 6 feet, with the listener and speaker facing each other.
3. Hearing loss often causes people to be more affected by background noise. Many persons with hearing loss (even when they are using hearing aids) have difficulty understanding speech in noisy situations or when more than one person is speaking.
4. Try to eliminate sources of background noise before engaging in conversation (e.g., turn down the television or radio, turn off the water, or move to a quieter area). Beware of hidden sources of noise that you barely notice (e.g., fans or machinery).
5. Clue the hearing-impaired person into the topic of the conversation.
6. Even the best speechreader cannot understand all of speech by visual cues alone. Here are some things you can do to help the speechreader:

   - Use natural gestures and facial expressions.
   - Avoid distracting movement such as chewing, eating, or covering your mouth when speaking.
   - Do not exaggerate your lip gestures when speaking.
   - Make sure there is sufficient light in the room where you are conversing.
   - Always face the hearing-impaired person when speaking and be sure that you have his or her attention before you begin to talk.

7. If communication breaks down,

   - Rephrase or repeat the message.
   - Say a key word from the message.
   - Spell or write a key word or the portion of the message that was missed.
   - Say each digit individually (for numbers).
   - Shorten or simplify the message.
   - Use code words (e.g., say, "F as in Frank").

Index

Audiometry, pure-tone—*continued*
    bone-conduction testing, 256–257
    interpretation, of hearing loss, 257–259
        degree, 257–258
        nature, 258–259
        shape, 258
    speech, 259–261
        detection threshold, 260
        most comfortable loudness level, 260–261
        recognition testing, 260
        recognition threshold, 259
        uncomfortable loudness level, 261
Auditory-evoked response, 267
    late, 268–269, 270
    middle latency, 267–268, 269
Auditory discrimination loss, 238–239
Auditory system, disorders and diseases of, 240–249. *See also* Ear, anatomy of; Hearing assessment; Hearing disorders
    causes of,
        acoustic trauma, 247
        encephalitis, 245
        erythroblastosis, 243
        fetal alcohol syndrome, 242–243
        fungal infections, 248
        measles, 244–245
        Meniere's disease, 246–247
        meningitis, 245
        mumps, 245
        neoplasms, 248
        noise, 248
        otitis media, 243–244
        otosclerosis, 245–246
        ototoxic agents, 246
        prenatal diseases, 241–242
            cytomegalovirus, 242
            rubella, 241–242
        prenatal genetic disorders, 240–241
        vestibular schwannoma, 247
    presbycusis, 248–249
Auditory threshold detection sensitivity, 228
Augmentative and alternative communication, 205–224. *See also* Severe speech (and physical) impairment (SSI, SSPI)
    culturally diverse, 222
    definition, 205
    family objections to, 212
    interdisciplinary team for, 212
    and job retention, 219–220
    specialists in, 221–222
Aural rehabilitation. *See* Hearing rehabilitation

"Baby talk," 54

Bilingualism
    and aphasia, 193–194
    and language development, 76–79
        code-mixing, 76
        code-switching, 76
        dominant language, 76–77
        interference errors, 77, 78
        passive, 77
Bloom and Lahey's content categories, 62–64
Bone-conduction testing, 256–257
Brain, anatomy of. *See* Cerebral cortex, organization of
Broca's aphasia, 191–193
Brown v. Board of Education of Topeka, 11
Brown's 14 morphemes, 66
Brown's stages of language development, 65–66

Cancer, laryngeal, 151–152
Central auditory processing disorder, 236–237
Cerebellopontine angle tumor, 247
Cerebral cortex, organization of, 185–187
    lobes, 186
Cerebrovascular accident, services for patients with, 36–37
Cholesteatoma, as cause of hearing loss, 248
Chomsky, Noam, biological theory of language development of, 11, 55
Citizen's Act, 7
Cleft palate, 153–155
Cochlear implants, 288, 289
Cognition, and language development, 51–53. *See also* Language learning, theories of, cognitive
Collaboration, professional, 24–25
Collaborative model, 97, 98–99
Communication board
    culturally appropriate symbols for, 214
    definition of, 206
Communication disorders
    future treatment of, predictions about, 19
    history of treatment of, 4–5, 8–17
        1900–1929, 8
        1930–1939, 8–9
        1940–1949, 9–10
        1950–1959, 10–11
        1960–1969, 11–12
        1970–1979, 13–14
        1980–1989, 14–15
        1990s, 15–17
    inclusion model and, 17–18, 19. *See also* Inclusion model
    prevalence of, 17
Communication system, definition of, 207
Consultation, professional, 24–25

Hearing disorders—*continued*
   central auditory processing disorder, 236–237
   classification of, parameters for, 229–231
      age of onset, 229–230
      degree of impairment, 229
      origin or cause, 230
      type of impairment, 230–231
   conductive, 235–236, 258
   impact of, variables that influence, 289–290
   mixed, 159
   normal hearing sensitivity range, 228–229
   otologist, role of, 227
   prevalence of, 253–256
      by age, 254, 255
      by race, 254–256
      by sex, 254
   sensorineural, 236, 258–259
   symptoms, syndromes, and signs linked to,
         237–238
      auditory discrimination loss, 238–239
      diplacusis, 239
      nystagmus, 239–240
      paracusis of Willis, 239
      recruitment, 238, 261
      speech and language disorders in chil-
            dren, 238
      tinnitus, 239
      vertigo, 240
Hearing impairment, prevalence of, 17
Hearing rehabilitation, 277–302
   in adults, 289–295
      auditory and auditory-visual training,
            292–293
      conversational approach, 293
      coping strategies, 293–294
      counseling, 294–295
      individual vs. group sessions, 291
      program content, 291
      speechreading, 291–292
   assistive devices, 286–288. *See also* Assistive
            devices for hearing impairment
   in children, 295–300
      communication methods, 296–297
         combination
            cued speech, 297, 298
            total communication, 297
         manual (American Sign Language),
               296–297
         oral, 297
      infants and preschoolers, 297, 299
      parents' involvement, 295
      school-age, 299–300
   cochlear implants, 288, 289
   hearing aids for, 278–286. *See also* Hearing
            aids

   multicultural perspectives and, 300–301
   professionals involved in, 277–278
   tactile aids, 289
Hooper Visual Organization Test, 199, 200
Hormonal disorders, as cause of vocal disor-
         ders, 152
Hyoid bone, 141
Hypernasality, vocal, 154–155
Hyperpituitarism, and low vocal pitch, 152

Illocutionary stage of language development,
         60
Impairment, definition of, 206
Inclusion model, 17–18, 19, 32–33, 97, 98–99,
         215
   collaboration in, 34–35
   vs. traditional pull-out programs, 33–34
Individual education plans (IEPs), 25
Individuals with Disabilities Education Act, 15–16
Infants. *See also* Language, development of, in
         infants
   factors contributing to disabilities in, 27–28
Inflectional markers, 46–47
Infrahyoid laryngeal muscles, 142

Language, 43–58. *See also* Language learning,
         theories of
   components of, 45–51
      morphology, 46–47
      phonology, 45–46
      pragmatics, 48–51. *See also* Pragmatics
      semantics, 47–48
      syntax, 47
   definition of, 43–45
   development of, 59–86. *See also* Phonologic
         development
      in adolescents, 81–82
         sentence length, 81–82
         use of abstract vocabulary, 82
         use of slang expressions, 82
      in infants, 60–61
      in preschoolers, 67–79
         nonstandard English speakers, 70–79
            African-American, 70–75. *See also*
               African-American English, fea-
               tures of
            bilingual children, 76–79. *See also*
               Bilingualism, and language
               development
         standard English speakers, 67–70
            conjoined independent clauses,
               68–69
            embedded and conjoined phrases
               and clauses, 68
            morphologic inflections, 68

Rubella, as cause of hearing disorder, 241–242

Scanning, definition of, 206
Schwannoma, vestibular, as cause of hearing loss, 247
Secondary school programs, for the disabled, 31–32
    problems associated with, 35
Semantics, 47–48
Severe speech (and physical) impairment (SSI, SSPI). *See also* Augmentative and alternative communication
    causes and extent of, 207–208
    education and, 213–218
        classroom assistive technology, 216
        classroom social interaction, 216–217
        early intervention, 213–214
        inclusion model, 215
        literacy development, 217–218
        transition to higher education, 218
    effect of on independent living and adult relationships, 220–221
    effect of on vocation, 218–220
        finding a job, 218–219
        keeping a job, 219–220
    family life and, 210–213
        attitude of family toward disability, intervention, and technology, 211–212
        cultural considerations, 213
        partnership with professionals, 212–213
    historical perspective, 208–209
    self-esteem and, 209–210
    terminology and, 206
    trends for individuals with, 221–222
        declining financial resources, 221
        technology advances, 221
Severe speech and physical impairment (SSPI). *See* Severe speech (and physical) impairment (SSI, SSPI)
Social Security Act, 7, 8
Soldier's Vocational Rehabilitation Act, 7
Spasmodic or spastic dysphonia, 157–158
Speech detection threshold, 260
Speech recognition threshold, 228, 259
Speech-language pathologists
    employment settings of, 25–26
    and individual education plans, 25
    professional development for, 25
    skills required of, 23
    transdisciplinary knowledge of, 23–24
Speechreading, 291–292
Spondee words, 228
Standardized tests, in assessment of language disorders, 94–95, 100–101

Stapedectomy, 246
Static compliance, 262, 264
Strategy, in SSI or SSPI, definition of, 206
Strauss syndrome, 9
Stroke
    as cause of aphasia, 188
    services for patients with, 36–37
Stuttering, 165–184
    among minority groups, 169–171
        African-Americans, 170–171
        Native Americans, 169–170
    coping with, 168–169
    definition of, 165
    development of, 167–168
    emotions underlying, 166
    identification of, 166–167
    incidence of, 169–170
    linguistic peculiarities of, 167
    treatment, 171–181
        in children, 181
        fluency, maintenance of, 180
        integrated approach to, 174–175
        social and cultural factors in, 175–176
        speak more fluently vs. stutter more fluently debate, 173–174
    techniques, 176–180
        attitudes and secondary behaviors, 176
        language and prosody, 177–178
            GILCU, 177
        overall speech change, 179
        physical speech targets, 179
        stuttered moment, 180
    theoretic approaches, 171–173
        anticipatory-struggle theories, 173
        breakdown theories, 172
        cybernetic theories, 173
        learning theories, 173
        repressed-need theories, 172
        shadowing, 171
Suprahyoid laryngeal muscles, 142
Symbol, definition of, 206
Syntax, 47

Technique, definition of, 206
Technology-Related Assistance for Individuals with Disabilities Act of 1989, 216
Teeth, and phonologic disorders, 122
Telephone device for the deaf (TDD), 288
Temporal patterning tests, 272
Terminology for disability, changes in, 5–6
Thyroid cartilage, 139–140
Tinnitus, 239
    from ototoxic agents, 246